MICROCIRCULATION

Blood-Vessel Interactions Systems in Special Tissues

1

MICROCIRCULATION

Volume 1: Blood-Vessel Interactions
Systems in Special Tissues

Volume 2: Transport Mechanisms
Disease States

MICROCIRCULATION

Blood-Vessel Interactions Systems in Special Tissues

1

Edited by

John Grayson and Walter Zingg

University of Toronto
Toronto, Canada

PLENUM PRESS · NEW YORK AND LONDON

Library of Congress Cataloging in Publication Data

World Congress for the Microcirculation, 1st, University of Toronto, 1975.
Microcirculation.

Sponsored by the Canadian Society for Microcirculation.
Includes bibliographies and index.
CONTENTS: v. 1. Blood-vessel interactions.—v. 2. Transport Mechanisms.
1. Microcirculation—Congresses. I. Grayson, John. II. Zingg, Walter, 1924-
III. Canadian Society for Microcirculation. IV. Title.
QP106.6.W67 1975 599'.01'1 76-26051
ISBN 0-306-37097-2 (v. 1)

Proceedings of the First World Congress for the Microcirculation held at the University of Toronto, Toronto, Canada, June 15-20, 1975 and sponsored by the Canadian Society for the Microcirculation, published in two volumes, of which this is volume one.

A Division of Plenum Publishing Corporation
227 West 17th Street, New York, N.Y. 10011

Printed in the United States of America

FIRST WORLD CONGRESS FOR THE MICROCIRCULATION

Toronto, June 1975

Symposia Chairmen and Section Editors:

David H. Lewis, *Linköping, Sweden*
James B. Bassingthwaighte, *Seattle, Washington*
Harry L. Goldsmith, *Montreal, Canada*
Stanley Rowlands, *Calgary, Canada*
Walter Zingg, *Toronto, Canada*

President of the Canadian Society:

Raymond O. Heimbecker, *London, Ontario, Canada*

Organizing and Coordinating Committee:

Secretary General: Glen A. Taylor, *Toronto, Canada*
Members: Glen A. Taylor, *Toronto, Canada*
Irving H. Koven, *Toronto, Canada*
John Grayson, *Toronto, Canada*
Raymond O. Heimbecker, *London, Ontario, Canada*
Walter Zingg, *Toronto, Canada*
James W. Davidson, *Hamilton, Canada*
Sean Moore, *Hamilton, Canada*
Harry L. Goldsmith, *Montreal, Canada*
Eugene M. Renkin, *Davis, California*
James B. Bassingthwaighte, *Seattle, Washington*
Harold J. Wayland, *La Jolla, California*
Adolphe Neetens, *Antwerp, Belgium*
David H. Lewis, *Linköping, Sweden*

Preface

The recognition of the microcirculation as an ideal interdisciplinary meeting place for the life sciences is really a postwar phenomenon. The European and the American Societies more than any other organizations launched the idea, and the success of the European Society's International Meetings gave impetus to a growth of interest from a handful of specialists to the wide interdisciplinary study which microcirculation now represents. The meeting held in Canada in June 1975 was, however, the first truly international meeting devoted to the microcirculation. It, too, was a success from every point of view, and the exchange of knowledge and new ideas was rewarding. It is our present hope that the tradition of European meetings with their characteristic European flavor will continue, but larded by larger, international congresses conceived on a worldwide basis.

For the present conference we were fortunate in the presence of Dr. B. Zweifach. He was once referred to as the "father of the microcirculation." This claim, unfortunately, I cannot accept. That honor probably belongs to Harvey, who by one of the most brilliant strokes of inductive reasoning in medical history inferred the existence of capillaries though he could not see them. Ben Zweifach's role was rather that of the midwife, presiding at the birth rather than the conception. The baby he delivered long years ago has since thriven lustily and its growth is in no small measure due to the continuing zeal of Zweifach and his associates.

The present volumes are a record of the proceedings of our recent meeting. They consist in part of the main symposium presentations with the exception of the platelet symposium held in Hamilton. The rest of the volumes consists of brief reports based on the free communications. Most of these describe new work, and their number and quality are perhaps the best testimony of all to the appeal of microcirculation in current medical and life sciences research.

Toronto J. Grayson

Contents

3. Red Cell Interactions with the Microcirculation

7. Lymphatics

II. Blood Flow in Special Tissues

9. Pulmonary Circulation

10. MyocardialBloodFlow

12. Blood Flow in Skeletal Muscle

13. Microcirculation in Other Tissues

Introduction

Opening Address: First World Congress for the Microcirculation

BENJAMIN W. ZWEIFACH

I think it is a tribute to all of you in the audience that a conference with such a breadth of coverage can be held in an area which not too many years ago was in every sense only a microscopic segment of physiology or pathophysiology. A page or two in textbooks was sufficient to cover our knowledge. I can recall some 25 years ago, when a number of people working in the field of capillary microscopy decided it was time to assert ourselves as a recognized discipline, that only a handful of perhaps 30 investigators were on hand to set up the first definitive microcirculation conference. At that time, the emphasis in the field was on anatomical details. Also on hand were a number of clinically oriented scientists who had long been convinced of the potential value of biomicroscopy as a diagnostic tool in man. Vascular physiologists concentrated their efforts in the main on the large blood vessels, so that only a few stragglers were present.

If one goes back to the literature of the time, it can be seen that almost all of the basic concepts which today are accepted as the mainstream of our thinking had already been formulated. Such leaders as August Krogh, Sir Thomas Lewis, Elliot and Eleanor Clark, and Eugene Landis were able to pinpoint the substantive issues in terms which we would have difficulty in improving on today. By the very nature of the instrumentation available, the approach had to rely on meticulous description. The motion picture was the ultimate medium of communication. Ingenious methods were developed to permit biomicroscopy of almost all the important tissues. The diversity of patterns which the microcirculation took in different tissues continued to amaze investigators.

BENJAMIN W. ZWEIFACH · Department of Bioengineering, University of California, San Diego, La Jolla, California.

To what then can we attribute the almost explosive growth of the field, especially in the past 15–20 years? In hindsight a number of factors can be distinguished, none of which by itself can, however, explain the revival of interest in microcirculatory phenomena. Just as in the case of the trend in modern biology where many of the answers to complex problems were found to lie in the biochemical and biophysical behavior of the cell, the unit building block of the body, many of the answers to the functional behavior of the circulatory system as a whole are to be found at the level of the fundamental structural unit of the cardiovascular system, the microcirculation.

One clue can be obtained by examining the subject matter covered in the papers presented here. The phenomenal increase in the number of individuals who have involved themselves in microcirculatory research can be traced to the influx of people from other disciplines—especially engineering, physics, and mathematics. Also, as was inevitable, the ubiquitous role of the microcirculation has begun to redirect the interests of an increasing number of physiologists.

The term "microcirculation" has come into common usage to replace older terms such as "capillary bed" and "terminal vascular bed" which served in a descriptive sense to refer to all vessels of microscopic dimensions. If one goes back to the work of Sir Thomas Lewis in the 1920s on the cutaneous vasculature, one finds that he was aware that all vessels of capillary dimensions are not structurally similar and he preferred to use the term "minute blood vessels." Although the existence of a discrete microvascular unit is generally accepted, its representation as a structural entity is not as well worked out.

The size of the network intervening between the arterioles and venules varies in different tissues—ranging from as few as four to six capillaries to as many as several hundred. The precise boundary limits of the microcirculation are of more than academic interest, since somewhere during this transition from large to minute blood vessels there must be an overlapping and then a separation of systemic as opposed to local regulatory mechanisms. The terms "arteriole" and "venule" are used in a somewhat loose context, so that it is difficult to define the afferent and efferent boundaries of the microvascular bed, particularly where whole organs are used to obtain such data. As one surveys the seemingly endless permutations displayed, it is evident that even the most detailed model for a specific tissue does not necessarily match that for any other tissue. The sophisticated data which are becoming increasingly available will be meaningful only if a structural frame of reference is provided onto which such information can then be fitted.

Current research has *not only* led to a more exact formulation of the problems being posed but has also made it abundantly clear that as the questions become more sophisticated there is a corresponding need to examine more critically the limitations of the methods used in microcirculatory research.

As the questions which are being posed become more sophisticated, the need to examine the limitations of the direct microscopic approach becomes of paramount importance. In the past, most workers were content to use simple visible indices as a means of determining the physiological state of the microcirculation—keeping track of the effects of general anesthesia, tissue handling, exposure to the atmosphere, etc. Among the criteria used were the difference in caliber of the paired terminal arterioles and venules, the presence of spontaneous vasomotion, the absence of leukocyte sticking, and the response of the muscular vessels to standardized threshold concentrations of vasoactive agents. In their day, these criteria were adequate, since changes in vasomotor behavior and exchange were being analyzed in a somewhat broad and qualitative context. Today as we delve deeper into fundamental biochemical and physical parameters and have the capability of measuring with reasonable precision many of the basic features of the system, it is quite clear that intravital procedures must include safeguards not to disturb the very tissue mechanisms on which local regulation depends.

Despite the major advances in our ability to record and to process information, and the application of computer techniques to analyze complex interactions, it is somewhat sobering to be reminded that many of the fundamental questions raised almost 40–50 years ago by August Krogh and Thomas Lewis still remain open-ended. In some ways, our ability to obtain data in this area is perhaps greater than is our capacity to digest the information.

We find on the one hand attempts to synthesize the activities of the microcirculation as a whole from observations of single vessels, and on the other hand attempts to interpolate from observations of the behavior of large masses of tissue to given elements within the black box. A major difficulty of relying solely on the latter approach stems from the fact that the microvessels are a heterogeneous group in which no single function is simply distributed.

In the main, two different approaches have been used to establish the dynamic characteristics of the microcirculation:

1. Considerable information has been obtained from the study of whole organs or masses of tissue under both *in vivo* and perfused

conditions. These, of course, are average or lumped values and, for the most part, are indirect manifestations of microcirculatory behavior.

2. Much more extensive has been the use of intravital microscopy in tissues which, because of their accessibility and thinness, lend themselves to such examination. Here again, two camps exist. One group favors the use of surgically exteriorized tissues because of the ease with which both invasive and noninvasive measurements can be made, and in addition because local environmental factors can be controlled. The other camp attempts to avoid the problems associated with general anesthesia and tissue handling through the study of special appendages such as the wing of the bat or the transparent ear chamber of the rabbit. Clearly each approach entails a compromise of some kind and no single preparation can provide all of the information necessary for a truly rigorous analysis.

It is obvious that in our haste to bring microcirculatory research out of the qualitative, purely descriptive realm into a more modern quantitative framework much has been left undone at the structural level—an approach which is out of fashion but which requires no new techniques, only perseverance. It has been found convenient to bypass areas of uncertainty by placing the blame on the fact that comparisons are difficult to make when some 10–15 different types of intravital preparations are in use. It is, however, equally challenging that, despite all of these differences, all terminal vascular beds are able to perform identical nutritive functions.

A substantial impact has been made by the application of electron microscopy, which has brought into clearer perspective the structural attributes of the capillary barrier. Ultrastructural details have made it possible to recognize wide differences in the makeup of capillaries in skeletal muscle, in skin, in glands, etc. The endothelial cell has emerged as something other than a remarkably thin lining for the vascular system. As this frontier continues to be pushed forward here, new and challenging questions are being raised—the significance of the numerous endothelial cell vesicles, the nature of intercellular binding forces, the physicochemical makeup of the basement membrane, the nature of the endocapillary lining material. The older concept of the microvessel wall as a fixed, readily definable porous sieve is no longer tenable. Instead, the operational characteristics of the vessel appear to reflect the dynamic properties of its structural components. If the challenging vesicle concept holds up as a generalized transport phenomenon, the permeability coefficient would represent the dynamic activity of the endothelial cell—no fixed pores are needed, but rather a continuously changing population of intracellular vesicles. What then dictates that the effective pore radius is maintained at

45 Å? Other interpretations favor transcapillary movement of materials via the intercellular route, but the need to reconcile ultrastructural with physiological evidence has brought a new perspective into this area.

Numerous attempts have been made to locate the precise sites where local adjustments have been made and to characterize the responsible mechanisms. We have been left a rich legacy in the concepts of vasomotion, the involvement of strategically located precapillary branches frequently identified as sphincters, myogenically mediated autoregulation, and smooth muscle contractility as opposed to endothelial cell contractility, to name but a few phenomena concerned with blood flow.

The basic mechanisms underlying blood-to-tissue exchange are continuously being revised. Only the broad outlines of the potential contribution of the rheological properties of the blood itself to tissue perfusion have been formulated so that its relevance to specific microcirculatory states remains to be documented.

Emphasis has, for the most part, been placed on the nutritive function of the microcirculation. Even more challenging are the vascular beds which serve specialized functions as in the case of the microvasculature in the kidney, the liver, the spleen, and glandular tissues. Most of what is usually discussed under the umbrella of the term "microcirculation" refers to the vessels in skeletal muscle, in skin, or in specialized appendages such as the mesentery, the bat wing, or the hamster cheek pouch. The circulation to the various organs which make up the splanchnic viscera is quite specialized and atypical, as is the microcirculation in tissues such as the brain and the lung, each of which has a unique organization whose details are only beginning to be documented.

Still ahead of us are the many solid tissues which are inaccessible to direct microscopy and which can at present be examined only on the basis of inflow–outflow information. The unraveling of the functional properties of the microcirculation in structures such as the myocardial muscle of the heart, most of splanchnic viscera, the liver, and the brain will depend on our ability to distill from the diversity of tissues accessible to direct microscopy those basic aspects of structure and function which may be common to all microvascular beds and which are essential for their role in local regulation. Much too much emphasis has been placed on the differences encountered in particular tissues.

On the whole, one feels intuitively that, with the almost explosive resurgence of the field, major advances in our understanding of microcirculatory homeostasis are in the offing. The organizers of this symposium are to be congratulated on the breadth and scope of the topics. I am certain that we will find ourselves both enriched and stimulated by the wealth of information displayed here.

I

Blood and Blood Vessel Interaction

1

Blood Rheology Interpreted through the Flow Properties of the Red Cell

1.1. Macroscopic Rheology and Tube Flow of Human Blood

GILES R. COKELET

The problem of quantitatively relating the bulk rheological properties of blood, as measured in a viscometer, to the flow behavior of that blood in *in vivo* systems, such as microcirculatory networks, has existed for quite some time. Indeed, this problem has also existed for *in vitro* systems of very small physical scale. If we mention the Fåhraeus-Lindqvist effect (Fåhraeus and Lindqvist, 1931) and the classical perfusion experiments of Whittaker and Winton (1933), we are reminded of early examples which appear to show that one cannot take bulk rheological data for blood and proceed to predict, by conventional methods, the flow behavior of that blood in *in vivo* situations. This apparent conflict has not been completely resolved.

We now understand a lot about the bulk (or macroscopic) rheological properties of blood, of how they change with changes in plasma composition, red cell aggregation, and deformability, and the mechanisms which govern these changes of properties. A number of comprehensive reviews on the subject of blood rheology and related subtopics are in the literature (Braasch, 1971; Charm and Kurland, 1974; Chien, 1975; Cokelet, 1972; Dintenfass, 1971; Goldsmith and Skalak, 1975; LaCelle and Weed, 1971; Merrill, 1968; Schmid-Schönbein and Wells, 1971; Wayland, 1967; Whitmore, 1968). In addition, the two following presentations, by Brooks and

GILES R. COKELET · Department of Chemical Engineering, Montana State University, Bozeman, Montana.

Skalak, deal in depth with red cell aggregation and red cell deformation, the two processes which primarily influence the rheological properties of blood. Consequently, I will pass on to the more clouded question of how we relate these macroscopic rheological properties to blood flow behavior in small-scale systems.

The discussion will involve only one elementary flow situation: the steady flow of human blood through small, rigid, impermeable, smooth-walled tubes. Many may argue that this is an irrelevant system, since, except for the smallness of the physical scale, it bears only the most superficial resemblance to an *in vivo* system. However, two factors prompt a discussion of this topic: (1) the relationships between the macroscopic rheological properties of blood and its flow behavior in this simple geometry are not clearly understood; (2) if the principles governing the fluid mechanical behavior of this simple system were quantitatively understood, they would certainly represent the most likely candidates to be the principles governing the more complicated *in vivo* systems.

1.1.1. Hematocrit of Flowing Blood

Studies of the macroscopic rheological properties of blood have repeatedly demonstrated the overwhelming importance of the blood's hematocrit in determining those properties. This reason alone would be sufficient for us to determine the average hematocrit of the blood flowing in a tube or vessel before trying to predict the relevant pressure drop–flow rate relationship from rheological data. In addition, hematocrit data are useful because they allow us to calculate, from mass balances on the red cells and the blood as a whole, other useful parameters. Consequently, this presentation will start by discussing various hematocrits and then will progress into the question of how to predict pressure drop–flow rate relationships and other matters.

Three hematocrits will be discussed. Figure 1 is a schematic representation which depicts the places where the three hematocrits are measured after steady flow conditions have been established. The various hematocrits are:

1. H_F, the average hematocrit of the blood in the reservoir feeding blood to the tube.
2. H_T, the average hematocrit of the blood inside the tube, called the tube or dynamic (Wayland, 1967) hematocrit. An operational definition of H_T is attained by suddenly stopping the steady flow, collecting all the blood components in the tube and mixing them

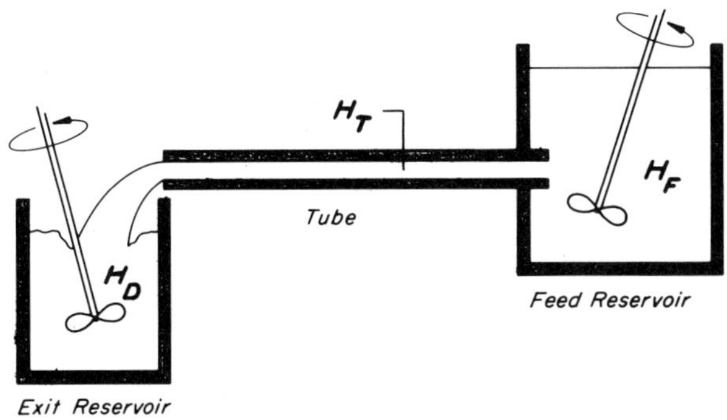

Figure 1. Diagram showing where the three hematocrits discussed in the text are measured. See text for explanation of how they are determined.

until the suspension is uniform, and then measuring the sample hematocrit, which would be H_T.

3. H_D, the discharge hematocrit, which is the average hematocrit of the blood flowing from the tube. The reservoir used to collect the outflowing blood must initially be empty and is not used to collect a sample of outflowing blood until after steady flow has been attained everywhere.

At steady state, mass balances tell us two things:

1. The discharge hematocrit, H_D, must be the hematocrit of the blood actually entering the tube; if it is less than the feed reservoir hematocrit, H_F, then some physical screening process which retards the entry of red cells into the tube (relative to plasma entry) must be occurring at the tube entrance.
2. The ratio of the discharge hematocrit to the tube hematocrit, H_D/H_T, is equal to the ratio of the red cell average velocity to the blood average velocity, $\bar{U}_C/\bar{U}_B$. Experimental data may show this velocity ratio to be a function of the tube hematocrit and the blood velocity, but the value of H_F used to establish the conditions in the tube will be immaterial to this relationship.

Consider first H_D, the discharge hematocrit. The experimental data for this quantity, obtained for tubes whose inside diameters are everywhere constant (even in the entrance section of the tube), are shown in Fig. 2, where H_D has been divided by H_F to give a relative discharge hematocrit. This ratio is equal to unity in larger tubes, at least up to feed

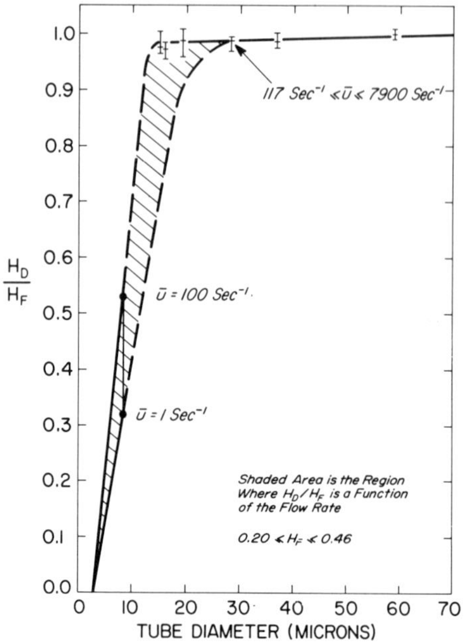

Figure 2. Variation of the relative discharge hematocrit with tube diameter and velocity. The velocities noted for the 8.1-μm tube are red cell average velocities; the larger tube velocities are blood average velocities. The crossbars indicate the range and mean values of all data obtained with a given tube size (number of samples per point ranged from 4 to 14).

hematocrits of about 0.55, and is independent of the blood flow rate (experimental range of flow rates $\bar{U}$ was 13–212 tube diameters per second for the 59-μm tube, and 0.3–110 tube diameters per second for larger tubes). In smaller tubes, this hematocrit ratio is a function of the flow rate: for the 8.1-μm tubes, when the red cell flow rate is 80–100 tube diameters per second, the hematocrit ratio averages to 0.53, while the corresponding average at flow rates of 0.8–3 tube diameters per second is 0.32. These results are independent of the feed hematocrit within the range indicated in the figure. The dashed curves are estimates of the expected behavior; the intercept on the abscissa is the theoretical minimum tube diameter (2.74 μm) through which a red cell can squeeze if its surface area stretches to the value it has just before osmotic hemolysis (the data of Evans and Fung, 1972, were used in this calculation).

The velocity dependency shown in Fig. 2 is due to the red cell flexibility and its influence on the ease with which a cell can enter the tube entrance. Obviously, the shape of the tube entrance also influences the curves in those regions where the relative discharge hematocrit is less than unity. Funnel-shaped entrances would show curves with steeper slopes in the region where the relative discharge hematocrit is less than 1. Decreases in cell flexibility would be expected to distort the curves so that the initial sections would rise at a lower angle. We have tried to obtain data with glutaraldehyde-hardened red cells but have not been able to maintain the necessary steady flows in tubes with diameters below 99 μm; in 99-μm and larger tubes, suspensions of hardened cells show the same behavior as normal cell suspensions (Barbee, 1973).

The other hematocrit of interest is the tube or dynamic hematocrit, H_T. Figure 3 shows how this hematocrit varies with tube diameter and H_F for tubes with inside diameters equal to or greater than 29 μm. The tube relative hematocrit, H_R, plotted as the ordinate, is defined as the ratio H_T/H_F. This ratio drops below unity for tubes smaller than about 300 μm, and the ratio for smaller tubes is a function of tube diameter and feed hematocrit. These data were found to be independent of flow rate and cell flexibility (for tubes greater than 99 μm in diameter with hardened red cells); they were also unaffected when the suspending phase was changed from plasma to isotonic saline.

Figure 4 shows how this tube relative hematocrit behaves in smaller tubes. The top two lines are from the previous figure. These data were obtained by making a series of microphotographs of the blood in a tube.

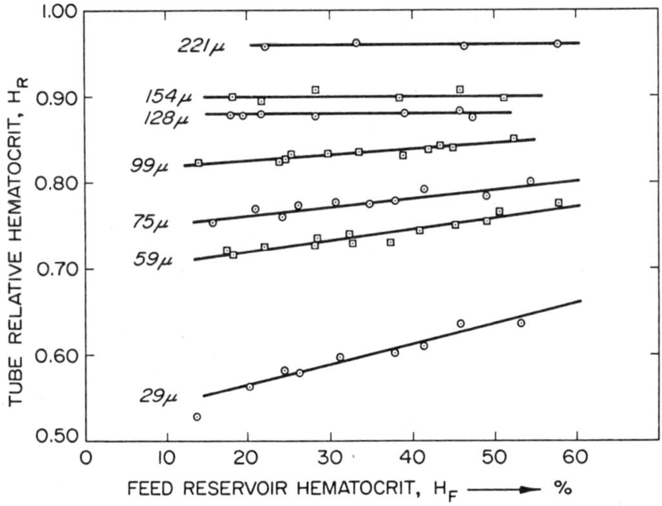

Figure 3. Variation in tube (or dynamic) relative hematocrit as a function of tube size and feed reservoir hematocrit. Reprinted from Barbee and Cokelet (1971*a*).

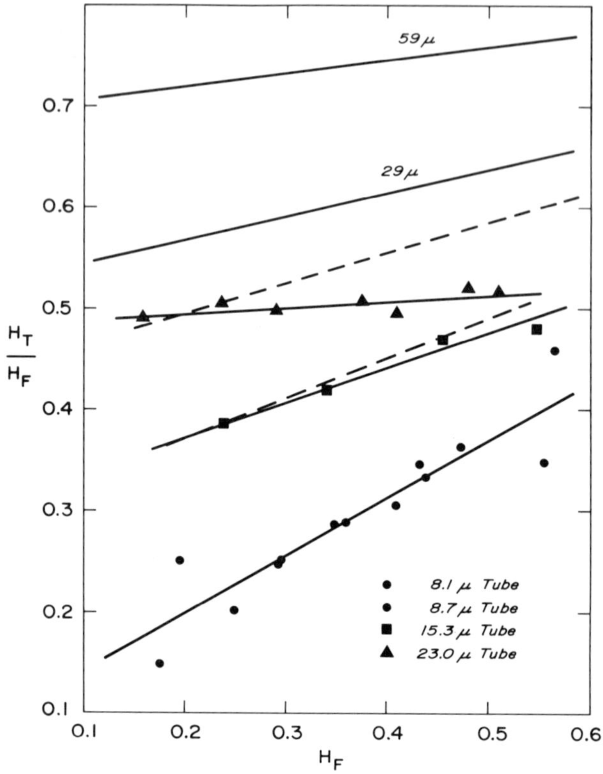

Figure 4. Variation in tube relative hematocrit as a function of tube size and feed reservoir hematocrit for smaller tubes. See text for explanation of dashed lines.

By determining the average number of cells per unit tube length from the photographs, one can calculate the average tube hematocrit, knowing the tube dimensions and the red cell average volume. The solid lines are least-squares fits through these data points. The lines for the 15.3- and 23.0-μm tubes have slopes markedly different from what one would expect by extrapolation of the data in the previous figure. If one crossplots the data in Fig. 3 along with the 8.1–8.7 μm tube line in this figure, and interpolates for the lines for the 15.3- and 23.0-μm tubes, one obtains the dashed lines shown in Fig. 4. Why this discrepancy for these two tubes? It is believed that the dashed lines are correct and the solid lines deviate from them because at higher hematocrits some cells are hidden from view by their neighbors and so are not counted when the microphotographs are viewed. All the cells in the 8.1–8.7 μm tubes are in view since the cells are forced to travel single file down the tube. At a feed hematocrit of 0.50, the difference between the two lines for the 23-μm tube indicates that 12.8% of the cells were hidden from view and not counted; with a corresponding tube hematocrit of 0.294, this seems possible. For the 15.3-μm tube, the corresponding values are 2.9% of the cells missed in counting, the tube average hematocrit being 0.245. We are now using high-speed cinemicrophotographs to resolve this difference: frame-by-frame analysis enables one to count cells as they are uncovered and come into view in sequential frames.

These data seem to be independent of flow rate, which is surprising. This will also be investigated with our high-speed cinemicrophotography work.

These data indicate a number of things. First, the fact that the relative discharge hematocrit can be 1 while the relative tube hematocrit is much less than 1 confirms the widely held idea that the red cells are not distributed uniformly across the tube cross-section. The local hematocrit must be higher than the average in regions where the local flow rate is higher than the average velocity, and *vice versa*. Second, collecting the blood flowing from a tube and measuring its average hematocrit generally does not tell what the average hematocrit is inside the flow channel. Third, from the information on H_T and H_D, the ratio of the average red cell velocity to the average blood velocity, $\bar{U}_C/\bar{U}_B$, can be determined. This velocity ratio will vary with the tube diameter and the hematocrit. As an example, this function is shown in Fig. 5 for the case of H_F held constant at a value of 0.40. The dots are experimental data; the dashed curves are based on the dashed curves of Figs. 2 and 4. The peaks are consistent with the observation that, for these conditions, red cells flow down the tube in a

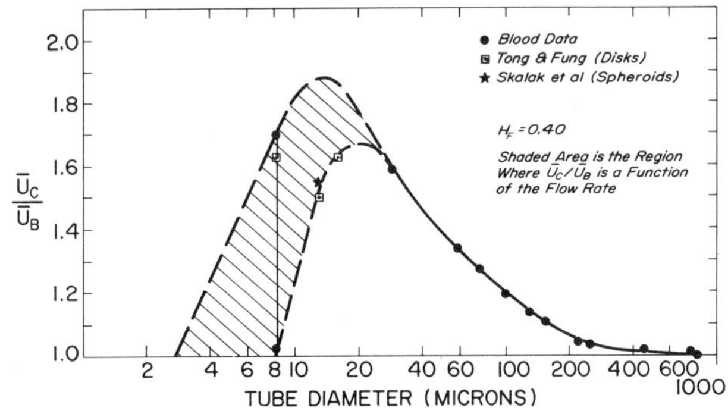

Figure 5. Dependence of the ratio of the average red cell velocity to the average blood velocity on the tube size and flow velocity, for the case where the feed reservoir hematocrit is held constant at 0.40.

single file until the tube diameter increases to between 12 and 15 μm at high flow rates and at very low flow rates the critical tube diameter is slightly greater than that. The high flow rate curve has an intercept at a tube diameter of 2.74 μm, the theoretical minimum tube diameter through which a red cell can flow, and the limiting low flow curve has an intercept slightly below 8 μm, the theoretical minimum tube size for flow of an undeformed red cell. Also shown in Fig. 1 are a few velocity ratios from model studies by Tong and Fung (1971) and Skalak *et al.* (1972). The peak velocity ratios are based on model predictions given in the latter reference. As pointed out by Skalak *et al.* (1972), the shape of the particle has very little influence on this velocity ratio; the ratio of the particle diameter to tube diameter is the factor with the most influence on the velocity ratio.

It appears, at least in tubes and vessels that are smaller than about 30 μm in diameter, that the average red cell velocity cannot be easily related to the blood flow rate. This is so because the red cell is deformable, causing the effective cell diameter to be a function of the vessel size and the flow rate. This in turn influences the critically important particle–tube diameter ratio. In *in vivo* systems, where the vessel diameter may vary appreciably with axial position because of the cellular nature of the wall, and the cross-section of the lumen is noncircular, the red cell–blood velocity ratio function will be even further complicated.

1.1.2. Hematocrit, Wall Shear Stress, and Flow Rate

The question arises, can we predict the pressure drop–flow rate relationship for blood flowing in a tube, given these hematocrit data? The answer is presented in graphical form, first in Fig. 6.

This figure is a plot of the wall shear stress, τ_W, vs. the blood bulk velocity divided by the tube diameter, $\bar{U}$. These two parameters are directly calculable from the measured pressure gradient, blood flow rate, and tube diameter. The reason for plotting pressure drop–flow rate data in this manner is that it can be shown that for steady, uniform, laminar flow of a fluid in a tube all the data for a given fluid will fall on a single curve, regardless of the dimensions of the tubes used in obtaining the data. Furthermore, from this plot, one can calculate the rheological properties of the fluid. The basis for these conclusions lies in the derivation of two flow functions, variously attributed to either Mooney, Rabinowitsch, or Weissenberg (see Markovitz, 1968, and especially Savins and Markovitz, 1968, for a discussion of the historical aspects of this question), and used, for example, by Metzner and Reed (1955), Oldroyd (1949), and Merrill *et al.* (1968).

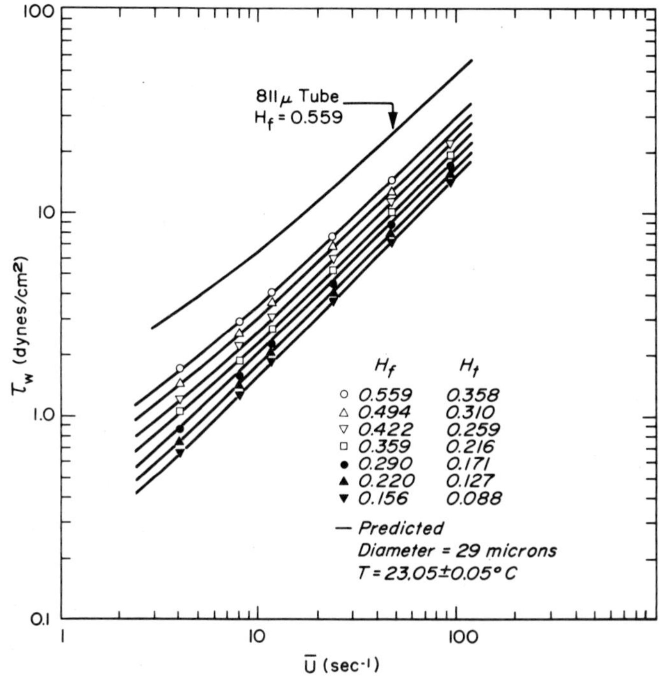

Figure 6. Relationship between wall shear stress and average blood velocity divided by the tube diameter. The points are experimental data obtained with 29-μm tubes; the curves represent data obtained with an 811-μm tube. When the curve (larger tube data) and points (smaller tube data) are close together, the dynamic hematocrits were equal. Reprinted from Barbee and Cokelet (1971*b*).

There is one restriction on this general method: it is applicable only to fluids for which the shear stress is a single function of the shear rate. We would not expect this requirement to be met in the case of blood flowing in a relatively small tube, because, as we have already noted, for tubes smaller than about 300 μm in diameter the hematocrit must vary with radial position, and since the hematocrit has a strong influence on the blood rheological properties we would not expect to find a single rheological relationship for all the blood in a tube. Also, in very small tubes, we would not expect it to work because the continuum model of blood (implied in the derivation) probably would fail (and certainly loses physical meaning) when the cell size and tube diameter become comparable in magnitude. Nevertheless, let us apply this general method to see how well it works.

In Fig. 6, the solid curves represent data obtained when blood flows through an 811-μm tube, a size sufficiently large that H_T equals H_F. Each curve is for a different hematocrit. The symbols represent data obtained with a 29-μm tube, where H_T is not equal to H_F, as indicated in the table in the figure. If we ignored the fact that H_T for the 29-μm tube is less than H_F and just assumed that H_T equals H_F, we would see the Fåhraeus-Lindqvist effect: e.g., compare the top curve for a 811-μm tube with H_F = 0.559 and the curve indicated by open circles, which represents data for a 29-μm tube with $H_F = 0.559$. At any given $\bar{U}$, the wall stress is less for the 29-μm tube than for the 811-μ tube. However, if we recognize that the blood in the 29-μm really has a hematocrit $H_T = 0.358$, and we obtain data with the 811-μm tube for $H_F = H_T = 0.358$, upon putting these data on the plot we find that they are represented by the solid curve which passes through the open circles. Similar agreement is shown at the other hematocrit levels; if we make sure that H_T is the same in all tubes, then the data for that blood do indeed fall on a single curve. Furthermore, we can

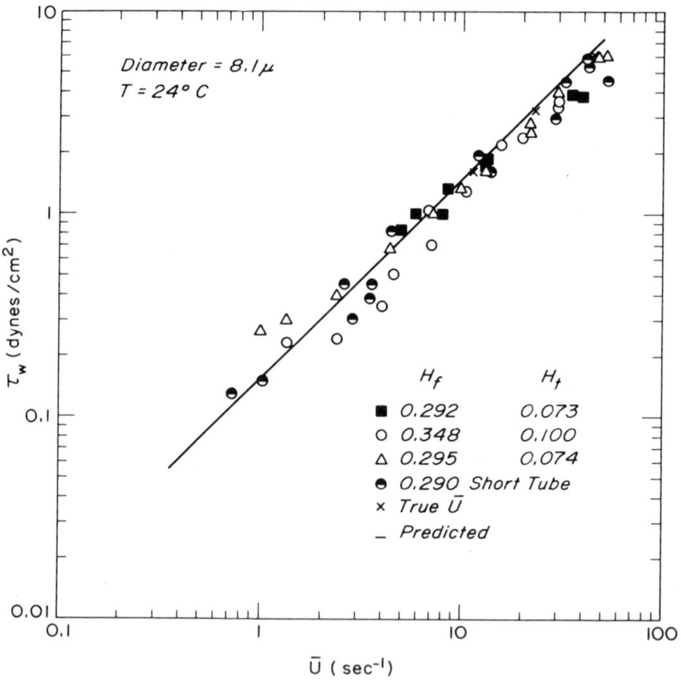

Figure 7. Comparison between the predicted and the experimental relationship between wall shear stress and reduced average velocity. The few crosses represent a few data plotted using the blood average velocity; the other points are plotted using the red cell average velocity. See text for explanation.

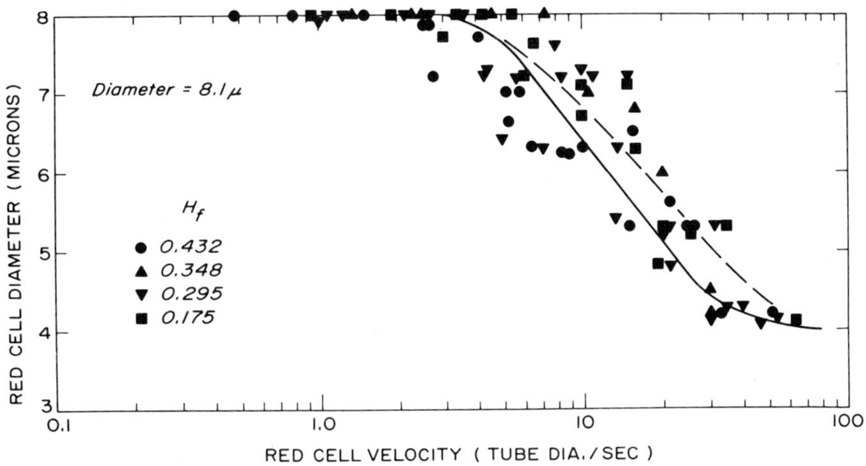

Figure 8. Silhouette diameter of human red cells as a function of red cell velocity for blood flow through a 8.1-μm tube. If the solid curve is taken as representative of the data, the dashed curve represents the predicted behavior for rigid particles with the same diameter as the silhouette diameter.

predict that curve from the macroscopic rheological properties of the blood.

It should be pointed out that this behavior is not peculiar to blood alone. Seshadri and Sutera (1970) have found the same behavior for suspensions of rigid spheres and discs flowing through tubes, for "hematocrits" below 0.30 and particle–tube diameter ratios below 0.10.

We have found the same behavior to be valid in 23.0-, 15.3-, and 8.1-μm tubes (for experimental range of H_T values between zero and an upper hematocrit level of 0.25 for the 23.0-μm tube size and 0.15 for the smallest tube size). Figure 7 shows some data obtained with 8.1-μm tubes. The line is the predicted behavior and the symbols (except for the crosses) are the data plotted as wall shear stress vs. the average *red cell* velocity divided by the tube diameter. This is an incorrect way to plot the data if we want to test the general predictive method described above: we should use the blood velocity, not the red cell velocity. These data are plotted this way to illustrate what happens when one does use the red cell velocity (easily measured by a photometric dual-slit device or by analysis of high-speed cinemicrophotographs). Characteristically, at low velocities the data seem to cluster on the predicted curve; at high flow rates the data fall below the curve. When one does plot the data correctly, using the blood velocity instead of the red cell velocity, the data points at low flow rates are not moved, but the high flow rate points shift to the left so that they also cluster on the predicted curve.

The reason for this shift of the points can be explained with the help of the data shown in Fig. 8. This is a plot of the diameter of the red cell silhouette as seen in a frame of a high-speed cinemicrophotograph, for blood flow in an 8.1-μm tube, as a function of the red cell velocity. As the red cell velocity increases, the cell becomes deformed. At low flow rates, it practically fills the lumen, acting as a plug or piston, so that effectively it and the blood have the same average velocity. At high flow rates, it is deformed and is in the center of the tube and so has a higher velocity than the blood as a whole. These red cell dimension data are essentially in agreement with the data of Hochmuth *et al.* (1970).

The two curves in Fig. 8 are meant to compare experimental data with the predictions of computer model studies by Skalak *et al.* (1972). If the solid curve is taken as representative of the experimental data, then

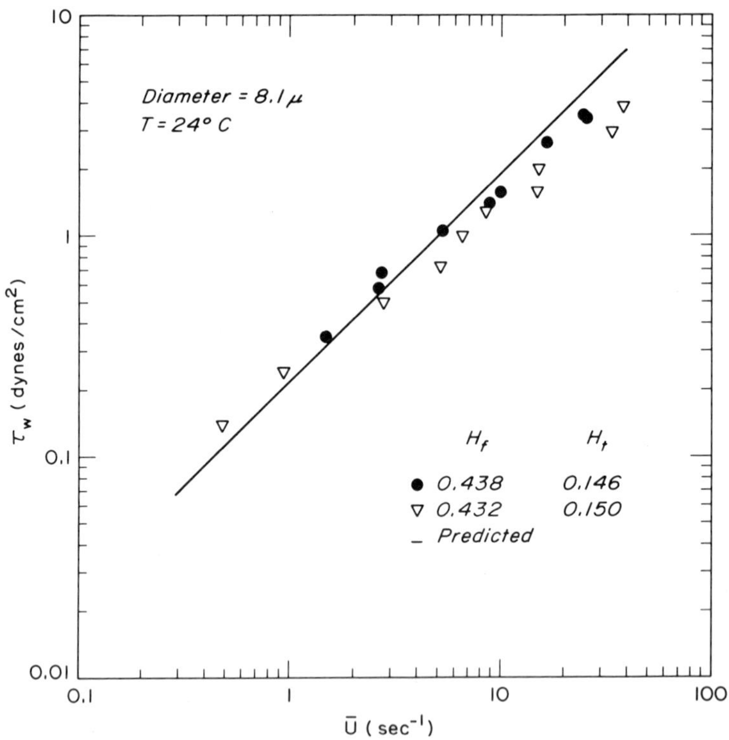

Figure 9. Same relationship as shown in Fig. 7, except that the hematocrit levels are higher.

the dashed curve represents the corresponding red cell diameter prediction from the models for rigid particles flowing down a tube.

Figure 9 shows more data, similar to those of Fig. 7, but for a higher hematocrit level. The comments made relative to Fig. 7 apply here as well. However, this agreement between experimental data and predictions based on a continuum model of the fluid and macroscopic rheological data, especially for these smallest tubes, is preposterous. There are many reasons that this predictive method should not work. For example, theoretical models based on the flow of suspensions of rigid particles in tubes predict that at a given particle flow rate the apparent viscosity of the suspension should increase linearly with hematocrit at low hematocrits, and then, at higher hematocrits, increase more slowly with increasing hematocrit, eventually becoming almost insensitive to hematocrit (Skalak *et al.* 1972). This is just the opposite of the trend shown by the blood bulk rheological properties, where the apparent viscosity increases roughly exponentially with hematocrit. The success of the predictive technique is obviously fortuitous, although useful, and is probably limited to low values of H_T in 8–10 μm tubes.

1.1.3. Hematocrit and Viscosity: Other Data

There are a number of literature references which contain data on blood flow in very small tubes (Barbee and Cokelet, 1971*a,b*; Barras, 1969; Bayliss, 1965; Braasch and Jenett, 1968; Fåhraeus, 1929; Fåhraeus and Lindqvist, 1931; Haynes and Burton, 1959; Jay *et al.*, 1972; Kümin, 1949). Generally, for each reported experiment, not all of the important variables were measured: usually the tube hematocrit, H_T, was not measured. This makes analysis of the literature data problematical, but one method of analysis will be presented to show that the techniques mentioned earlier are supported by the literature data.

For purpose of illustration, some of the data of Braasch and Jenett (1968) have been selected. They pumped suspensions of pig red cells in serum through slightly conical tubes in a pulsatile manner, at a mean wall shear stress of 50 dyn/cm^2, which is sufficiently high to make the flow appear to be Newtonian. It is believed that they calculated their relative viscosity data by effectively dividing the cell suspension viscosity by the viscosity of water, so the liberty has been taken of converting their data to a relative viscosity based on the serum viscosity (which they reported). These data are shown in Fig. 10.

In this figure, the lower curve represents data obtained for various diameter tubes while H_F was constant at 0.43; the upper curve is similar except that H_F is 0.63. These data are another demonstration of the Fåhraeus-Lindqvist effect.

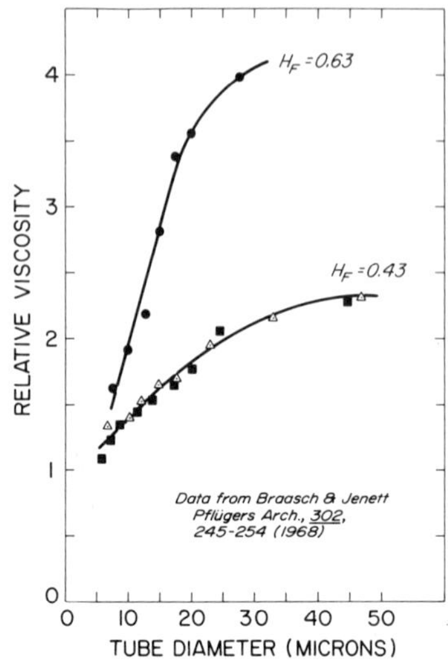

Figure 10. Relative viscosity of suspensions of pig red cells in pig serum as a function of tube diameter and at two feed reservoir hematocrit levels. These data illustrate the Fåhraeus-Lindqvist effect.

We recognize that while H_F is constant for the data along one of these curves, H_T is progressively decreasing as the tube diameter decreases. If we take into account this variation in dynamic hematocrit, can we predict these apparent viscosity data from macroscopic rheological data? To answer this question, we need two relationships: one for H_T as a function of the tube diameter, and one for the high shear rate relative viscosity of the cell suspension as a function of hematocrit. Having neither of these relationships for pig red cells in serum, we have to fall back on some general expressions based on human cell suspensions.

1. For a fixed value of H_F, the ratio H_T/H_F is a linear function of the logarithm of the tube diameter D:

$$H_T/H_F = a_0 + a_1 \ln D \tag{1}$$

   where A_0 and A_1 are functions of h_F.
2. At high shear rates and for hematocrits below about 0.40, the relative viscosity is an exponential function of the hematocrit:

$$\begin{aligned}\ln \eta_r &\equiv \ln (\eta/\eta_0) \\ &= bH\end{aligned} \tag{2}$$

   where B is a constant.

Combining these two equations yields

$$\ln \eta_r = (a_1 b H_F) \ln D + (a_0 b H_F) \tag{3}$$

which says that a plot of the logarithm of the relative viscosity vs. the logarithm of the tube diameter should be a straight line if H_F is held constant. Such a plot for the Braasch-Jenett data is shown in Fig. 11, where the lines are least-squares regression lines.

These data indeed seem to verify the linear relationship predicted by equation (3). Skeptics would frown upon this demonstration, however, since "everyone knows that any set of data plotted on a log–log graph gives a straight line." To satisfy such critics, the constants of equations (1), (2), and (3) were evaluated from human red cell suspension data for the case where H_F is constant at a value of 0.43. The appropriate equations are

$$H_T/H_F = 0.218 \ln D - 0.130$$

where D is in micrometers, and

$$\ln \eta_r = 2.59\, H$$

where H is in decimal form. Combining these gives

$$\ln \eta_r = 0.2431 \ln D - 0.148 \tag{4}$$

An analogous equation for the case of H_F constant at 0.63 is not reported because data for evaluating the constants in equation (1) are not available and extrapolation of existing data is of questionable validity.

The appropriate data and the graphical presentation of equation (4) are shown in Fig. 12. While the line representing equation (4) does not fit

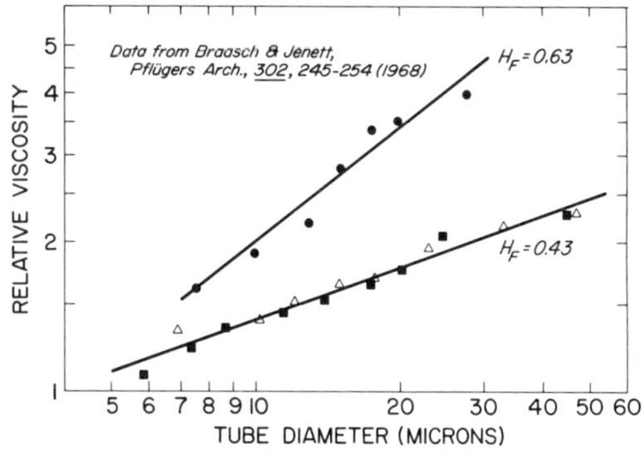

Figure 11. Data of Fig. 10 plotted on a log–log graph to test equation (3). The lines are least-squares fits to each set of data.

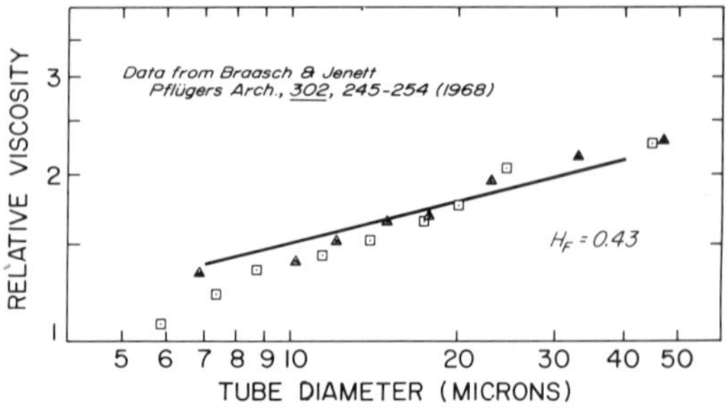

Figure 12. A test of equation (4). The line is drawn only for the range for which equation (4) is known to be valid for human blood.

the data as well as the corresponding least-squares line in Fig. 11, the agreement is sufficient to be encouraging (how much of the discrepancy may be due to differences between human and pig red cells is unknown).

Except for the data of Jay *et al.* (1972), similar analyses of the literature data previously cited lead to the same general conclusions, so it appears that if the dynamic hematocrit, H_T, is known, the pressure drop–flow rate relationship for the tube flow of blood can be predicted from macroscopic rheological data, at least in the range of H_T values so far investigated.

Jay *et al.* (1972) studied blood flow in tubes with diameters between 4 and 15 μm and with flow rates from 0 to 1000 μm per second. They reported that "a single erythrocyte flowing through the tubes increases the flow resistance and the apparent viscosity by about 30% over that of the suspending medium alone" and "the apparent viscosity of whole blood even at hematocrits of over 80% is only 55% higher than the viscosity of plasma." These results would seem to conflict both with the experimental results discussed previously and, on a quantitative plane, with the model results of Skalak *et al.* (1972). However, this conflict is probably only apparent.

Jay *et al.* (1972) used red cell velocity as a measure of flow for cell suspensions, and used the velocity of 1–2 μm latex microspheres (introduced into cell-free plasma or water) as a measure of flow for cell-free fluids. The translation of such particle velocities into suspension or fluid average velocities is not straightforward.

1.1.4. Models of Blood Flow in Tubes

Up to this point, the discussion has looked at the tube flow of blood in terms of overall or average-value parameters, a miniscale viewpoint. One is tempted to see if microscale parameters, such as the red cell radial distribution and the velocity profile, can be predicted from macroscopic rheological properties and miniscale parameters. There are innumerable literature reports of attempts to make such analyses; only three will be referred to here: Thomas (1962), Gazley (1972), and Baker (1972).

Thomas recognized that the hematocrit is not constant across the tube cross-section. He used the common two-phase model: a wall layer of plasma and a core of uniform-hematocrit blood. The plasma layer was taken to have Newtonian flow properties. Thomas, realizing that the blood in the core region was non-Newtonian, used a form of the Mooney-Rabinowitsch-Weissenberg equation (referred to earlier) in his analysis. The necessary rheological data had to be experimentally determined and he obtained them by an extrapolation of tube flow data. In addition, his analysis used the principles of the conservation of mass (of cells and of the suspending medium) and the equations of motion (conservation of momentum). Thomas applied his analysis to two sets of data:

1. Kümin's data (Kümin, 1949). These data for defibrinated ox blood were for a single H_F value of 0.40, and covered the tube diameter range of 58–4554 μm, with the smaller tube sizes at 58, 102, 178, and 390 μm. Using some of Kümin's data to get the necessary macroscopic rheological function, Thomas then calculated the wall layer thickness for the smaller tubes. The calculated thickness ranged between 1.5 and 5.0 μm; within the limits of estimated error, all tubes showed a limiting value of 1.5 μm at low shear rates, with limiting high shear rate values between 3.8 and 5.0 μm. There is a suggestion from the calculated values that the wall layer thickness decreases as tube diameter decreases.
2. Fåhraeus's data (Fåhraeus, 1929). These data consisted of H_T as a function of tube diameter for a single value of H_F and for tube diameters ranging from 50 to 1100 μm. All flows were presumably at very high rates. Thomas used these data (and the same macroscopic rheological data as used to analyze Kümin's data) to calculate the plasma wall layer thickness. This thickness was between 3.3 and 9.3 μm, generally showing an increase with decreasing diameter (a trend contrary to that found from Kümin's data). While Thomas speculated on this difference in behavior of the calculated plasma layer thickness with changes in the tube diameter, he indicated that one cannot draw firm conclusions about the cause of the difference.

Thomas's analysis is noteworthy for the fact that it recognized the radial variation of hematocrit, the non-Newtonian rheological behavior of the blood, and the fact that H_T and H_F are not equal. A significant feature of his results is the smallness of the plasma layer thickness.

Gazley (1972) limited his analysis to very high flow rates. He also used a two-phase fluid model to describe blood flow through tubes; this model consisted of a wall layer of blood, of a uniform hematocrit which may be zero or nonzero, and a core fluid, also of uniform hematocrit. Both phases were assumed to be Newtonian, since the analysis is only for very high flow rates. Like Thomas's, his analysis used the principles of the conservation of mass and momentum. From the data of Barbee (1971), which covered human blood flow in tubes with diameters between 29 and 811 μm, and H_F values from 0.15 to 0.55 (and which are included in some earlier figures), Gazley calculated the following:

1. The wall layer thickness is 4.45 μm, independent of tube diameter or hematocrit.
2. The wall layer hematocrit, H_W, is proportional to the square of H_F

$$H_W = 0.4H_F^2$$

3. As shown in Fig. 13, the core fluid shows essentially the same viscosity–hematocrit relationship as bulk blood, but the viscosity–

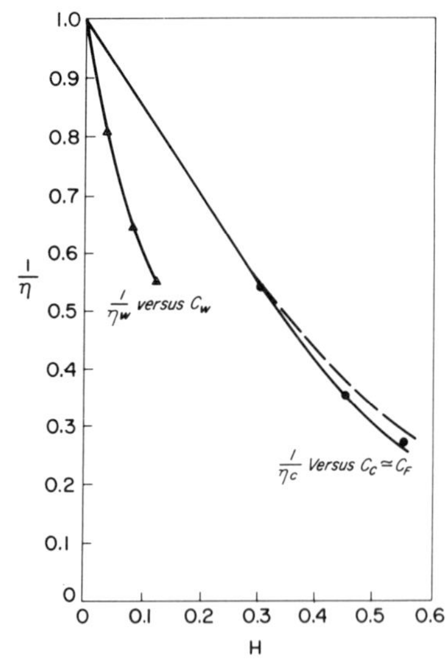

Figure 13. Apparent fluidity (reciprocal apparent viscosity η) vs. hematocrit for the wall layer blood and the core blood, as determined by Gazley (1972) from his model of high-velocity blood flow in tubes. The dashed curve represents the experimental macroscopic rheological properties of the same human blood. Reprinted from Gazley (1972).

hematocrit relationships for the wall layer blood are markedly different, because of the close proximity of the tube's smooth wall. Gazley also used the data of Fåhraeus and Lindqvist (1931) to confirm aspects of his analysis, but the data were too few to permit a complete analysis. This unique approach produced some interesting information, in addition to indicating the thinness of the wall layer of fluid.

The last analysis of tube blood flow to be mentioned here is that of Baker (1972), and is the most ambitious: she used the continuum equations of motion and several other necessary constraints to predict the pressure drop–flow rate relationship, the hematocrit relationships, and the fluid velocity profiles. Basically, she started with the equations of motion and analytical expressions representing experimental macroscopic rheological data for blood as functions of hematocrit and shear rate. It was necessary to know the hematocrit profile in the tube; this has not been measured, but after considering the information available in the literature, she decided to try the general hematocrit relationship

$$H = H^*[1 - (r/R)^E] \tag{5}$$

where r is the radial distance to the position of interest, R is the tube radius, and both H^* and E are constants. Two contraints which were imposed were

$$H_T = \frac{2}{R^2}\int_0^R Hr\,dr \tag{6}$$

which is a mass balance on red cells, and which, from use of equation (5), gives

$$H^* = \left(\frac{E+2}{E}\right)H_T$$

and, as the second constraint, the mass balance,

$$\bar{U}(2\pi R^3) = 2\pi\int_0^R vr\,dr \tag{7}$$

where v is the local velocity. In practice, one picks a tube size R, H_F, and $\bar{U}$; the corresponding H_T is obtained from experimental data. One then guesses a value of E and proceeds to perform the integrations indicated by equations (6) and (7), the velocity profile having been calculated by integration of the equation of motion with the use of the macroscopic rheological properties of blood with a hematocrit H [which varies with position according to equation (5); it should be noted that Baker uses a 4-μm-thick plasma wall layer in her calculations]. The calculated $\bar{U}$ value from equation (7) must match the experimental $\bar{U}$ value when the correct value of E has been guesses.

Except for cases where the hematocrit H_T was very low, the value of E was always greater than 15, usually between 40 and 50. This indicates that the hematocrit profiles show a constant hematocrit across most of the tube cross-section, decreasing only immediately next to the wall.

The velocity profiles predicted by these calculations agreed very well with the experimental profiles which Baker measured (tube size range 71.9–142.5 μm, H_F range 0.135–0.58, blood velocity range 1.94–164.4 tube diameters per second), as well as those reported by Gaehtgens *et al.* (1970) and Bugliarello and co-workers (Bugliarello and Hayden, 1963; Bugliarello *et al.*, 1963; Bugliarello and Sevilla, 1970) for somewhat smaller tubes. Thus it would appear that at least in the intermediate tube sizes the continuum approach combined with the appropriate macroscopic rheological properties yields considerable information even on a micro-scale.

However, so far in her analysis, Baker had not utilized all the available experimental data. Having determined both the velocity and hematocrit profiles by the procedure outlined above, she next calculated the discharge hematocrit, H_D. She found that the calculated H_D values did not equal H_F (as shown experimentally) but were usually closer to H_T than H_F. In an effort to overcome this difficulty, she used three different general hematocrit distribution functions: (1) a profile which had a peak at some radius intermediate between the tube centerline and wall, (2) a profile which was flat until close to the wall, and (3) a profile which showed the hematocrit inversely proportional to the local velocity but finite at the wall. None of these hematocrit profiles resulted in a complete reconciliation between predictions and experimental data. Additional attempts to match predicted and experimental data also failed. Baker concluded that all the microscale behavior of blood flow in tubes could not be predicted from macroscopic parameters and the continuum model.

1.1.5. Conclusions

In conclusion, three ideas may be summarized:

1. The Fåhraeus-Lindqvist effect does exist, but is due to the fact that the hematocrit of the blood flowing in a tube decreases as the tube diameter decreases. Once the significance of the dynamic hematocrit is recognized, it is possible to predict the pressure drop–flow

rate relationship for blood flow through a tube from bulk rheological data which may be obtained from conventional viscometers. This statement is, of course, limited to the range of tube sizes and hematocrits discussed here. Satisfactory velocity and hematocrit profiles cannot be predicted.

2. In a series of vessels of decreasing diameter, the dynamic hematocrit will decrease as vessel diameter decreases, even in the absence of inward fluid transfer across the vessel wall.
3. The ratio of the average red cell velocity to the average blood velocity is a nonlinear function of tube diameter and hematocrit and for the smaller tubes (diameter less than 25–30 μm) is also a function of the flow rate (especially in the cell velocity range 1–100 tube diameters per second). Unfortunately, the sensitivity of this velocity ratio to changes in velocity is greatest where it is easiest to reliably measure the average red cell velocity by use of photometric dual-slit methods or by frame-by-frame analysis of cinemicrophotographs.

ACKNOWLEDGMENTS

It is a pleasure to acknowledge the contributions of Dr. James Barbee, Ann Berg Cicale, and Kauo-Rong John Sun, who obtained many of the data reported here. This work was supported by United States Public Health Service Research Grant HL-12723.

References

Baker, M., 1972, Double-slit photometric measurement of velocity profiles for blood in microvessels and capillary tubes, Ph.D. thesis, California Institute of Technology, Pasadena.

Barbee, J., 1971, The flow of human blood through capillary tubes with inside diameters between 8.7 and 221 microns, Ph.D. thesis, California Institute of Technology, Pasadena.

Barbee, J., 1973, Concentration reduction and dilatant flow behavior in suspensions of hardened human red cells, *Trans. Soc. Rheol.* **17**:413.

Barbee, J. H., and Cokelet, G. R., 1971*a*, The Fåhraeus effect, *Microvasc. Res.* **3**:6.

Barbee, J. H., and Cokelet, G. R., 1971*b*, Prediction of blood flow in tubes with diameters as small as 29 microns, *Microvasc. Res.* **3**:17.

Barras, J. P., 1969, Blood rheology—General review, *Bibl. Haematol.* **33**:277.

Bayliss, L. E., 1965, The flow of suspensions of red blood cells in capillary tubes: Changes in the "cell-free" marginal sheath with changes in the shearing stress, *J. Physiol. (London)* **179**:1.

Braasch, D., 1971, Red cell deformability and capillary blood flow, *Physiol. Rev.* **51**:679.

Braasch, D., and Jenett, W., 1968, Erythrocytenflexibilität, Hämokonzentration und Reibungswiderstand in Glascapillaren mit Durchmessern zwischen 6 bis 50μm, *Pfluegers Arch.* **302**:245.

Bugliarello, G., and Hayden, J. W., 1963, Detailed characteristics of the flow of blood *in vitro, Trans. Soc. Rheol.* **7**:209.

Bugliarello, G., and Sevilla, J., 1970, Velocity distribution and other characteristics of steady and pulsatile blood flow in fine glass tubes, *Biorheology* **7**:85.

Bugliarello, G., Kapur, C., and Hsiao, G., 1963, The profile viscosity and other characteristics of blood flow in an non-uniform shear field, in: *Proceedings of the Fourth International Conference on Rheology,* Part 4 (A. L. Copley, ed.), pp. 351–369, Interscience, New York.

Charm, S. E., and Kurland, G. S., 1974, *Blood Flow and Microcirculation,* Interscience, New York.

Chien, S., 1975, Biophysical behaviour of red cells in suspensions, in: *The Red Blood Cells,* Vol. 2 (D. N. Surgenor, ed.), pp. 1031–1133, Academic Press, New York.

Cokelet, G. R., 1972, The rheology of human blood, in: *Biomechanics: Its Foundations and Objectives* (Y. C. Fung, N. Perrone, and M. Anliker, eds.), pp. 63–103, Prentice-Hall, Englewood Cliffs, N.J.

Dintenfass, L., 1971, *Blood Microrheology—Viscosity Factors in Blood Flow, Ischaemia and Thrombosis,* Appleton-Century-Crofts, New York.

Evans, E., and Fung, Y.-C., 1972, Improved measurements of the erythrocyte geometry, *Microvasc. Res.* **4**:335.

Fåhraeus, R., 1929, The suspension stability of the blood, *Physiol. Rev.* **9**:241.

Fåhraeus, R., and Lindqvist, R., 1931, Viscosity of blood in narrow capillary tubes, *Am. J. Physiol.* **96**:562.

Gaehtgens, P., Meiselman, H. J., and Wayland, J., 1970, Velocity profiles of human blood at normal and reduced hematocrit in glass tubes up to 130 μ diameter, *Microvasc. Res.* **2**:13.

Gazley, C., 1972, Small-scale phenomena in the flow of dispersions, in: *Proceedings of the Fourth All-Union Heat and Mass Transfer Conference, Minsk, BSSR,* Vol. 9, p. 3; also Report p-4796, Rand Corp., Santa Monica, Calif.

Goldsmith, H. L., and Skalak, R., 1975, Hemodynamics, *Annu. Rev. Fluid Mech.* **7**:213.

Haynes, R. H., and Burton, A. C., 1959, Role of the non-Newtonian behaviour of blood in hemodynamics, *Am. J. Physiol.* **197**:943.

Hochmuth, R. M., Marple, R. N; and Sutera, S. P., 1970, Capillary blood flow. 1. Erythrocyte deformation in glass capillaries, *Microvasc. Res.* **2**:409.

Jay, A. W. L., Rowlands, S., and Skibo, L., 1972, The resistance to blood flow in capillaries, *Can. J. Physiol.* **50**:1007.

Kümin, K., 1949, Bestimmung de Zähigkeitskoeffizienten für Rinderblut bei Newtonscher Strömung in verschiden weiten Röhren und Capillaren bei physiologischer Temperatur, dissertation, Universität Bern.

LaCelle, P. L., and Weed, R. I., 1971, The contribution of normal and pathologic erythrocytes to blood rheology, *Prog. Hematol.* **7**:1.

Markovitz, H., 1968, The emergence of rheology, *Physics Today* **21(4)**23.

Merrill, E. W., 1968, Rheology of blood, *Physiol. Rev.* **49**:863.

Merrill, E. W., Benis, A. M., Gilliland, E. R., Sherwood, T. K., and Salzman, E. W., 1968, Pressure–flow relations of human blood in hollow fibers at low flow rates, *J. Appl. Physiol.* **20**:954.

Metzner, A. B., and Reed, J. C., 1955, Flow of non-Newtonian fluids—Correlation of the laminar, transition, and turbulent-flow regions, *AIChE J.* **1**:434.

Oldroyd, J. G., 1949, The interpretation of observed pressure gradients in laminar flow of non-Newtonian liquids through tubes, *J. Colloid Sci.* **4**:333.

Savins, J. G., and Markovitz, H., 1968, Letter to the Editor and Authors' Reply, *Physics Today* **21(8):**13.

Schmid-Schönbein, H., and Wells, R. E., 1971, Rheological properties of human erythrocytes and their influence upon the anomalous viscosity of blood, *Ergeb. Physiol.* **63:**146.

Seshadri, V., and Sutera, S. P., 1970, Apparent viscosity of coarse, concentrated suspensions in tube flow, *Trans. Soc. Rheol.* **14:**351.

Skalak, R., Chen, P. H., and Chien, S., 1972, Effect of hematocrit and rouleaux on apparent viscosity in capillaries, *Biorheology* **9:**67.

Thomas, H. W., 1962, The wall effect in capillary instruments: An improved analysis suitable for application to blood and other particulate suspensions, *Biorheology* **1:**41.

Tong, P., and Fung, Y.-C., 1971, Slow particulate viscous flow in channels and tubes—Application to biomechanics, *J. Appl. Mech.* **38:**721.

Wayland, H., 1967, Rheology and the microcirculation, *Gastroenterology* **52:**342.

Whitmore, R. L., 1968, *Rheology of the Circulation,* Pergamon Press, Oxford.

Whittaker, S. R. F., and Winton, F. R., 1933, The apparent viscosity of blood flowing in the isolated hindlimb of the dog, and its variation with corpuscular concentration, *J. Physiol. (London)* **78:**339.

1.2. Red Cell Interactions in Low Flow States

D. E. BROOKS

In vitro viscometric studies have shown that anticoagulated whole blood behaves as a complex non-Newtonian fluid. Its complexity derives from the unique way in which erythrocytes—the principal constituents of the dispersed phase—interact in shear flow with the suspending medium and with each other to produce the shear-dependent apparent viscosities commonly observed. The most important element in these interactions is the erythrocyte membrane. It is the purpose of this discussion to focus on those properties of the membrane that we believe are responsible for the rheological behavior of whole blood in low flow states.

As has been known since the introduction of low shear rate viscometers into the field of biorheology, the apparent viscosity of anticoagulated whole blood, or of suspensions of erythrocytes in plasma, increases strongly with decreasing shear rate below about 10 s^{-1} (Merrill *et al.*, 1963). The increase is much larger in the presence of physiological concentrations of fibrinogen than it is if serum or saline is used as the suspending medium. Typical data taken from Brooks *et al.* (1970) are shown for human erythrocyte suspensions in Fig. 1. If such suspensions are examined microscopically at zero shear rate, those which contain physiological concentrations of fibrinogen are observed to be extensively aggregated, while those in which serum or saline constitutes the suspending medium exhibit no clumping. This observation is the basis for the widely held belief that the high viscosities measured for whole blood at low shear rates are due to the presence of cellular aggregation. In what follows I shall summarize briefly our work on the mechanisms involved in erythrocyte aggregation–disaggregation reactions and on a method for obtaining a quantitative measure of the degree of aggregation present in cell suspensions.

When suspended in physiological media, whether in the presence or absence of plasma proteins, erythrocytes bear a net negative surface charge (Seaman, 1975). A diffuse cloud of counterions, called the ionic double layer, forms in solution adjacent to the cell surface, attracted by the membrane charge. The double layer bears a net charge equal and opposite to that of the cell. Because of thermal agitation and the reduced magnitude of electrostatic forces in media of high dielectric constant such

D. E. BROOKS · Departments of Pathology and Chemistry, University of British Columbia, Vancouver, British Columbia, Canada.

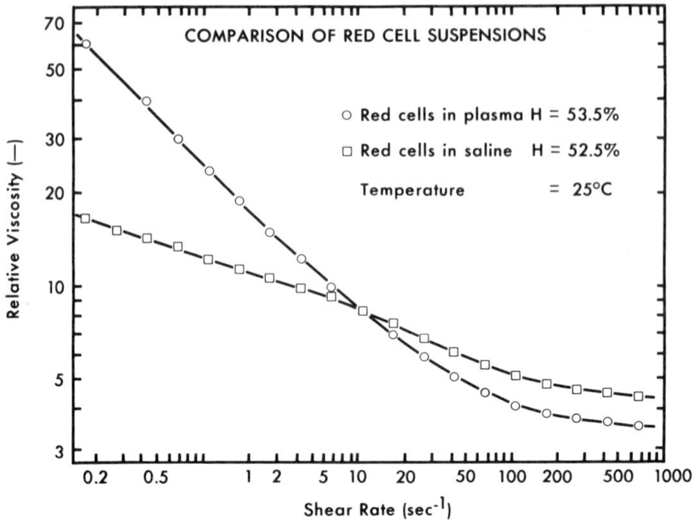

Figure 1. Relative viscosity as a function of applied shear rate for washed human erythrocytes resuspended in either homologous ACD plasma or 0.145 M NaCl, pH 7.2 ± 0.2. Data were obtained using a Weissenberg rheogoniometer. T = 25°C.

as water, the ionic double layer extends some tens of angstroms out from the cell surface. If two cells, bearing similar surface charges, approach within approximately 200 Å of each other, their charged double layers begin to overlap. Since the overlapping double layers contain net charges of the same sign, they tend to repel each other electrostatically, preventing the cells from making contact. There are attractive forces due to van der Waals interactions which also act between cells and effectively reduce the magnitude of the intercellular repulsion, but these are of insufficient magnitude to overcome the electrostatic forces and cause erythrocytes to aggregate. It is the cell surface charge, then, with its neutralizing ionic double layer, which is probably responsible for maintaining erythrocytes as single cell suspensions of relatively low viscosity in simple media such as physiological saline.

When fibrinogen is present in the suspending medium at physiological concentrations, erythrocyte aggregates (rouleaux) are clearly observed, however. Hence either the repulsive forces acting between cells have been reduced or the attractive forces have been increased. The red cell surface charge density is higher in plasma than in saline (Seaman *et al.*, 1962), probably because of protein adsorption, so electrostatic repulsion between cells should be if anything stronger when fibrinogen is present. Van der Waals attractive forces will be effectively reduced by the presence of protein in the aqueous phase, even if it adsorbs to the cell surface (Kiefer *et al.*, 1975). It appears, therefore, that an additional source of intercellular attraction is present in media containing fibrinogen. Since other blood cellular elements such as platelets do not necessarily aggregate in plasma, it is believed that the effect resides in an interaction of fibrinogen with the erythrocyte surface—presumably adsorption, since fibrinogen should not penetrate the cell membrane.

Fibrinogen is not the only macromolecule that can induce erythrocyte aggregation. Early work by Fåhraeus (1929) and Thorsén and Hint (1950) on erythrocyte sedimentation rates indicated that a variety of polymers and polypeptides were capable of clumping cells. We therefore decided, in order to have broader control over the chemical properties of the aggregating species and to minimize charge effects, to study in some detail the interaction of a neutral polymer, dextran, with human erythrocytes. As well as providing a general model for macromolecule-induced cellular interactions, dextran is of intrinsic interest because of its widespread use as a plasma expander. The results of our adsorption, electrokinetic, and rheological studies have provided some insight into the operative mechanisms in this system.

1.2.1. Dextran–Erythrocyte Interactions

1.2.1.1. Conditions for Aggregation at Physiological Ionic Strength

Fresh thrice-washed human erythrocytes were suspended in solutions of physiological saline which contained different concentrations of a series of sharply cut dextran fractions (kindly supplied by Pharmacia Fine Chemicals, Uppsala). The suspensions were examined microscopically and the degree of aggregation present at equilibrium was graded visually on a scale of 0 to 4+ (see original publication for details: Brooks, 1973*c*). The results are represented in Fig. 2 as a kind of phase diagram; each point represents a concentration and molecular weight of dextran at which the degree of cellular aggregation present was estimated. Suspensions containing those concentrations and molecular weights within the shaded region showed evidence of aggregation of the degrees indicated. There are several points of interest:

1. At physiological ionic strength, dextran fractions of low molecular weight could not induce aggregation at any concentration. Above molecular weights of about 41,000, however, clumping of some degree could be observed at certain concentrations. Hence a minimum molecular size was required for the aggregating agent to be effective.

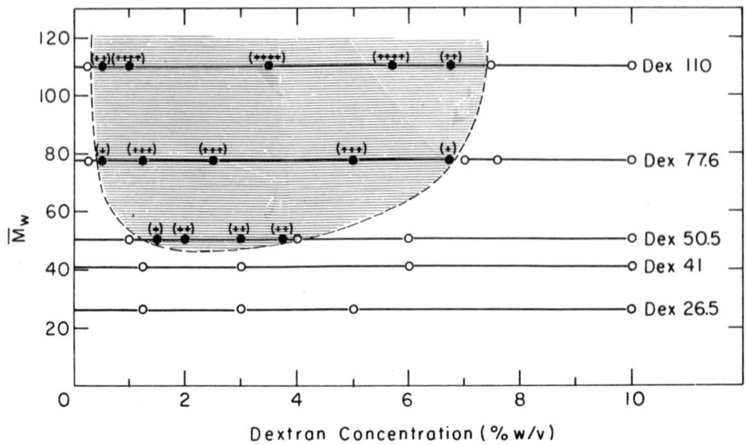

Figure 2. Concentrations and molecular weights of dextran which produced aggregation in saline suspensions of human erythrocytes. Aggregation of some degree was present for conditions within shaded region. Typical degrees of aggregation are shown for conditions given by solid points. Dextran weight-average molecular weights are given by 10^3 times fraction number. Reprinted by permission of Academic Press from Brooks (1973*c*).

2. For molecular weights greater than 41,000, a critical concentration above which aggregation occurred could be defined for each dextran fraction. This critical aggregation concentration was a monotonically decreasing function of molecular weight. That is, the larger the molecule the lower the concentration required to induce cell aggregation. In fact, at any fixed concentration the degree of aggregation increases with increasing molecular weight.
3. For a given molecular weight, the degree of aggregation initially increases rapidly as the concentration is increased. At higher concentrations, however, the degree of aggregation begins to decrease until at a second critical concentration the suspensions were found to be disaggregated and remain so no matter how much more polymer is added. The critical concentration for disaggregation is larger the higher the molecular weight.

It is convenient to discuss these results in terms of the following: first, the mechanism of dextran-induced aggregation; second, a quantitative technique for the measurement of the degree of aggregation present; and third, the mechanism of disaggregation.

1.2.1.2. The Aggregation Mechanism: Macromolecular Bridging

As was described in the opening of this report, red cells suspended in physiological saline probably remain disaggregated because of the ionic double layer which is set up adjacent to a charged cell surface. This cloud of counterions forms a zone which cannot be easily penetrated by the double layer of a second charged surface. Aggregation can occur either if very strong short-range forces are present which can bring the cell together in spite of electrostatic repulsion or if attractive forces are present which can act at distances greater than the effective extension of the ionic double layers. Macromolecular dimensions are frequently considerably greater than double layer thicknesses. If there is a tendency for a species of macromolecule to adsorb to cells, individual molecules can adsorb simultaneously to two adjacent surfaces, bridging the intercellular gap and tying the cells together at separations which are sufficiently great that double layer repulsion is small. This macromolecular bridging mechanism was first suggested to operate in colloidal dispersions flocculated by high polymers (Lamer and Smellie, 1956) and was later shown to occur in red cell suspensions clumped by polylysine (Katchalsky *et al.,* 1959). We believe macromolecular bridging to be the cause of aggregation in the dextran–erythrocyte systems as well, for the following reasons:

1. Dextran has been shown to adsorb to red cells from physiological salt solutions (Brooks, 1973*b*). Although adsorption is weak, the binding capacity of the membrane is high since no saturation occurs at concentrations up to 10 g/100 ml.
2. The minimum molecular weight requirement for aggregation is suggestive of this mechanism. Too small a molecule would be unable to span the intercellular gap.
3. There is evidence from the adsorption isotherm that strongly supports the bridging model. Figure 3 shows the concentration dependence of adsorption of dextran 77.6 (weight-average molecular weight, $\bar{M}_w$, is 77,600) to washed human erythrocytes in physiological saline (Brooks, 1973*b*). The adsorption isotherm is linear from 0.001 to about 7 g/100 ml. Above 7 g/100 ml, however, the amount of polymer adsorbed per cell increases sharply. The increase is seen at almost exactly the same concentration at which disaggregation is first observed when the dextran concentration is increased (Fig. 2). As shown in the inset of Fig. 3, correspondence between the critical disaggregation concentration and that at which an increased adsorption occurs strongly supports the macromolecular bridging model. Disaggregation should free some of the sites

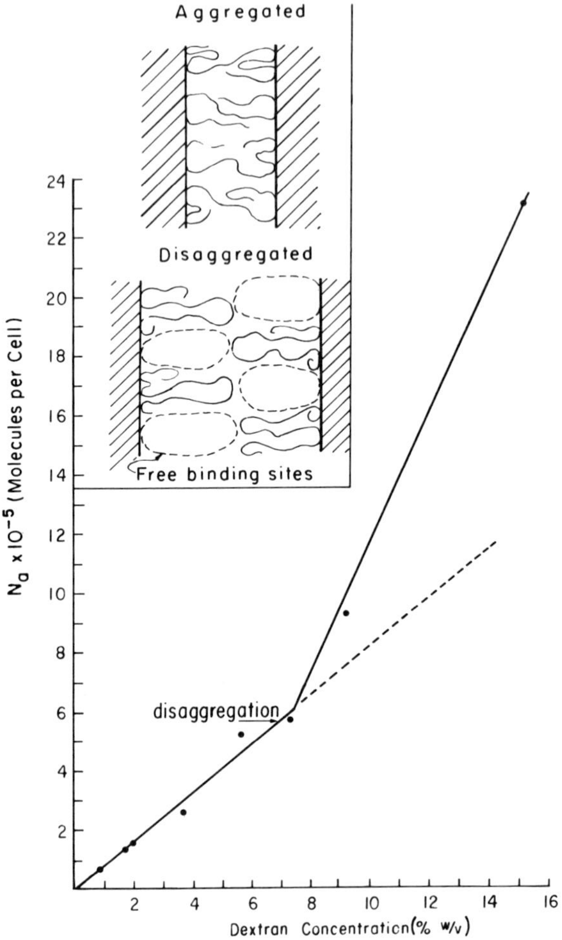

Figure 3. Isotherm of dextran 77.6 adsorption to human erythrocytes at physiological ionic strength in terms of the number of molecules adsorbed per cell, N_a. T = 25°C. Reprinted by permission of Academic Press from Brooks (1973*c*).

on the membrane to which bridging molecules were adsorbed. Occupation of these sites by nonbridging molecules increases the number of molecules per cell relative to the number which would be present if the cells were aggregated. This is the best supporting evidence for the bridging model currently available.

The cell membrane is an important element in this aggregation reaction as it forms the substrate to which the bridging macromolecules adsorb. While in some systems such as lectin-induced aggregation (Nicolson, 1974) or immunological agglutination (Roitt, 1974) much is known about the binding sites for bridging molecules, we at present have little information regarding the dextran–membrane interaction. The interaction is certainly weak, however, and since the adsorptive capacity is so large it is probably of a nonspecific nature. Nonetheless, these weak interactions are capable of markedly altering the flow characteristics of cell suspensions in which they occur.

1.2.1.3. A Quantitative Index of Cellular Aggregation

To study the details of the cellular aggregation reaction in our model system or to be able to apply the information gained here to whole blood, a quantitative measure of the degree of aggregation present in a given suspension is clearly desirable. Ideally, one would like to know the maximum force or energy required to separate two aggregated cells. Such an absolute measurement has not yet been a parameter from bulk suspension measurements which will faithfully reflect conditions at the cellular level.

A number of approaches have been used: sedimentation rate studies (Thorsén and Hint, 1950), low shear rate viscosity measurements (Chien *et al.*, 1970), viscometric (Cokelet *et al.*, 1963) and static (Charm and Kurland, 1967) yield stress measurements, optical transmittance (Born, 1962) and reflectance (Usami and Chien, 1973) techniques, and a variety of objective (Jan and Chien, 1973) and subjective (Brooks, 1973*c*) procedures based on the microscopic appearance of cell suspensions. None of these parameters provides a measure of only the forces acting between cells, however. Sedimentation rate measurements, even when corrected for density, viscosity, and hematocrit, will depend on cell size and shape as well as tube dimensions. Yield stress estimations vary widely depending on the technique used. Optical techniques sense variations in the size and shape of cell aggregates; it is not all clear how these parameters depend on intercellular forces. The objective microscopic aggregation index of Jan and Chien (1973) can be used only at low hematocrit and does not give results which agree with other methods applied at higher hematocrits (Chien and Jan, 1973). Subjective visual grading is very useful for crude determinations, but again the estimate is based largely on the size and shape of cell aggregates and there is no theory connecting these parameters with the forces and free energies of interest.

The above objections apply in general to viscometric techniques as well. There is some theoretical work available, however, which allows in some circumstances calculation of interparticle forces from the results of rheological experiments (Albers and Overbeek, 1960; Curtis and Hocking,

1970). Such calculations are based on the fact that in shear flow suspended aggregates are subject to local shear stresses. If these local shear stresses are small compared to intercellular forces, the aggregates will move as single units under their influence. If the shear stresses are large enough, however, they can act in such a way as to pull the cells apart (Goldsmith and Mason, 1967). Hence, if the local shear stresses acting on an aggregate were known under the conditions at which aggregate breakdown occurred, an estimate of the intercellular forces could be made. However, the problem of calculating local shear stresses from the shear rate and shear stress measured viscometrically for concentrated cell suspensions is extremely complicated and has not yet been solved. Viscosity determinations on suspensions concentrated enough to give good data cannot therefore be interpreted in terms of intercellular forces at present.

Although viscosity measurements have no absolute meaning in terms of cell–cell interactions, they may be used to provide a relative estimate of the degree of aggregation present in a suspension. In general, for concentrated suspensions to flow, intercellular associations, if present, must be continually broken down. Energy will necessarily be expended during this process. Since the apparent viscosity, η, is proportional to the rate of energy dissipation at any shear rate, aggregated suspensions should have higher viscosities than those in which no intercellular links have to be broken down, provided that the other energy dissipation mechanisms present are equal in the two cases. Under these conditions, the ratio of the apparent viscosities of aggregated and disaggregated suspensions of equal hematocrit should provide a measure of the degree of aggregation present. Moreover, this ratio should be a direct reflection of the amount of energy required per unit time to break intercellular bonds. It is possible that shape factors could be different in the two cases, which would also contribute to the viscosity difference, but it seems likely that at high hematocrits where the cells are in continual contact with one another shape effects should be small.

If the continuous phase viscosities, η_0, differ in the suspensions to be compared, the ratio of relative viscosities, η/η_0, should provide the necessary information, again assuming that η_0 differences do not affect the other modes of energy dissipation present. Red cell suspensions do not satisfy this assumption, however, because contributions to the apparent viscosity associated with cellular deformability vary with changes in η_0 (Brooks *et al.*, 1970). These contributions should be minimized at low shear rates, however, where the local shear stresses responsible for deformation are small. We therefore anticipated that the relative viscosity ratio, *R*, would provide a quantitative index of the degree of aggregation

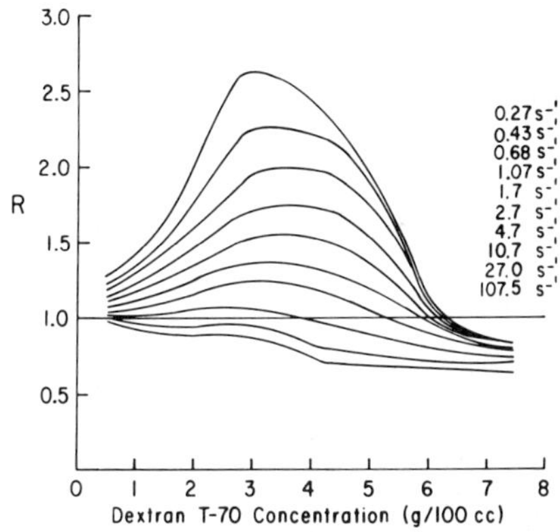

Figure 4. Relative viscosity ratio R (see text for definition) as a function of dextran T70 concentration for washed human erythrocytes in saline–EDTA, measured at the shear rates indicated. Hematocrit 30%, $T = 25°C$.

present if it were evaluated at a sufficiently low rate of shear (Brooks *et al.*, 1974).

Figure 4 shows the variation of R for suspensions of washed human erythrocytes at 30% volume concentration in saline–EDTA (0.15 M NaCl, 5 mM $NaHCO_3$, 1 mM Na_2 EDTA) plus various concentrations of dextran T70, $\bar{M}_w \simeq 70{,}000$. Here

$$R = \frac{(\eta/\eta_0)_{dex}}{(\eta/\eta_0)_{sal}}$$

where $(\eta/\eta_0)_{dex}$ is the relative viscosity of red cells in dextran and $(\eta/\eta_0)_{sal}$ is the relative viscosity of red cells in saline–EDTA. At the highest shear rates, R is less than 1 at all dextran concentrations. That is, the relative viscosities of suspensions containing dextran, which have higher continuous phase viscosities, are all less than those in saline–EDTA under these conditions. This reflects both the absence of aggregation at high shear rates and the increased cellular deformation which occurs in media more viscous than saline–EDTA. As the shear rate, $\dot{\gamma}$, is decreased, values of R greater than 1 begin to appear at some concentrations, implying that energy dissipation due to intercellular bond breaking is relatively more important than the decreased dissipation associated with cellular deformation. At lower shear rates, the range of dextran concentrations, and hence of η_0, over which R is greater than 1 increases. For $\dot{\gamma} \leq 0.68$, however, no further increase is found in the range of polymer concentrations for which R is greater than 1. By this criterion, then, there should be no

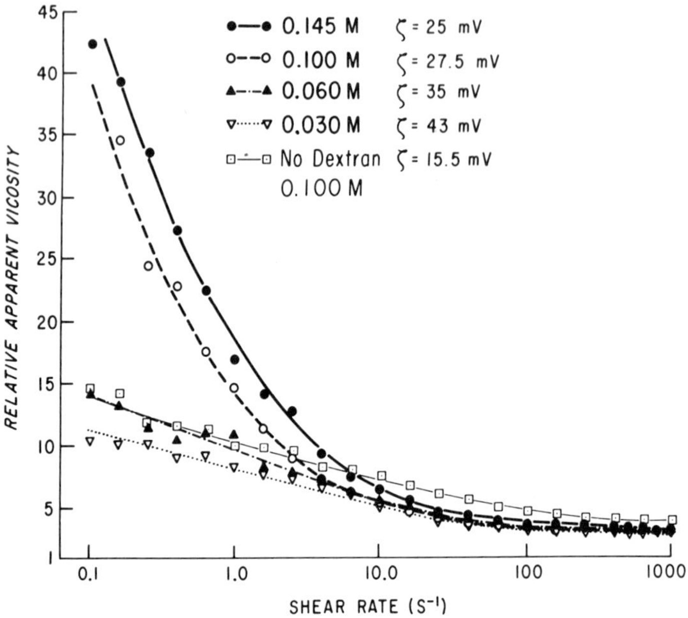

Figure 5. Relative viscosity as a function of shear rate for washed human erythrocytes at the ionic strengths indicated. Dextran T70 concentration 3 g/100 ml, hematocrit 50.0 ± 0.2%, T = 25°C. Reprinted by permission of Pergamon Press from Brooks *et al.* (1974).

aggregation present above about 6% dextran T70, and in fact microscopic examination of static suspensions confirms that this is the case.

The use of R as an aggregation index can be further examined by varying the ionic strength of the medium (maintaining isotonicity with sorbitol) at constant dextran concentration. Figure 5 shows the (η/η_0) vs. $\dot{\gamma}$ curves for 50% hematocrit suspensions of erythrocytes in 3% dextran T70 ($\bar{M}_w$ = 69,500) and various concentrations of NaCl. Deferring for the moment a discussion of why these curves differ, it seems clear that in 0.145 and 0.10 M NaCl plus 3% dextran T70 there is evidence of aggregation. Analyzing these and similar data using the relative viscosity ratio calculated at a series of shear rates provides the plots in Fig. 6. Below $\dot{\gamma} = 0.3\ s^{-1}$ the intercepts with $R = 1$ are independent of shear rate, so by our earlier reasoning values of R at such shear rates should provide an index of the degree of aggregation present. These values are given in Fig. 7 for $\dot{\gamma} = 0.17\ s^{-1}$. They are interpreted to mean that aggregation is more severe, and occurs over a wider dextran concentration range, the higher is the ionic strength. From the R values there is no evidence of any aggregation occurring in 0.03 M NaCl at any polymer concentration.

Although there is no absolute technique against which the results in Fig. 7 can be checked, it is possible to at least compare the critical dextran concentrations for aggregation and disaggregation as given by the concentrations at which R equals 1 with those at which microscopic examination of static suspensions indicates aggregation is absent. This comparison is made in Fig. 8, where another aggregation diagram is given, the shaded regions again indicating conditions under which aggregation was observed visually. It is clear that in every system the solid points around the boundary, which are the concentrations at which R equals 1, coincide with the visually estimated conditions indicated by the open ellipsoids. Near the critical aggregation–disaggregation conditions, then, the relative viscosity ratio must accurately reflect the degree of aggregation present, provided that it is evaluated at a shear rate low enough that the conditions for $R = 1$ are independent of $\dot{\gamma}$. The magnitude of R at such shear rates provides a quantitative index at aggregation which probably mirrors the strength of intercellular associations under near zero flow conditions.

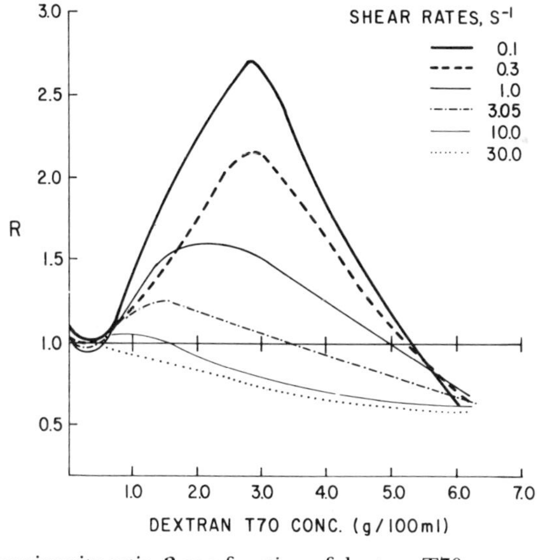

Figure 6. Relative viscosity ratio R as a function of dextran T70 concentration measured at the shear rates indicated for washed human erythrocytes. Ionic strength 0.10 M, hematocrit 50.0 ± 0.2%, T = 25.0°C. Reprinted by permission of Pergamon Press from Brooks *et al.* (1974).

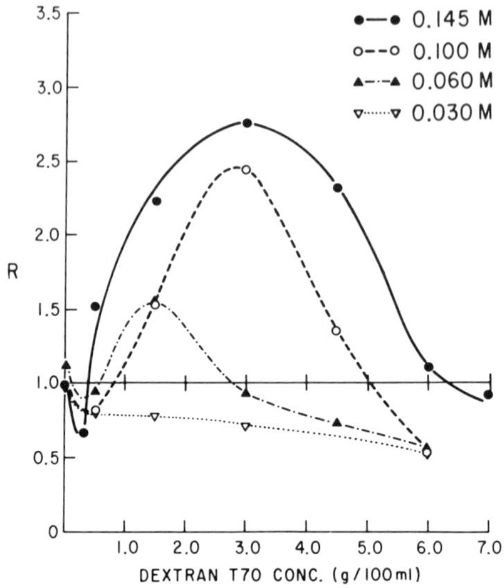

Figure 7. Relative viscosity ratio R as a function of dextran T70 concentration for washed human erythrocytes suspended in media of the ionic strengths indicated. Hematocrit 50.0 ± 0.2%, shear rate 0.17 s^{-1}, T = 25°C. Reprinted by permission of Pergamon Press from Brooks *et al.* (1974).

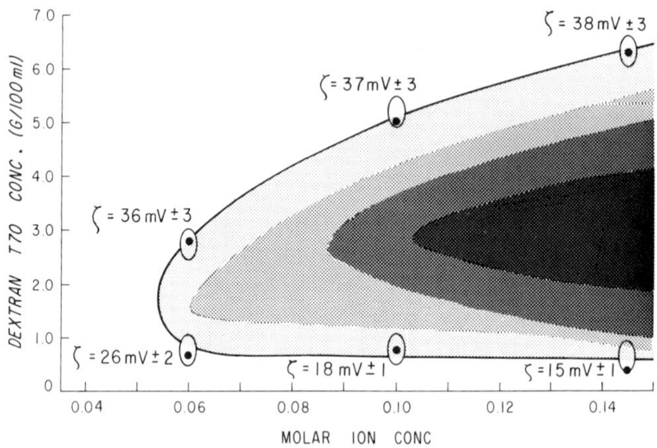

Figure 8. Conditions of dextran T70 concentration and ionic strength under which washed human erythrocytes were aggregated. The presence and degree of aggregation are indicated by the presence and degree of shading. Solid points are conditions for which R = 1 in Fig. 7; open ellipsoids represent estimates of critical conditions by optical microscopy. The ζ potentials given are for the conditions indicated by solid points. Reprinted by permission of Pergamon Press from Brooks *et al.* (1974).

1.2.1.4. An Example: Role of Membrane Deformability in Aggregation

As an example of the application of R as a relative measure of the degree of aggregation, we might consider the results of our studies on aldehyde-fixed erythrocytes in dextran solutions (Knox *et al.,* 1975). These cells are rigid under shear and cannot deform to provide the large areas of contact and maximum numbers of intercellular bonds necessary for tight aggregation. This effect is clearly seen in the plots of R as a function of dextran T70 concentration and shear rate given in Fig. 9. Comparison with Fig. 4 shows that the deformable cell suspensions are characterized by peak R values which are more than twice as large (relative to the $R = 1$ baseline) as those for fixed cells at the lowest shear rates. Hence the maximum degree of aggregation appears to be much greater in the normal than in the fixed suspensions. These results are consistent with the idea that large areas of contact, which can only occur if cells can deform out of their biconcave discoid shape under the influence of intercellular tension generated by bridging macromolecules, are necessary to achieve maximum aggregation in any given macromolecular solution. While there are other minor contributing factors involved (Knox *et al.,* 1975), we believe that these results effectively illustrate the role that membrane deformability can play in cellular aggregation.

1.2.1.5. The Mechanism of Disaggregation: Electrostatic Repulsion

Although dextran is a neutral, non-ionogenic polysaccharide, it imparts an unexpected increase in surface electrostatic potential to cells with which it is in equilibrium (Ponder, 1957). The potential at the

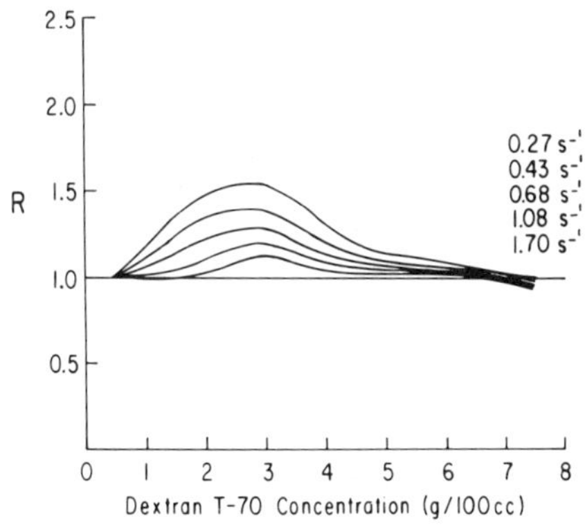

Figure 9. Relative viscosity ratio R as a function of dextran T70 concentration. Conditions were the same as for Fig. 4 except that cells were fixed in formaldehyde. Fixed cell volume concentration 30%.

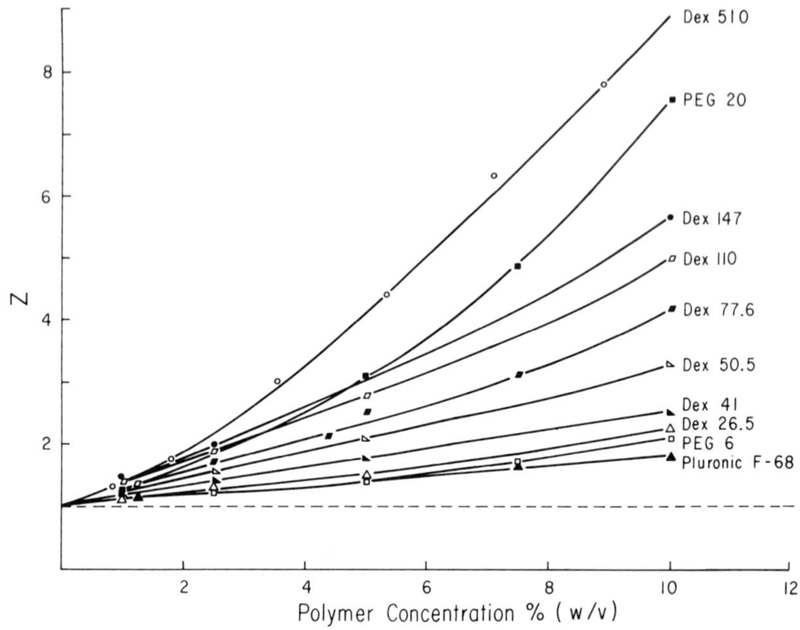

Figure 10. Relative ζ potential as a function of neutral polymer concentration in saline suspensions of washed human erythrocytes. Dextran (Dex) and polyethylene glycol (PEG) molecular weights are given by 10^3 times fraction number. T = 25°C. Reprinted by permission of Academic Press from Brooks and Seaman (1973).

hydrodynamic surface of the cell, known as the ζ potential, can be calculated from the results of cell electrophoretic mobility determinations (see Seaman, 1975, for a review). Dextran has been found to increase the cellular ζ potential as a function of both concentration and molecular weight of the polymer. Figure 10 illustrates this phenomenon, where the relative ζ potential of washed human erythrocytes, Z (Z is the ζ potential in the presence of polymer divided by that in its absence), is plotted as a function of concentration for a variety of dextran fractions and other neutral polymers dissolved in physiological saline. It is seen that every molecular weight and concentration of dextran is associated with a well-defined value of Z greater than 1. We have elsewhere discussed in detail the possible artifacts associated with these measurements (Brooks and Seaman, 1973) and have shown that the results cannot be due to ion adsorption to the adsorbed polymer, dielectric constant effects, or membrane rearrangements. We have proposed a model for the effect that is consistent with the available evidence (Brooks, 1973*a*). In this model, the ζ potential increase turns out to be due to an expansion of the ionic double layer resulting from interactions between counterions and the layer of neutral polymer adsorbed at the cell surface. Physically, the effect arises from the preference of the counterions to be solvated by water molecules rather than by adsorbed polymer segments. Hence they tend on average not to occupy sites immediately adjacent to the adsorbed polymer. The resulting ion exclusion effect increases the thickness of the ionic double layer, and, since the cell surface charge is not altered by the presence of adsorbed neutral polymer, the surface potential increases. The model also predicts that, because of double layer expansion, if two similar cells bearing adsorbed polymer were to approach each other closely, the electrostatic repulsion due to double layer overlap could be orders of magnitude larger than it would have been in the absence of polymer. Intercellular electrostatic repulsion should therefore be markedly enhanced in the presence of dextran.

The above discussion immediately suggests that erythrocyte aggregation observed at high dextran concentrations is due to enhanced electrostatic repulsion between cells. It therefore becomes of interest to cast the aggregation data of Fig. 2 in terms of the ζ potential of the cells rather than the dextran concentration in which they are suspended. Figure 11 is the aggregation diagram plotted in this way; the disaggregation conditions are seen to be characterized by a critical disaggregation potential which is an increasing function of molecular weight.

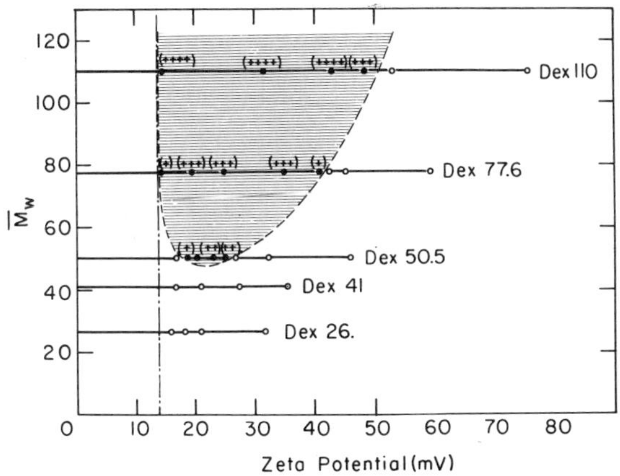

Figure 11. Aggregation diagram of Fig. 2 replotted in terms of the cellular ζ potential instead of dextran concentration. The length of each line indicates the ζ potential produced by 10 g/100 ml of fraction indicated. Reprinted by permission of Academic Press from Brooks (1973*c*).

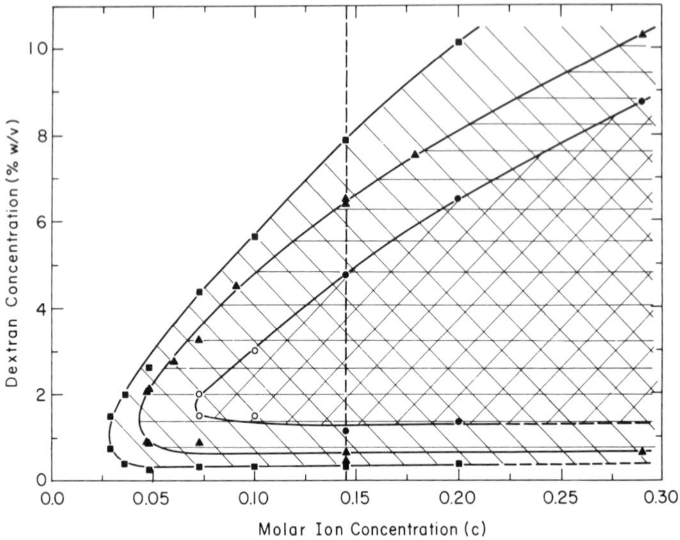

Figure 12. Concentrations of dextran and NaCl which produced detectable aggregation in human erythrocyte suspensions. Solid curves are critical conditions for aggregation; open points indicate very weak aggregation; vertical line indicates physiological ionic strength. Dextran fractions: ■, dextran 101; ▲, dextran 63; ● dextran 45. Reprinted by permission of Academic Press from Brooks (1973*c*).

While this explanation is very appealing, there are other possible mechanisms by which the disaggregation could occur (Brooks, 1973*c*). There is strong supporting evidence for an electrostatic effect, however. First, if the cell surface potential is drastically reduced by methylation (Brooks, 1973*c*) or neuraminidase treatment (Jan and Chien, 1973), disaggregation does not occur at high dextran concentrations, even for fractions of molecular weight too low to induce aggregation of normal cells. Second, if the double layer is expanded partly by lowering the ionic strength as well as by increasing dextran concentration, disaggregation occurs at lower levels of polymer. This point is demonstrated in Figs. 7 and 12, where aggregation diagrams for combinations of ionic strength and polymer concentrations of different dextran fractions are presented. The disaggregation concentrations are seen to change drastically with changes in ionic strength, but in such a way as to be characterized by a roughly constant critical ζ potential. It is extremely difficult to explain these results by any but an electrostatic mechanism. The constant critical potential for disaggregation is reasonable; it probably reflects the minimum separation that cells can tolerate without aggregating in the presence of polymer. Dextran at a given molecular weight will only be able to maintain a stable bridging configuration over a finite range of surface separations. Since there is no evidence from the adsorption isotherm of intermolecular interactions, this allowable separation range should be independent of dextran concentration in the adsorbed layer, and hence independent of its solution concentration. It seems likely that the critical disaggregation potential characterizes the repulsion which is just large enough to keep cell separations greater than the bridging range of the molecules involved. Higher molecular weights could span greater separations and hence would be characterized by higher critical disaggregation potentials, as seen in Fig. 11.

1.2.2. Erythrocyte Aggregation in Whole Blood

One of the purposes of the above study was to model some of the possible reactions which cause red cell aggregation in normal and pathological blood. As was brought out briefly in the opening paragraphs, fibrinogen has been shown to be necessary for normal rouleaux formation. Since it has been shown to adsorb to red cells (Müller and Gramlich, 1965) and since it has a high molecular weight, fibrinogen seems very likely to cause red cell aggregation by the mechanism of macromolecular bridging. While this is certainly not a new idea, and while there is some more supporting evidence for this model (Merrill *et al.,* 1969), it should be pointed out that none of the evidence is conclusive and other mechanisms are possible. Furthermore, bridging may not be the only role fibrinogen plays in erythrocyte interactions. It has been suggested, for instance, that fibrinogen increases the deformability of normal cells (Rampling and Sirs, 1972). The definitive statement on the roles of fibrinogen in erythrocyte interactions may therefore not yet have been made.

It might be noted in passing that although dextrans appear to be good materials with which to model red cell aggregation in whole blood there is one significant difference between the two systems. High concentrations of fibrinogen do not cause disaggregation, even though the erythrocyte ζ potential is elevated (Brooks, unpublished). This could be due to the extreme size of the molecule, a high binding constant for its adsorption, or some other factor, but it is clear that at high concentrations the actions of dextran and fibrinogen differ in this important aspect.

1.2.3. Summary

Suspensions of washed human erythrocytes in saline solutions of dextran were examined as a model of the cellular aggregation reactions believed to be responsible for the viscometric behavior of blood at low rates of shear. Good evidence was obtained for the mechanism of macromolecular bridging as the cause of aggregation in these systems. The disaggregation observed at high dextran concentrations was shown to be caused by intercellular electrostatic repulsion transmitted via ionic double layer overlap. A rheological technique is described based on analysis of the relative viscosity ratio which provides a quantitative index of aggregation and which is believed to provide a measure of the strength of intercellular attachments. Three properties of the red cell membrane are shown to be of importance in determining the degree of aggregation present:

1. The ability of the membrane to act as a set of binding sites for macromolecular adsorption.
2. The deformability of the membrane, which permits large areas of close membrane apposition, permitting in turn the maximum amount of intercellular bridging.
3. The membrane surface charge density, which is responsible for electrostatic repulsion between cells, the force that modifies most cellular interactions and that in the presence of high concentrations of dextran can be sufficiently strong to prevent stable intercellular attachments from forming.

ACKNOWLEDGMENTS

I thank Dr. R. J. Knox and Dr. G. V. F. Seaman for helpful discussions. Parts of this work were completed while the author was a Centennial Fellow of the Medical Research Council of Canada.

References

Albers, W., and Overbeek, J. T. G., 1960, Stability of emulsions of water in oil. III. Flocculation and redispersion of water droplets covered by amphipolar monolayers, *J. Colloid Sci.* **15:**498.

Born, G. V. R., 1962, Aggregation of blood platelets by adenosine diphosphate and its reversal, *Nature (London)* **194:**927.

Brooks, D. E., 1973*a*, The effect of neutral polymers on the electrokinetic potential of cells and other charged particles. II. A model for the effect of adsorbed polymer on the diffuse double layer, *J. Colloid Interface Sci.* **43:**687.

Brooks, D. E., 1973*b*, The effect of neutral polymers on the electrokinetic potential of cells and other charged particles. III. Experimental studies on the dextran/erythrocyte system, *J. Colloid Interface Sci.* **43:**700.

Brooks, D. E., 1973*c*, The effect of neutral polymers on the electrokinetic potential of cells and other charged particles. IV. Electrostatic effects in dextran-mediated cellular interactions, *J. Colloid Interface Sci.* **43:**714.

Brooks, D. E., and Seaman, G. V. F., 1973, The effect of neutral polymers on the electrokinetic potential of cells and other charged particles. I. Models for the zeta potential increase, *J. Colloid Interface Sci.* **43:**670.

Brooks, D. E., Goodwin, J. W., and Seaman, G. V. F., 1970, Interactions among erythrocytes under shear, *J. Appl. Physiol.* **28:**172.

Brooks, D. E., Goodwin, J. W., and Seaman, G. V. F., 1974, Rheology of erythrocyte suspensions: electrostatic factors in the dextran-mediated aggregation of erythrocytes. *Biorheology* **11:**69.

Charm, S. E., and Kurland, G. S., 1967, Static method for determining blood yield stress, *Nature (London)* **216:**1121.

Chien, S., and Jan, K.-M., 1973, Red cell aggregation by macromolecules: Roles of surface adsorption and electrostatic repulsion, *J. Supramol. Struct.* **1:**385.

Chien, S., Usami, S., Dellenback, J., and Gregersen, M. I., 1970, Shear-dependent interactions of plasma proteins with erythrocytes in blood rheology, *Am. J. Physiol.* **219:**143.

Cokelet, G. R., Merrill, E. W., Gilliland, E. R., Shin, H., Britten, A., and Wells, R. E., 1963, The rheology of human blood-measurement near and at zero shear rate, *Trans. Soc. Rheol.* **7:**303.

Curtis, A. S. G., and Hocking, L., 1970, Collision efficiency of equal spherical particles in a shear flow, *Trans. Faraday Soc.* **66:**1381.

Fåhraeus, R., 1929, The suspension stability of the blood, *Physiol. Rev.* **9:**241.

Goldsmith, H. L., and Mason, S. G., 1967, The microrheology of dispersions, in: *Rheology*, Vol. 4 (F. Eirick, ed.), pp. 85–250, Academic Press, New York.

Jan, K.-M., and Chien, S., 1973, Role of surface electric charge in red blood cell interactions, *J. Gen. Physiol.* **61:**638.

Katchalsky, A., Danon, D , Nevo, A., and DeVries, A., 1959, Interactions of basic polyelectrolytes with red blood cell. II. Agglutination of red blood cells by polymeric bases, *Biochim. Biophys. Acta* **33:**120.

Kiefer, J. E., Parsegian, V. A., and Weiss, G. H., 1975, Model for van der Waals attraction between spherical particles with non-uniform adsorbed polymer, *J. Colloid Interface Sci.* **51:**543.

Knox, R. J., Brooks, D. E., Nordt, F. J., and Seaman, G. V. F., 1975, Rheology of normal and aldehyde-treated erythrocytes in dextran T-70 solutions, *Biorheology* **12:**89.

Lamer, V. K., and Smellie, R. H., Jr., 1956, Flocculation, subsidence, and filtration of phosphate slimes. I. General, *J. Colloid Sci.* **11:**704.

Merrill, E. W., Cokelet, G. C., Britten, A., and Wells, R. E., 1963, Non-Newtonian rheology of human blood—Effect of fibrinogen deduced by subtraction, *Circ. Res.* **13:**48.

Merrill, E. W., Cheng, C. S., and Pelletier, G. A., 1969, Yield stress of normal human blood as a function of endogenous fibrinogen, *J. Appl. Physiol.* **26:**1.

Müller, H. E., and Gramlich, F., 1965, Ueber den plasma-protein Film an der Oberflache menschlicher Erythrocyten, *Acta Haematol.* **34:**239.

Nicolson, G. L., 1974, The interactions of lectins with animal cell surfaces, in: *International Review of Cytology*, Vol. 39 (G. H. Bourne and J. F. Danielli, eds.), pp. 89–190, Academic Press, New York.

Ponder, E., 1957, Revetements des plaquettes humains et des globules rouges par les dextranes, *Rev. Hematol.* **12:**11.

Rampling, M., and Sirs, J. A., 1972, The interactions of fibrinogen and dextrans with erythrocytes, *J. Physiol. (London)* **223:**199.

Roitt, I. M., 1974, *Essential Immunology*, Blackwell, Oxford.

Seaman, G. V. F., 1975, Electrokinetic behaviour of red cells, in: *The Red Blood Cell,* Vol. II, 2nd ed. (R. Surgenor, ed.), pp. 1135–1229, Academic Press, New York.

Seaman, G. V. F., Kok, D'A., and Heard, D. H., 1962, The electrophoretic mobility of human red cells re-suspended in their native serum, *Clin. Sci.* **23:**1.

Thorsén, G., and Hint, H., 1950, Aggregation, sedimentation and intravascular sludging, *Acta Chir. Scand. Suppl.* **154:**1.

Usami, S., and Chien, S., 1973, Optical reflectometry of red cell aggregation under shear flow, *Bibl. Anat.* **11:**91.

1.3. Rheology of Red Blood Cell Membrane

RICHARD SKALAK

Knowledge of the rheology of the red blood cell membrane is being currently advanced at a rapid rate and the entire picture is not yet clear. Nevertheless, the main outlines of the mechanical material properties of the membrane are fairly distinct, and this brief review will attempt to summarize the current state of affairs.

An important recent advance in thinking about the red blood cell membrane is that it behaves very differently depending on how it is stressed. Any isotropic stress which tends to increase the area of the membrane encounters a stiff elastic response. Under isotropic stresses, the membrane is like a nearly incompressible fluid in a two-dimensional sense. On the other hand, the elastic modulus for a change of shape or shearing stress at constant area is comparatively small. The distinctions between isotropic and shearing stresses and deformations are important and will be discussed in more detail in the next section.

Considerations of the elasticity of the red blood cell membrane must include bending stresses for a complete treatment of shapes such as the biconcave disc. Bending is associated with small forces and small energies, but is important if accurate shapes are to be computed.

The red blood cell membrane also exhibits viscous behavior. This response is again very different for isotropic deformations as compared to purely shearing motions. The membrane is comparatively fluid under shearing stresses but is highly viscous and distends very slowly under isotropic tension. The combination of viscous and elastic responses makes the red blood cell membrane a viscoelastic material in any case.

At sufficiently high stresses, the red blood cell membrane shows plastic behavior, meaning that it suffers a permanent, irrecoverable deformation. Such behavior is observed, for example, when so-called tethers are formed and in some sickled–unsickled cells. Once again, striking differences are found under different states of stress. A definite and low-yield stress is observed in shear, and very large plastic deformations may result prior to rupture. In isotropic tension, the membrane is not plastic. No distinct yield stress is observed, but fracture appears to occur in a more or less brittle manner at an extension of only a few percent.

RICHARD SKALAK · Department of Civil Engineering and Engineering Mechanics, Columbia University, New York, N.Y.

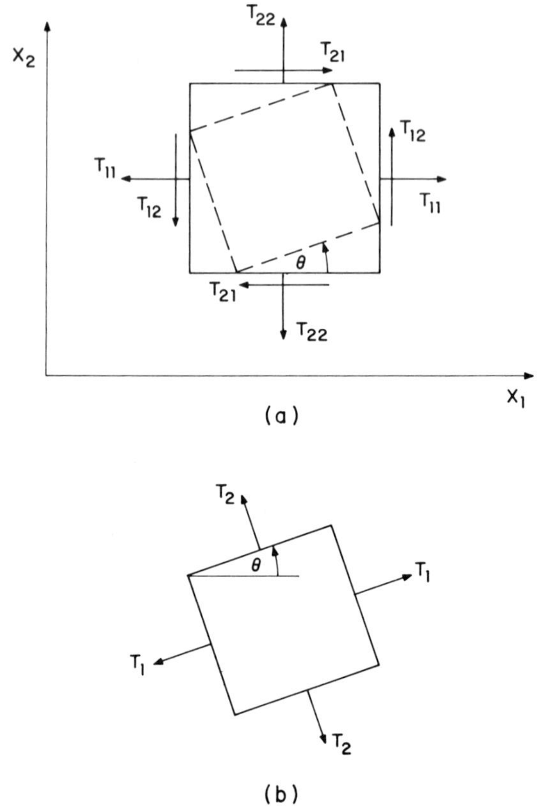

Figure 1. Membrane stress resultants. (a) General case. (b) Stress resultants in principal axes.

The present article will not treat the mechanics of fracture of the red blood cell membrane as in osmotic hemolysis or destruction by high shear rates. Fracture is logically included as part of the rheology of the membrane, but it is not a property which affects the gross rheology of blood in most of circulation. Fracture is a very important aspect in the life cycle of the red blood cell and in the flow of blood in contact with artificial surfaces inside or outside the body. There are several previous reviews on these subjects (Blackshear, 1972; Leverett *et al.*, 1972).

1.3.1. Stress and Strain

In the description of stresses in a thin shell such as the red blood cell membrane, it is convenient to deal directly with resultant forces per unit length, such as surface tension, on any cross-section of the membrane rather than the detailed stresses which are forces per unit area. Neglecting bending effects, the general scheme of membrane stress resultants, T_{ij}, is shown in Fig. 1a. Here T_{11} is the force per unit length (dyn/cm) in the x_1 direction as shown. In a homogeneous material, the stress resultant, T_{11}, would be equal to the average stress, σ_{11}(dyn/cm^2), times the thickness, h, of the membrane. The red blood cell membrane is not a homogeneous material, and the use of stress resultants, T_{ij}, avoids the discussion of molecular level forces and the need for knowledge of the thickness of the membrane.

In addition to the tensions T_{11} and T_{22}, there may be a shear stress T_{12} acting on the edge of a membrane element as shown in Fig. 1a. The units of T_{12} are also dyn/cm. T_{12} represents a force per unit length acting parallel to the edge of the element. It may be shown that, in general, the two shear resultants are equal, i.e., $T_{12} = T_{21}$.

In any case, there always exist at least two perpendicular directions (shown at angle θ to x_1,x_2 in Fig. 1a) for which the shear resultants are zero, as shown in Fig. 1b. The normal stresses in these axes are called the principal stresses, T_1 and T_2. It is convenient to continue the discussion in these principal axes (Fig. 2a).

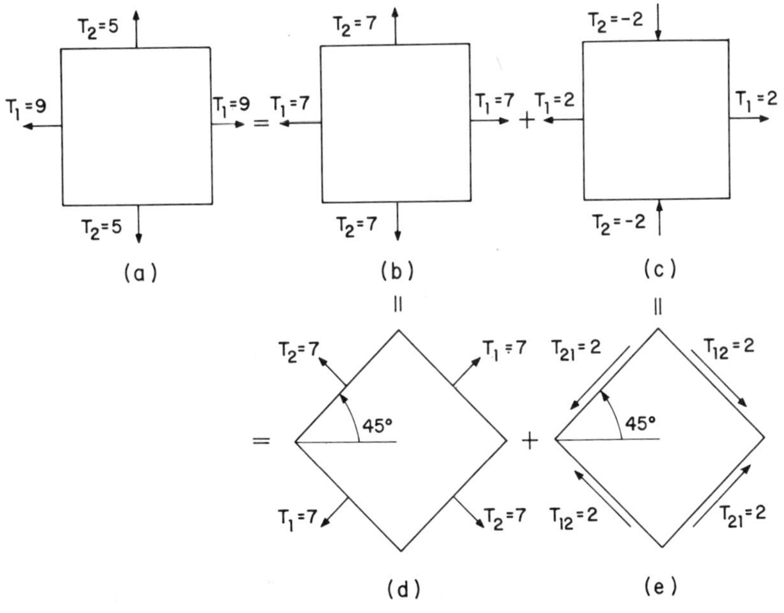

Figure 2. Resolution of principal tensions. (b, d) Isotropic part of (a). (c, e) Deviatoric or shear stress part of (a).

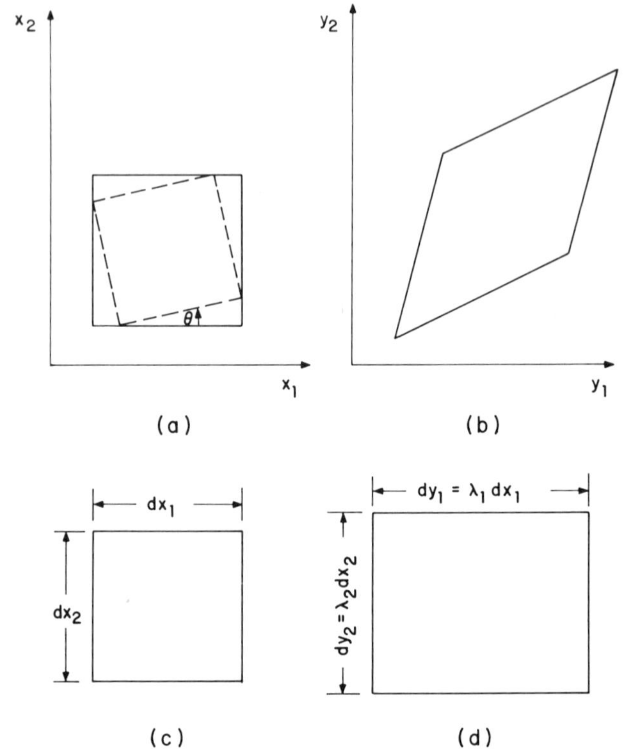

Figure 3. Deformation of a membrane element. (b) General deformation of (a). (d) General deformation of (c) in principal axes of strain.

The two principal tensions, T_1 and T_2 (Fig. 2a), will not be equal in general in a membrane with some rigidity. The general field may be resolved into a purely isotropic part (Fig. 2b) plus a so-called deviatoric part (Fig. 2c) which has a zero average and is equivalent to a pure shear (Fig. 2e). Figure 2 shows a particular numerical case. The stress systems in Fig. 2d,e are equivalent to those in Fig. 2b,c; the system (a) is equal to (b) plus (c) or (d) plus (e).

A similar resolution may be obtained for deformations. A square element (Fig. 3a) may in general be deformed to a parallelogram (Fig. 3b) in which both the shape and area have changed. However, principal axes at angle θ in Fig. 3a exist for which the square element (Fig. 3c) is deformed into a rectangle (Fig. 3d). In Fig. 4a, a particular case of a general deformation in principal axes is shown. The initial unit square shown dotted is assumed to have the final rectangular shape shown in solid lines. Figure 4b shows the isotropic part of the deformation which is an equal extension in all directions and produces the same area change as in Fig. 4a. A deformation from the expanded square (dotted lines) to the final shape (solid lines) is shown in Fig. 4a. No area change is involved in Fig. 4c. An equivalent sequence of deformations is shown in Fig. 4d,e. Considering a unit element inclined at 45° to the principal axes, Fig. 4d shows the isotropic area change and Fig. 4e shows a shearing deformation without change of area. The deformation in (a) is equivalent to (b) followed by (c) or (d) followed by (e).

The deformation shown from Fig. 3a to Fig. 3b may be described by specifying the final coordinates y_1,y_2 of any point as a function of initial coordinates, x_1,x_2. The strain tensor e_{ij} (usually called Green's strain tensor) is defined as

$$e_{ij} = \frac{1}{2}\left(\frac{\partial y_k}{\partial x_i}\frac{\partial y_k}{\partial x_j} - \delta_{ij}\right) \tag{1}$$

where δ_{ij} is the Kronecker delta and i,j,k range over 1,2 with summation

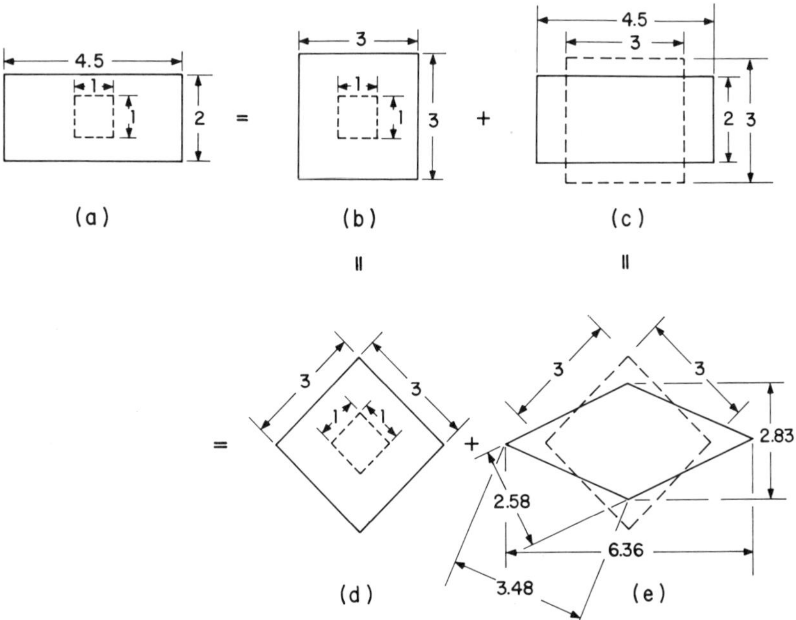

Figure 4. Deformation of a membrane element (a) resolved into an isotropic change of area, (b) or (d), plus a change in shape at constant area, (d) or (e).

indicated by repeated indices as usual. In principal axes (Fig. 3c,d), the strain components are

$$e_{11} = \frac{1}{2}\left[\left(\frac{\partial y_1}{\partial x_1}\right)^2 - 1\right] \qquad e_{22} = \frac{1}{2}\left[\left(\frac{\partial y_2}{\partial x_2}\right)^2 - 1\right] \tag{2}$$

It is convenient to define extension or stretch ratios in principal coordinates by

$$\lambda_1 = dy_1/dx_1 \qquad \lambda_2 = dy_2/dx_2 \tag{3}$$

Referring equation (3) to Fig. 3c,d indicates that λ_i is the final length of a line element divided by its initial length. From equations (2) and (3), it follows that

$$e_{11} = \tfrac{1}{2}(\lambda_1{}^2 - 1) \qquad e_{22} = \tfrac{1}{2}(\lambda_2{}^2 - 1) \tag{4}$$

In a continuous motion, the coordinates y_i will be functions of time, t, as well as of x_i. Then the velocity components of any point are

$$u_1 = \partial y_1/\partial t \qquad u_2 = \partial y_2/\partial t \tag{5}$$

In dealing with viscous behavior, it is conventional to use a rate of deformation tensor, E_{ij}, defined by

$$E_{ij} = \frac{1}{2}\left(\frac{\partial u_i}{\partial y_j} + \frac{\partial u_j}{\partial y_i}\right) \qquad i,j = 1,2 \tag{6}$$

In principal axes of E_{ij},

$$E_{11} = \partial u_1/\partial y_1 \qquad E_{22} = \partial u_2/\partial y_2 \qquad E_{12} = 0 \tag{7}$$

If a deformation takes place at constant area as in Fig. 4c or 4e, then

$$\lambda_1\lambda_2 = 1 \tag{8}$$

and for a continuous motion

$$\frac{\partial u_1}{\partial y_1} + \frac{\partial u_2}{\partial y_2} = 0 \tag{9}$$

Equations (8) and (9) are equivalent for a continuous motion at constant area.

1.3.2. Elastic Properties of Red Blood Cell Membrane

The notion of elastic stresses implies that a strain energy function exists. It represents stored elastic energy. Let W_m be the strain energy per unit of initial area (dyn/cm) associated with the stresses T_{ij}. It has been shown (Skalak *et al.*, 1973) that these stresses may be calculated as follows.

First, the Piola-Kirchhoff stresses, S_{ij}, are given by

$$S_{ij} = \partial W_m / \partial e_{ij} \tag{10}$$

These S_{ij} are referred to initial coordinates. Then

$$T_{ij} = \frac{1}{J} S_{kl} \frac{\partial y_i}{\partial x_k} \frac{\partial y_j}{\partial x_l} \tag{11}$$

where J is the determinant

$$J = \left| \frac{\partial y_i}{\partial x_j} \right| = \lambda_1 \lambda_2 \tag{12}$$

In general, for a membrane which is isotropic with respect to directions in the plane of the membrane, it can be shown that W_m must be a function of the invariants I_1, I_2 of the Green's strain tensor e_{ij}. The particular forms of invariants used here are

$$I_1 = 2(e_{11} + e_{22}) = \lambda_1{}^2 + \lambda_2{}^2 - 2 \tag{13}$$

$$I_2 = 2(e_{11} + e_{22}) + 4(e_{11}e_{22} - e_{12}{}^2) \tag{14}$$

I_2 may also be written

$$I_2 = \lambda_1{}^2\lambda_2{}^2 - 1 = (A/A_0)^2 - 1 \tag{15}$$

where A and A_0 are the final and initial areas of an element.

The particular functional form of W_m suggested (Skalak *et al.*, 1973) is

$$W_m = \frac{B}{4}\left(\tfrac{1}{2}I_1^2 + I_1 - I_2\right) + \frac{C}{8} I_2^2 \tag{16}$$

where B and C are elastic moduli, $B = 0.005$ dyn/cm and $C = 100$ dyn/cm. These values are based on experimental data by Hochmuth and Mohandas (1972) for B and by Evans (1975) for C. The modulus C controls the response when area is increased, and B is similar to a shear modulus. The large value of C provides a large resistance to area changes. The resulting expressions for principal tensions are

$$T_1 = [B(\lambda_1{}^2 - 1) + C\lambda_2{}^2 I_2]\lambda_1/2\lambda_2 \tag{17}$$

$$T_2 = [B(\lambda_2{}^2 - 1) + C\lambda_1{}^2 I_2]\lambda_2/2\lambda_1 \tag{18}$$

An interesting limiting approximation (Skalak *et al.*, 1973) is the case of $C \to \infty$ in which, for any finite stresses, the area remains constant ($\lambda_1\lambda_2 = 1$). In this case, a first approximation to equations (17) and (18) is, for small strains,

$$T_1 = Be_{11} + T_0 \tag{19}$$

$$T_2 = Be_{22} + T_0 \tag{20}$$

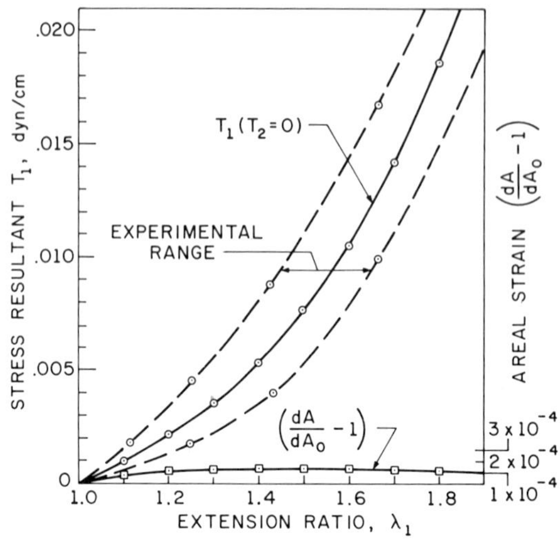

Figure 5. Stress–strain curve in uniaxial tension for red blood cell membrane. Note that areal strain is nearly zero (right-hand scale).

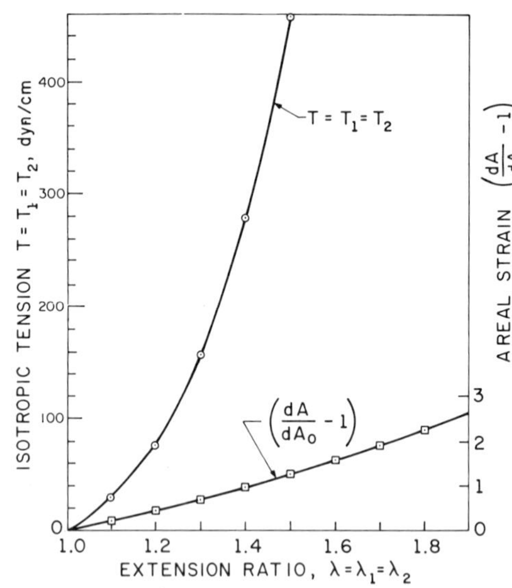

Figure 6. Stress–strain curve in isotropic tension for red blood cell membrane. Note that areal strain and tension are much larger than in uniaxial tension, Fig. 5.

where T_0 is an isotropic stress, similar to the pressure in an incompressible liquid. This was suggested also by Evans (1973).

The stresses that result from equations (17) and (18) are shown in Figs. 5 and 6 for the cases of uniaxial tension ($T_2 = 0$) and isotropic tension ($T_1 = T_2$). The slopes of these curves at the origin may be interpreted as initial elastic moduli. Assuming a thickness of the membrane of 100 Å, Fig. 5 gives a Young's modulus of 10^4 dyn/cm^2 and Fig. 6 gives an areal modulus of 10^8 dyn/cm^2.

All of the above discussion in terms of Cartesian coordinates x_i and y_i implies that the membrane is initially plane and remains plane. However, the discussion applies to curved membranes as well if we consider that the above relations are valid for the membrane stresses locally at any point. For curved membranes, bending stresses may also come into play. In the present discussion, only axisymmetrical cases will be considered.

Bending moments may be expressed in terms of a bending strain energy function, W_B (Zarda, 1974). The principal bending moments, M_1 in the azimuthal plane (Fig. 7) and M_2 in the circumferential direction, are given by

$$M_1 = \frac{1}{\lambda_2}\frac{\partial W_B}{\partial K_1} \qquad M_2 = \frac{1}{\lambda_1}\frac{\partial W_B}{\partial K_2} \tag{21}$$

where K_1 and K_2 are measures of the bending strains. In terms of the initial coordinates $\mathring{r},\mathring{\theta}$ and final coordinates r,θ shown in Fig. 8, the

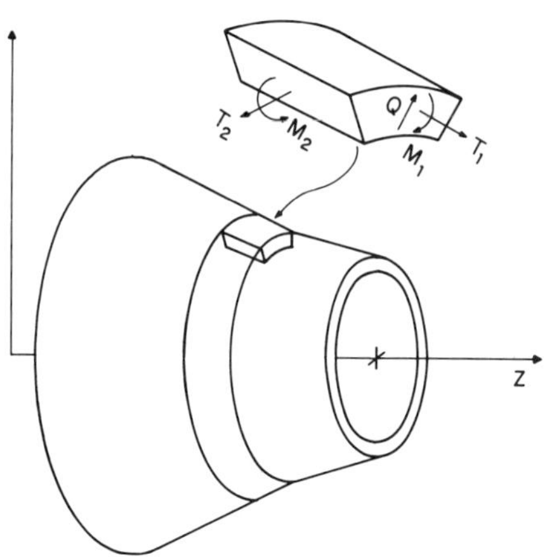

Figure 7. Bending moments in principal axes.

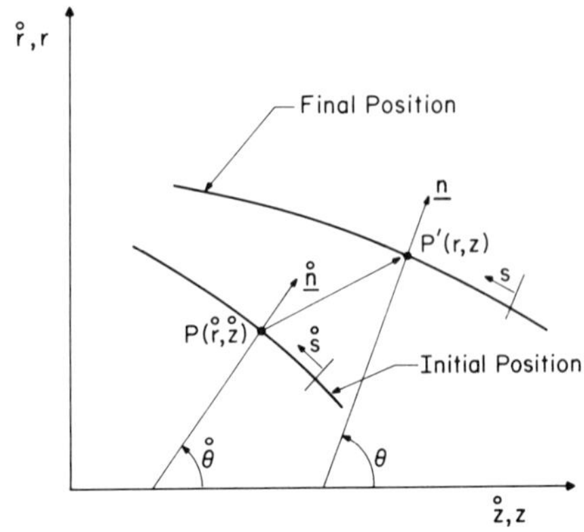

Figure 8. Definition of initial and final coordinates used in computing curvatures K_1 and K_2.

curvatures K_1 and K_2 are

$$K_1 = \frac{d\theta}{dS} - \frac{d\mathring{\theta}}{d\mathring{S}} \qquad K_2 = \frac{\sin\theta}{r} - \frac{\sin\mathring{\theta}}{\mathring{r}} \tag{22}$$

The bending strain energy function, W_B, is not known from any direct measurements, but a suggested form is (Zarda, 1974)

$$W_B = D(K_1{}^2 + 2\nu K_1 K_2 + K_2{}^2)/2 \tag{23}$$

where D is a bending stiffness which is here regarded as a single membrane property. The constant ν is also a material property which is similar to a Poisson's ratio. The above formulation leads to the usual theory of thin elastic shells under small deflections and strains. For such a shell, if it is of a homogeneous elastic material, the bending stiffness D would be $D = Eh^3/12(1 - \nu^2)$, where E is Young's modulus, h is the membrane thickness, and ν is Poisson's ratio. The red blood cell membrane is not regarded as homogeneous, but the constants D and ν are assumed directly as $\nu = \frac{1}{2}$ and $D = 2.72 \times 10^{-11}$ dyn·cm. This bending stiffness is suggested by computations on the sphering and formation of red blood cells (Zarda *et al.*, 1975). If the thickness of the red blood cell membrane is taken to be 100 Å, then the above values of ν and D correspond to a uniform material with Young's modulus $E = 2.55 \times 10^8$ dyn/cm² and $\nu = \frac{1}{2}$.

1.3.3. Viscoelasticity

Viscoelastic behavior of the red blood cell membrane was suggested by Katchalsky *et al.* (1960) to explain data on osmotic hemolysis. Rand (1964) also used a viscoelastic model to explain the gradual changes of stress and strain observed prior to hemolysis in pipette experiments on red blood cells. In both cases, the stresses near hemolysis are comparatively large and isotropic and the rates of change of the stresses and strains are comparatively slow, i.e., on the order of minutes. On the other hand, experiments by Hoeber and Hochmuth (1970) in which a red blood cell is rapidly ejected from a pipette show a recovery time of about $\frac{1}{3}$ s. Such recovery takes place at essentially constant surface area, and a viscous component of the membrane stresses associated with the rate of shearing deformation is to be expected.

The viscosity exhibited by the red blood cell membrane in shear may be anticipated to be much smaller than in isotropic deformation on the basis of the small stresses and short time scales associated with shearing. Hence it is logical to again separate these effects theoretically. A general approach to this end is given by Skalak (1973). The stresses discussed in the previous section are now given a superscript e to indicate that they are elastic in origin and the total stress at any instant S_{ij} is

$$S_{ij} = S_{ij}^{e} + S_{ij}^{v} \tag{24}$$

where S_{ij}^{v} is the viscous stress. The isotropic and deviatoric parts of S_{ij} may be written as $\bar{S}_{ij}$ and $\tilde{S}_{ij}$:

$$\bar{S}_{ij} = \tfrac{1}{2} S_{kk}\delta_{ij} \tag{25}$$

$$\tilde{S}_{ij} = S_{ij} - \bar{S}_{ij} \tag{26}$$

Each of the stress fields S_{ij}^{e} and S_{ij}^{v} may be similarly resolved. A broad class of viscoelastic behaviors which are generalizations of equation (24) may be described by (Skalak, 1973)

$$S_{ij} = \int_{-\infty}^{t} \{\tfrac{1}{2}[G_2(t-\tau) - G_1(t-\tau)]\delta_{ij}\dot{S}_{kk}^{e} + G_1(t-\tau)\dot{S}_{ij}^{e}\}\, d\tau \tag{27}$$

in which G_1 and G_2 are generalized relaxation functions of the type usually used in linear viscoelasticity (Flügge, 1967). In equation (27), the $\dot{S}_{ij}^{e}$ stands for the time rate of change of S_{ij}^{e}; the role of $\dot{S}_{ij}^{e}$ in equation (27) is analogous to that of the strain rate $\dot{e}_{ij}$ in linear theory. The relaxation functions G_1 and G_2 are associated with the deviatoric and isotropic parts of the stress, respectively. This can be seen by observing that the isotropic part of equation (27) is

$$\bar{S}_{ij} = \int_{-\infty}^{t} G_2(t - \tau)\dot{\bar{S}}^e_{ij}\, d\tau \qquad (28)$$

Next, subtracting equation (28) from equation (27), it follows that

$$\tilde{S}_{ij} = \int_{-\infty}^{t} G_1(t - \tau)\dot{\tilde{S}}^e_{ij}\, d\tau \qquad (29)$$

The inverse of equation (27) may be written

$$S^e_{ij} = \int_{-\infty}^{t} \{\tfrac{1}{2}[J_2(t - \tau) - J_1(t - \tau)]\delta_{ij}\dot{S}_{kk} + J_1(t - \tau)\dot{S}_{ij}\}\, d\tau \qquad (30)$$

where J_2 and J_1 are reduced creep functions for the isotropic and deviatoric parts of the stress; J_1 and J_2 are inverse to G_1 and G_2.

Available experimental data do not permit a precise evaluation of the functions G_1,G_2 or J_1,J_2 at this time, but some order of magnitude estimates are possible, assuming simple models. For example, a Kelvin model (a spring and a dashpot in series) for the deviatoric stress is represented by

$$G_1(t - \tau) = 1 + \frac{2\mu_1}{K_1}\delta(t - \tau) \qquad (31)$$

and for the isotropic stress by

$$G_2(t - \tau) = 1 + \frac{2\mu_2}{K_2}\delta(t - \tau) \qquad (32)$$

The first term (unity) on the right-hand sides of equations (33) and (34) gives rise to the elastic stress term in equation (24) when equations (31) and (32) are substituted into equation (27). The Dirac delta terms, $\delta(t - \tau)$, in equations (31) and (32) give rise to viscous stress terms which form S^v_{ij} in equation (24). The constants K_1 and K_2 in equations (31) and (32) are representative of the stiffness of the membrane in shear and isotropic tension. If equation (16) is used to describe the elastic stresses, K_1 and K_2 would be chosen to be B and C, respectively. The constants μ_1 and μ_2 are the viscosities to be associated with shearing deformation rates and rate of area expansion, respectively. The characteristic relaxation times associated with the deviatoric and isotropic parts of the stress are

$$t_1 = 2\mu_1/K_1 \qquad t_2 = 2\mu_2/K_2 \qquad (33)$$

The Kelvin model was introduced to discuss the isotropic tension in osmotic hemolysis by Katchalsky *et al.* (1960). Based on a membrane thickness of 100 Å, their estimates of the elastic and viscous constants correspond to $K_2 = 3.1$ dyn/cm and $\mu_2 = 27$–270 dyn·s/cm. These values give the time constant t_2 in the range of 17–170 s. Rand's data (1964) bear out this order of magnitude estimate for the relaxation time in isotropic tension.

Evans and Hochmuth (1975*a*) have used the Kelvin model to derive an estimate of the viscosity μ_1 associated with shearing. Their model is contained in the general scheme above by considering the membrane to be inextensible in regard to changes of area. Then the principal elastic stresses are given by equations (19) and (20), and, setting $G_2 = 0$, it may be shown that equation (27) leads to the formulation, in principal axes

$$T_1 = K_1 e_{11} + 2\mu_1 E_{11} + T_0 \tag{34}$$

$$T_2 = K_1 e_{22} + 2\mu_1 E_{22} + T_0 \tag{35}$$

In equations (34) and (35), the elastic constant B in equations (19) and (20) has been replaced by K_1 in the present notation and T_0 is an unknown isotropic tension. It should be noted that the viscous stresses in equations (34) and (35) are proportional to the rate of deformation E_{ij} defined by equation (6). This form of the viscous stress is analogous to a Newtonian incompressible fluid. This was introduced by Evans and Hochmuth (1975*a*) directly but follows here from the equivalent assumption (equation 31). The rate of deformation tensor E_{ij} appears through its relation to the time rate of change of the strain, $\dot{e}_{ij}$ (*cf*. Prager, 1961):

$$E_{ij} = \dot{e}_{kl} \frac{\partial x_i}{\partial y_k} \frac{\partial x_j}{\partial y_l} \tag{36}$$

From an analysis of the decay of the deformation of a red blood cell partially drawn into a pipette, Evans and Hochmuth (1975*a*) have estimated that the decay time t_1 is 0.2 s and from this that μ_1 is of the order of 10^{-3} dyn·s/cm.

More complex models of the red blood cell membrane viscoelasticity may be developed by the appropriate choice of functions G_1 and G_2 in equation (27). Rand (1964) introduced a four-element model for isotropic tension and obtained a good fitting of his data interpreted as isotropic tension. As more detailed data become available, the models may be refined.

1.3.4. Plasticity

Plastic behavior of a material is associated with permanent deformations which occur if sufficiently high stresses are applied. The critical stress state is called a yield condition and at or above this stress a variety of different behaviors may occur. For example, in a so-called viscoplastic or Bingham body, the rate of deformation after yielding is assumed proportional to the excess of the stress above its critical value.

In considering the plasticity of the red blood cell membrane, distinction must be made again between isotropic and shear stresses. In isotropic stress such as occurs in osmotic sphering, the membrane extends only a few percent before rupture. Rand (1964), in analyzing such experiments, has particularly remarked that no distinct yield stress or plastic flow appears. On the other hand, permanent deformations of red blood cells have been observed under a variety of conditions such as pipette experiments, sickling and unsickling cycles, and the formation of long tethers when a red cell adheres to a boundary and then is subjected to a shear stress. Such plastic deformations are presumably due to yielding associated with shear stresses.

The formation and growth of red blood cell membrane tethers have been described by Hochmuth *et al.* (1973) and have been interpreted as a viscoplastic behavior in shear by Evans and Hochmuth (1975*b*). In this analysis, the isotropic deformation is neglected and the membrane is assumed to hold its area constant so that $\lambda_1\lambda_2 = 1$. The yield criterion is taken to be whether or not the maximum shear stress in the membrane exceeds a critical value T_0 which is the yield stress of the membrane. The maximum shear stress at any point is conveniently expressed as half the difference of the principal tensions T_1 and T_2, i.e., $(T_1 - T_2)/2$. Then, in principal axes, the viscoplastic flow law adopted may be expressed as

$$E_{11} = 0 \qquad \text{if} \qquad (T_1 - T_2)/2 < T_0 \tag{37}$$

$$E_{11} = \frac{1}{2\mu_p}(T_1 - T_2)/2 \qquad \text{if} \qquad (T_1 - T_2) > 0 \tag{38}$$

where E_{11} is the deformation rate defined by equation (6) and μ_p is a viscosity associated with the plastic deformation. Under the assumption of constant area, it can be shown that

$$E_{11} = -E_{22} = \dot{\lambda}_1/\lambda_1 = -\dot{\lambda}_2/\lambda_2 \tag{39}$$

so that equations (37) and (38) define the plastic flow process completely. In equation (39), $\dot{\lambda}_1$ denotes the time rate of change of λ_1.

The analysis of tether formation by Evans and Hochmuth (1975*b*) assumes that an elastic deformation precedes the plastic flow and produces an initial cylindrical shape. The plastic flow due to excessive stress draws out the tether from the elastic diameter down to some minimum radius of the order of 100–500 Å. When the tether is steadily growing, membrane material flows from the main part of the cell through the plastic zone to form additional tether. The minimum tether radius is somehow determined by the membrane properties, but the details are not clear. Experimentally, tethers may be 100–200 μm long and appear to be of uniform diameter. The plastic flow analysis permits estimates to be made of both the critical shear stress T_0 and the viscosity μ_p which define the plastic behavior. The estimates derived are

$$T_0 = 0.016\text{–}0.08 \text{ dyn/cm} \tag{40}$$

$$\mu_p = 8 \times 10^{-3} \text{ dyn·s/cm} \tag{41}$$

The value of μ_p is somewhat larger than the shear viscosity μ_1 associated with viscous action during elastic deformation in equations (34) and (35). These two viscosities need not be equal, but the fact that they are of the same order of magnitude lends credence to the analyses. It should also be noted that the viscosity μ_2 associated with isotropic stress in equation (32) is about 3 orders of magnitude greater than μ_1 and μ_p. Evans and Hochmuth (1975*a,b*) have interpreted this behavior in terms of the detailed structure of the red blood cell membrane. The lipid bilayer which forms the bulk of the membrane is regarded as relatively fluid. The elastic, viscous, and plastic properties are attributed primarily to a structural protein layer, mostly spectrin, attached to the lipid bilayer. In particular, the large viscosity μ_2 apparent in isotropic tension may be due to gradual relaxation of crosslinking of this matrix. The plastic flow in shear may also be associated with deformation of this matrix since the shear viscosities are much greater than estimates for the bilipid layer alone.

1.3.5. Applications and Summary

The above descriptions of the various red blood cell membrane properties have not yet been widely used for any applications, although they now give a fairly comprehensive picture of the membrane behavior. Experimental data have mostly led to interpretations in terms of material properties rather than *vice versa*. However, in the future, predictions based on analyses using the fundamental membrane properties may be expected to be useful in predicting and interpreting experimental data. In the latter case, clinical use may be achieved in interpreting macroscopic observations in terms of microscopic mechanisms.

The applications that have been carried out are of exploratory rather than clinical interest. The osmotic sphering and the initial formation of the biconcave shape of the human red blood cell have been discussed on the basis of the elastic properties of the membrane by Zarda *et al.* (1975). It is shown that the red blood cell shape is produced if the initial shape is assumed to be a sphere and then the interior volume is reduced. The reduction in volume is supposed to represent the expulsion of the nucleus from the immature red blood cell.

Another interesting application has been given by Zarda (1974) for capillary blood flow. Using the above elastic model, the shape of the red blood cells in capillaries has been computed and shown to resemble closely the shapes observed *in vivo* (Branemark, 1969).

The bulk behavior of blood has been shown to be viscoelastic in oscillatory flow in tubes (Thurston, 1973) and in oscillatory shear flows (Chien *et al.*, 1975) in the rheogoniometer. The existence of the elastic component of the complex viscosity of whole blood depends on the elasticity of the red blood cell membrane since there is no other elastic element present. A model of red blood cell suspensions which incorporates this elastic effect at high hematocrits has been given by Tözeren *et al.* (1975).

Sieving tests (Chien *et al.*, 1971) may also be interpreted in terms of membrane properties. In these tests, red blood cells are forced to flow through fine cylindrical pores in polycarbonate sieves. The pressure required rises dramatically below a critical diameter of about 2.8 μm. In this range, the area of the red blood cell membrane must increase to allow the cell to pass through the sieve intact. This is one of the clearest demonstrations that the stiffness of the membrane is much larger in isotropic tension than in shear.

The viscosity and plasticity of the membrane itself have not been included in most modeling carried out to date. The viscosity of the membrane affects the bulk viscosity of blood, but the extent of this influence is not yet clear because it is masked by the viscosity of the fluids inside and outside the cell. Similarly, the plasticity presumably plays a role in the progressive stages leading to hemolysis in shear flows, but no detailed analyses are available.

Another application which can be forecast is the formation and disaggregation of rouleaux of red blood cells. The experiments and analyses of Chien and Jan (1973) and Brooks (this volume) make it clear that the binding force of adsorption of macromolecules, the repulsive forces of electrostatic charges, and the elastic forces of the red blood cell membrane all interact in a complex way to produce aggregation or disaggregation in the presence of a shearing stress. The degree of aggregation, in turn, has a strong effect on the macroscopic viscosity of blood (Chien *et al.*, 1973).

In summary, representative values of the rheological properties of the

Table I. Material Properties of Red Blood Cell Membrane[a]

Elasticity:	Shear	5×10^{-3}	dyn/cm
	Dilatation	100	dyn/cm
	Bending	2.72×10^{-11}	dyn·cm
Viscosity:	Shear	1×10^{-3}	dyn·s/cm
	Dilatation	27	dyn·s/cm
Plasticity:	Shear, yield stress	0.048	dyn/cm
	Shear, viscosity	8×10^{-3}	dyn·s/cm

[a] Values are representative and are not known precisely.

human red blood cell membrane have been established. Typical values have been collected in Table I. These are representative in the sense that they are not known accurately at this time, but at least the orders of magnitude are clear and form a significant pattern. The red blood cell membrane under isotropic tension is quite stiff and exhibits a slow (viscous) creep without any plastic behavior. By contrast, under shearing stresses, the red blood cell membrane is quite compliant, and exhibits a moderate viscosity and a very extensive plasticity under the proper circumstances. Because of this combination of properties, the red blood cell membrane may be often considered as deforming at constant area under low shearing stresses. This simplifies the mathematical analysis and is quite realistic in the typical shear flows that occur in the circulation.

ACKNOWLEDGMENTS

This research was sponsored by the U.S. National Institutes of Health, Heart and Lung Institute Grant HL-16851. Discussions with Professors Shu Chien, M. P. Bieniek, E. A. Evans, and R. M. Hochmuth have been most helpful.

References

Blackshear, P. L., 1972, Mechanical hemolysis in flowing blood, in: *Biomechanics: Its Foundations and Objectives* (Y. C. Fung., N. Perrone, and M. Anliker, eds.), pp. 501–528, Prentice-Hall, Englewood Cliffs, N.J.

Branemark, P.-I., 1969, *Intravascular Anatomy of Blood Cells in Man,* Karger, Basel.

Chien, S., and Jan, K.-M., 1973, Red cell aggregation by macromolecules: Roles of surface adsorption and electrostatic repulsion, *J. Supramol. Struct.* **1**:385.

Chien, S., Luse, S. A., and Bryant, C. A., 1971, Hemolysis during filtration through micropores: A scanning electron microscopic and hemorheologic correlation, *Microvasc. Res.* **3**:183.

Chien, S., Usami, S., Jan, K.-M., and Skalak, R., 1973, Macrorheological and microrheological correlation of blood flow in the macrocirculation and microcirculation, in: *Rheology of Biological Systems* (H. L. Gabelnick and M. Litt, eds.), pp. 12–48, Thomas, Springfield, Ill.

Chien, S., King, W., Skalak, R., Usami, S., and Copley, A. L., 1975, Viscoelastic properties of human blood and red cell suspensions, *Biorheology* (in press).

Evans, E. A., 1973, A new material concept for the red cell membrane, *Biophys. J.* **13**:926.

Evans, E. A., 1975, Elastic free energy, failure and dissipation in plasma membranes, in: *Fifth International Biophysics Congress,* August 4–9, 1975, Copenhagen, International Union for Pure and Applied Biophysics, abstracts, p. 25.

Evans, E. A., and Hochmuth, R. M., 1975*a*, Membrane viscoelasticity, *Biophys. J.* (in press).

Evans, E. A., and Hochmuth, R. M., 1975*b*, Membrane viscoplastic flow, *Biophys. J.* (in press).

Flügge, W., 1967, *Viscoelasticity,* Blaisdell, Waltham, Mass.

Hochmuth, R. M., and Mohandas, N., 1972, Uniaxial loading of the red cell membrane, *J. Biomech.* **5**:501.

Hochmuth, R. M., Mohandas, N., and Blackshear, P. L., 1973, Measurement of the elastic modulus for red cell membrane using a fluid mechanical technique, *Biophys. J.* **13**:747.

Hoeber, T. W., and Hochmuth, R. M., 1970, Measurement of red cell modulus of elasticity by *in-vitro* and model cell experiments, American Society of Mechanical Engineers, Paper No. 70-BHF-4, New York.

Katchalsky, A., Kedem, O., Klibansky, C., and DeVries, A., 1960, Rheological considerations of the haemolysing red blood cell, in: *Flow Properties of Blood and Other Biological Systems* (A. L. Copley and G. Stainsby, eds.), pp. 155–164, Pregamon Press, New York.

Leverett, L. B., Hellums, J. D., Alfrey, C. P., and Lynch, E. C., 1972, Red blood cell damage by shear stress, *Biophys. J.* **12(3)**:257.

Prager, W., 1961, *Introduction to Mechanics of Continua,* Ginn, New York.

Rand, R. P., 1964, Mechanical properties of the red cell membrane. II. Viscoelastic breakdown of the membrane, *Biophys. J.* **4**:303.

Skalak, R., 1973, Modelling the mechanical behavior of red blood cells, *Biorheology* **10**:229.

Skalak, R., Tözeren, A., Zarda, R. P., and Chien, S., 1973, Strain energy function of red blood cell membranes, *Biophys. J.* **13**:245.

Thurston, G. B., 1973, Frequency and shear rate dependence of viscoelasticity of human blood, *Biorheology* **10**:375.

Tözeren, A., Chien, S., and Skalak, R., 1975, Viscoelasticity of human blood, Euromech Colloquium 68, Varna, Bulgaria, September 15–18, 1975. To appear in *J. Biomech.,* Sofia, Bulgaria.

Zarda, P. R., 1974, Large deformations of an elastic shell in a viscous fluid, doctoral dissertation, Columbia University, New York.

Zarda, P. R., Chien, S., and Skalak, R., 1975, Sphering and formation of red blood cells, in: *1975 Biomechanics Symposium,* Vol. 10 (R. Skalak and R. M. Nerem, eds.), pp. 48–52, A.S.M.E., A.M.D., New York.

1.4. Pressure–Flow Relationships in the *in Vivo* Microcirculation

MARCOS INTAGLIETTA

The intrinsic flow properties of blood determined in *in vitro* experiments (Cokelet *et al.,* 1963) as well as the effective pressure–flow relationship measured in passive whole organs (Green *et al.,* 1944) indicate that the effective and/or functional viscosity of blood increases as the shear rate and/or flow velocity decreases. This behavior is believed to be a consequence of the tendency of red blood cells to aggregate and the distensibility of the vascular tree. The extension of the understanding of the flow properties of blood to the microcirculation is of considerable importance because at this level of the circulatory system the pressure gradients and corresponding flow velocities are small. Direct extrapolation to the microscopic behavior of the microcirculation suggests that the non-Newtonian behavior of blood should not be a significant factor since the shear rates attain the peak values in the capillaries, and their mechanical properties are such that they can be considered to be rigid tubes. However, a number of factors not contemplated in *in vitro* rheological studies and whole organ experiments indicate that the direct extrapolation from macroscopic measurements to the *in vivo* microscopic conditions might not yield the expected results. In effect, in the capillary system, blood becomes a two-phase fluid as the vessel lumen tends toward the red blood cell dimensions; bifurcations of the vessels are frequent, pulsatile effects persist throughout the network, and the surface inhomogeneity of the cellular lining of the vessel cannot be considered negligible relative to the dimension of the conduits.

The direct study of microscopic *in vivo* flow properties is presently under way as a consequence of the development of a number of key techniques with which to measure the appropriate variables for rheological analysis, namely, flow, pressure, and geometry. A description of current methods follows.

MARCOS INTAGLIETTA · AMES-Bioengineering, University of California, San Diego, La Jolla, California.

1.4.1. Instrumentation

1.4.1.1. Pressure

The current most reliable method with which to measure local pressures, and pressure gradients in vessels of 15–20 μm diameter and smaller, is the so-called resistance servonulling method originally developed by Wiederhielm *et al.* (1964). For the purpose of rheological studies, single pressure determinations are not sufficient, since the significant parameter is the pressure gradient. Dual simultaneous pressure measurements require the use of two independent systems utilized in conjunction with two separate microcannulas (Intaglietta, 1973).

The use of two independent pressure-measuring systems is particularly suited for characterizing the morphological properties which shape the pulsatile waveforms in the microcirculation. These data are contained in the variation of pulse amplitude and the speed of propagation of the pressure and flow perturbations. Sequential measurement in the microvascular tree was carried out by Zweifach (1974) to characterize the effects at branching points.

A particularly significant parameter is the propagation time of the fundamental, which can be measured directly from the experimental waveforms by the method of Intaglietta (1973) based on cross-correlation.

1.4.1.2. Flow

Measurements of blood flow in microscopic blood vessels is accomplished by indirect techniques based on the measurement of velocity of the flowing cellular elements. The principal technique is that devised by Wayland and Johnson (1967), where the image of the vessel under study is projected onto two detectors aligned in the direction of flow and the delay between optical signatures is measured by a special-purpose correlator (Tompkins *et al.*, 1974). More recently, we have extended this technique to video methods through the development of special purpose dual-channel video densitometers which measure the scene brightness in selectable areas of the video image and special-purpose pulse synchronization generators which allows one to increase the video framing rate.

The conversion of flow velocity to volumetric flow requires that special consideration be given to exact location of the source of photometric signals. This problem has been analyzed by Baker and Wayland (1974). The photometric method provides additional information on the structure of the flow, as shown by the study of Silva and Intaglietta (1974) in which it was found that the decay of cross-correlation between photometric signals as a function of detector separation is related to flow velocity and vessel diameter. In given circumstances, the cross-correlation function provides information on the size of the aggregates that are present in blood. This is noted from the presence of a second peak in the correlogram. In capillaries where cells flow in single file, the second peak is found to correspond to the size of the red cells. In the microcirculation of tumors, the second peak is found to correspond to aggregates of 12–15 μm.

1.4.1.3. Pulsatile Microhemodynamics

Up to the present time, the assumption has been made that the pulsatility in the macroscopic hemodynamics is damped out—by the compliance of the vasculature and the dissipation in the flow—to produce a steady flow in the microvessels.

The development of the resistance servonulling method for the measurement of pressure and the dual-slit technique for flow velocity measurement provided solid evidence for the persistence of pulsatile effects throughout the microvasculature. The pulsatile effects in both flow and pressure were characterized by Intaglietta *et al.* (1971). These studies were conducted in the cat omentum (Fig. 1), and it was shown that pulsatile effects propagate with a velocity lower than that which can be predicted from the known elastic properties of the microvasculature.

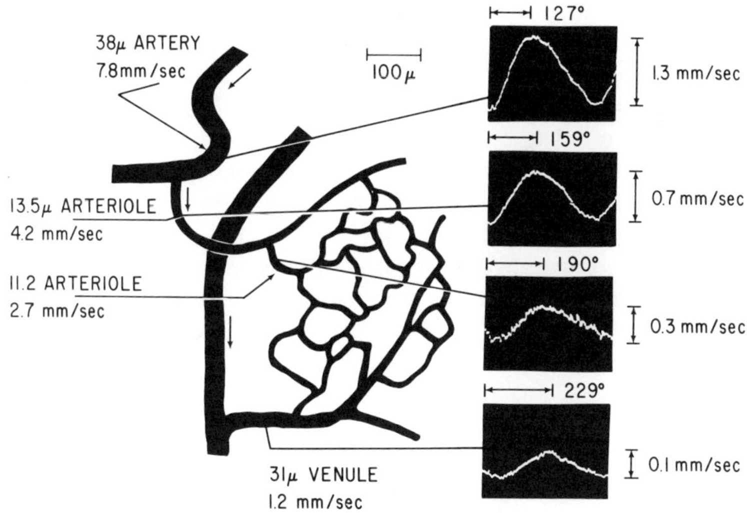

Figure 1. Pulsatile flow velocity in the microvasculature of the cat omentum. The waveforms are referenced to the fundamental component of the arterial pulse pressure measured in the carotid artery, approximately 5 cm from the heart. The waveforms are obtained by signal averaging, utilizing the systematic pulse pressure as a reference.

These conclusions were arrived at by measuring the phase shift in the fundamental as the pulses progress through the microcirculation.

Utilizing a method of signal recovery in which the signal that is buried in noise is repetitively added, utilizing the heartbeat as a reference, it was found possible to measure pulsatile effects in the venular microcirculation, and to relate the phase to the corresponding arteriolar events. The direct relationship between these effects was further established by noting that the phase shift measured between an arteriole and the corresponding venule would increase under the influence of a vasoconstrictor and *vice versa*.

1.4.2. Effect of Bifurcations

The continuous branching pattern exhibited by the microcirculation had to the present been assumed to cause negligible effects on the pressure–flow relationships in the microcirculation because of the low Reynolds number prevalent in this circuit. Studies by Zweifach (1974) have shown that branching has a profound effect on the presure distribution in the microcirculation, which ranges from pressure drops of the order of 15 cm of water when the ratio of branch to parent vessel is 0.2 to 3–5 cm for a ratio of 0.9.

A similar phenomenon has been observed in studying how flow pulses are propagated through the microcirculation. In this and previous studies, we have repeatedly measured phase shifts in the fundamental of the order of 60–80° (2–2.5 beats/min heart rate). This value is comparatively high when related to the presumed structural properties of the microvasculature. Furthermore, we found that even in comparatively long arteriolar vessels (300–500 μm) it was not possible to measure phase shifts between the ends. The latter finding was in part foreseen as a consequence of the comparative stiffness of these vessels. In our study, we noted that measurable phase shifts occurred across bifurcations, where the changes of waveform and phase shift in the fundamental were more pronounced as the branching ratio decreased.

1.4.3. Discussion

The pressure maps of the terminal vascular bed show that the most substantial pressure drop in the circulation occurs between vessels of 100 and 15 μm in diameter (see Fronek and Zweifach, 1975). This phenomenon has been attributed to the geometrical properties of the arteriolar vessels, which determine the noted increase in hydraulic resistance. On the basis of current measurements, it is apparent that there exist significant hemodynamic effects at the bifurcations of the microvascular network. These effects, which manifest themselves as pressure drops and changes in pulsatile conditions, appear to be as substantial as those which can be deduced on the basis of rheological considerations applied to unbranched tubes.

The fact that flow is pulsatile throughout the vessels where the major pressure drops occur is another factor which must be considered. The studies of Coulter and Singh (1971), among others, indicate that the apparent or effective viscosity of blood is affected by pulsatile conditions and increases as much as 40% at pulsatile frequencies of the order of 6 Hz. While this is outside of the normal range of the heart rate, it is well within the range of the higher harmonics contained in the pressure and flow pulses, and therefore could be a contributing factor.

ACKNOWLEDGMENT

This work was supported by United States Public Health Service Grant HL 12493.

References

Baker, M., and Wayland, H., 1974, On-line volume flow rate and velocity profile measurement for blood in microvessels, *Microvasc. Res.* **7**:131.

Cokelet, G. R., Merrill, E. W., Gilliland, E. D., Shin, H., Britten, A., and Wells, R. E., 1963, The rheology of human blood-measurement near and at zero shear rate, *Trans. Soc. Rheol.* **7**:303.

Coulter, N. A., and Singh, M., 1971, Frequency dependence of blood viscosity in oscillatory flow, *Biorheology* **8**:115.

Fronek, K., and Zweifach, B. W., 1975, Microvascular pressure distribution in skeletal muscle and the effect of vasodilation, *Am. J. Physiol.* **228**:791.

Green, H. D., Lewis, R. N., Nickerson, N. D., and Heller, A. L., 1944, Blood flow, peripheral resistance and vascular tonus, with observations on the relationship between blood flow and cutaneous temperature, *Am. J. Physiol.* **141**:518.

Intaglietta, M., 1973, Pressure measurements in the microcirculation with active and passive transducers, *Microvasc. Res.* **5**:317.

Intaglietta, M., Richardson, D. R., and Tompkins, W. R., 1971, Blood pressure, flow and elastic properties in microvessels of cat omentum, *Am. J. Physiol.* **221**:922.

Silva, J., and Intaglietta, M., (1974), The correlation of photometric signals derived from *in-vivo* red blood cell flow in microvessels, *Microvasc. Res.* **7**:156.

Tompkins, W. R., Monti, R., and Intaglietta, M., 1974, Velocity measurements by self tracking correlator, *Rev. Sci. Instrum.* **45**:647.

Wayland, H., and Johnson, P. C., 1967, Erythrocyte velocity measurements in microvessels by a two slit photometric method, *J. Appl. Physiol.* **22**:333.

Wiederhielm, C. A., Woodbury, J. W., Kirk, S., and Rushmer, R. F., 1964, Pulsatile pressure in the microcirculation of the frog's mesentery, *Am. J. Physiol.* **207**:173.

Zweifach, B. W., 1974, Quantitative studies of microcirculatory structure and function. I. Analysis of pressure distribution in the terminal vascular bed in cat mesentery, *Circ. Res.* **34**:843.

2

Methods for the Investigation of the Microcirculation

2.1. Noninvasive Measurement of Compliance of Small Arteries

RYU NAKAYAMA and KIYOJI KIMURA

A noninvasive method is presented for the measurement of the digital arterial compliance (C_s and C_d) by use of a pneumatic cuff (Gaertner capsule) as a gasket when inflated and a fingertip pneumoplethysmograph. The compliance is obtained from the mean amplitude of the volume pulse waves ($\Delta\bar{v}_i$ and $\Delta\bar{v}_j$) under the effect of the cuff pressures (P_{0-i} and P_{0-j}) by

$$C_s = C_i = 3\Delta\bar{v}_i/(P_s - P_{0-i})$$

$$C_s = C_j = \Delta\bar{v}_j/(P_s - P_{0-j})$$

$$C_d = C_{i-j} = 3(\Delta\bar{v}_j - \Delta\bar{v}_i)/(P_{0-i} - P_{0-j})$$

during the dicrotic phase defined in this study. The value C_s (= C_d) obtained from the data during the dicrotic phase is regarded as the compliance. As the cuff pressure is lowered to less than the systolic pressure, the coincident cuff pressure at the moment when the pulse wave begins to appear is regarded as the systolic pressure (P_s). The series of the pulse wave changes following the cuff pressure change is classified into five stages, i.e., A, B, C, D, and E. Stage D (dicrotic phase) is the successive stage after C and is characterized by the fact that the value C_s is equal to the value C_d and the pulse waves have the dicrotic notch. During the dicrotic phase, the venous pressure, the capillary pressure, and the diastolic pressure of arterioles in the segment distal to the compressed

RYU NAKAYAMA and KIYOJI KIMURA · Department of Internal Medicine, National Cancer Center Hospital, Tokyo, Japan.

area approximate the cuff pressure (P_0). Simultaneous recording of the venous occlusion plethysmogram with the volume pulse wave plethysmogram reveals that no inflow to the distal segment occurs during the dicrotic phase. Those facts indicate that the mean amplitude of volume pulse wave ($\Delta\bar{v}$) obtained in stage D is due to the mean pressure difference between the pressure in the vessel and that outside of it, i.e., $(P_s - P_0)/3$. This is why the value C_s (or C_d) obtained during the dicrotic phase can be regarded as the compliance. The mean value and standard deviation of compliance obtained from 100 healthy subjects was $6.0 \pm 3.3 \times 10^{-5}$ cm^3/mm Hg.

2.2. Measurement of Endothelial Strength Using Saline Jets

DALI J. PATEL, RAMESH N. VAISHNAV, H. BULENT ATABEK, and FRED PLOWMAN

Understanding the process of transport of blood lipoproteins and other macromolecules across the blood–vascular interface is of great importance in the study of the pathogenesis of atherosclerosis (Fry, 1973; Patel *et al.*, 1974). It is therefore important to quantify the strength of the endothelium which forms a part of the barrier controlling the flux of the macromolecules. To this end, experiments were carried out wherein jets of physiological saline were impinged normally on the endothelium of freshly excised segments of middle thoracic aortas of dogs. Typically, an aortic segment is slit open longitudinally and stretched to *in vivo* dimensions. The specimen is then submerged in a bath of saline and the bath is placed on the platform of the jet apparatus, which consists of a microscope with turret-mounted objectives, one objective being replaced by a brass objective with a nozzle at the end (diameter 0.4 mm). A chosen location on the blood vessel is then brought under an optical objective, the tissue is focused upon, and the jet is brought in place. A jet of a chosen strength (Re = 1000–3000) is allowed to strike the tissue for a chosen duration (10–60 s). The procedure is repeated for several locations. The tissue is then removed from the bath and Evans blue dye is gently poured on the endothelium. The dye is absorbed by the areas damaged by the jet, thus producing characteristic lesions, the most interesting type of which is an annular one (Patel and Vaishnav, 1974). In this lesion in the region where the jet strikes, there is no damage, attesting to the ability of the endothelium to withstand high normal stresses. The annular region where the shear stresses are high is damaged. Finally, the outer region where the shear stress is low is undamaged. The shear stress at the boundaries of the annular region is thus the shear strength of the endothelium.

The lesion is not quite circular. This hints at anisotropy of strength. The size of the lesion increases with the duration of impingement. This implies that the shear strength is lower for sustained shear stresses than for shear stresses of short duration.

The shear strength is being quantified as a function of radial distance

DALI J. PATEL, RAMESH N. VAISHNAV, H. BULENT ATABEK, and FRED PLOWMAN · National Heart and Lung Institute, The National Institutes of Health, Bethesda, Maryland, and The Catholic University of America, Washington, D.C.

by a hot-film anemometric technique using a 10× model of the jet. The method will thus provide an estimate of local endothelial strength under application of shear stresses of various durations.

References

Fry, D. L., 1973, Responses of the arterial wall to certain physical factors, in: *Atherogenesis: Initiating Factors,* Ciba Foundation Symposium 12 (new series), pp. 93–125, Associated Scientific Publishers, Amsterdam.

Patel, D. J., and Vaishnav, R. N., 1974, Some recent studies on the mechanical behavior of large arteries, in: *Proceedings of the Seventh Southeastern Conference on Theoretical and Applied Mechanics,* pp. 323–331, The Catholic University of America, Washington, D.C.

Patel, D. J., Vaishnav, R. N., Gow, B. S., and Kot, P. A., 1974, Hemodynamics, *Annu. Rev. Physiol.* **36:**125.

2.3. A Method of Determining Resistances from Pressure–Flow Measurements with Microvascular Occlusions

STEPHEN H. NELLIS

Open-circuit impedance functions were used to analyze the microcirculation. No specific structure need be assumed except a two-port, two-terminal network (Sabbagh, 1961) where the major artery and vein supplying the tissue are the input port. The two ends of the microvessel under study are the output port. The open-circuit measurements were made by occluding microvessels in the exteriorized omentum of anesthetized rabbits. The pressure upstream and downstream of the occlusion defines the source pressure of a Thevenin's equivalent circuit. The equivalent resistance value was calculated by plotting the flow through a given microvessel against the pressure developed across a gradual occlusion. The changes in pressure vs. the changes in flow during a slow occlusion were found to be linearly related. The Thevenin's equivalent resistance was maximum on the downstream of an occluded artery and on the upstream of the occluded vein. Within the capillary network, source pressures fell consistently within a narrow range. Topically applied norepinephrine resulted in drastic changes in source resistance and no changes in source pressures. Systemic norepinephrine resulted in changes in source pressures, but minimal changes in source resistance, even though a substantial change in microvascular resistance was indicated when arterial pressure minus micropressure divided by microvessel flow was used as a calculation for resistance. This method defines the functional characteristics of the distributing vessels in terms of two pressures and two equivalent resistances and is a procedure relatively easy to perform. The technique permits determination of the vascular components involved in the response to a particular stimulus.

References

Sabbagh, E., 1961, *Circuit Analysis,* Ronald Press, New York.

STEPHEN H. NELLIS · Cardiology Division, Milton S. Hershey Medical Center, Pennsylvania State University College of Medicine, Hershey, Pennsylvania.

2.4. Image Degradation in Magnification Radiology by Phase Shifts

JOEL E. GRAY and MARTIN TREFLER

With the advent of microfocus X-ray tubes and high-resolution recording media, both film and electronic detectors (Milne, 1974), the use of radiological imaging techniques for the visualization of small vessels has become more practical. High-resolution recording media are generally used in contact with the specimen, while small focal spots are used to greatest advantage in magnification. However, geometric magnification introduces severe degradation in the image due to the finite size and the intensity distribution of the focal spot (Takahashi and Yoshida, 1957) (Fig. 1a, b). The 0.3-mm focal spot used in our research (Fig. 1c) exhibits both the asymmetry and the splitting typical of most X-ray sources. The finite size of such sources produces edge gradients and loss of contrast (Milne, 1971). The splitting of the source and its asymmetry are manifested in more subtle ways. These can be best understood by a consideration of the phase transfer function (PTF)—a quantitative measure of the imaging characteristics of a system. To illustrate these effects, we have chosen to model an opacified blood vessel by a high-contrast, tapering lead foil. We have shown (Gray and Trefler, 1976) that the split in the source intensity distribution results in a value of the PTF of $\pm 180°$ which is associated with the negative values of the optical transfer function. These "phase shifts" are manifested in the image by spurious bifurcations and are best observed when the object is aligned parallel to the anode–cathode axis of the X-ray tube (Fig. 1d). We have also calculated the PTF for various degrees of focal spot asymmetry. Figure 1e shows the PTF as a function of spatial frequency. It can be seen that increasing asymmetry results in a phase shift that varies nonlinearly with frequency. The asymmetry also results in a loss of image contrast as compared to the case of a symmetrical focal spot. The nonlinear phase effects are manifested in the image by shifts of the intensity contours within the limits of the whole image envelope. These are best seen, as in Fig. 1f, when the object is aligned at 45° to the anode–cathode axis and appear as bends or "wows" in the image.

In summary, the properties of microfocal X-ray tubes are taken to best advantage with a geometric magnification technique. However, the

JOEL E. GRAY and MARTIN TREFLER · Radiological Research Laboratories, University of Toronto, Toronto, Ontario, Canada.

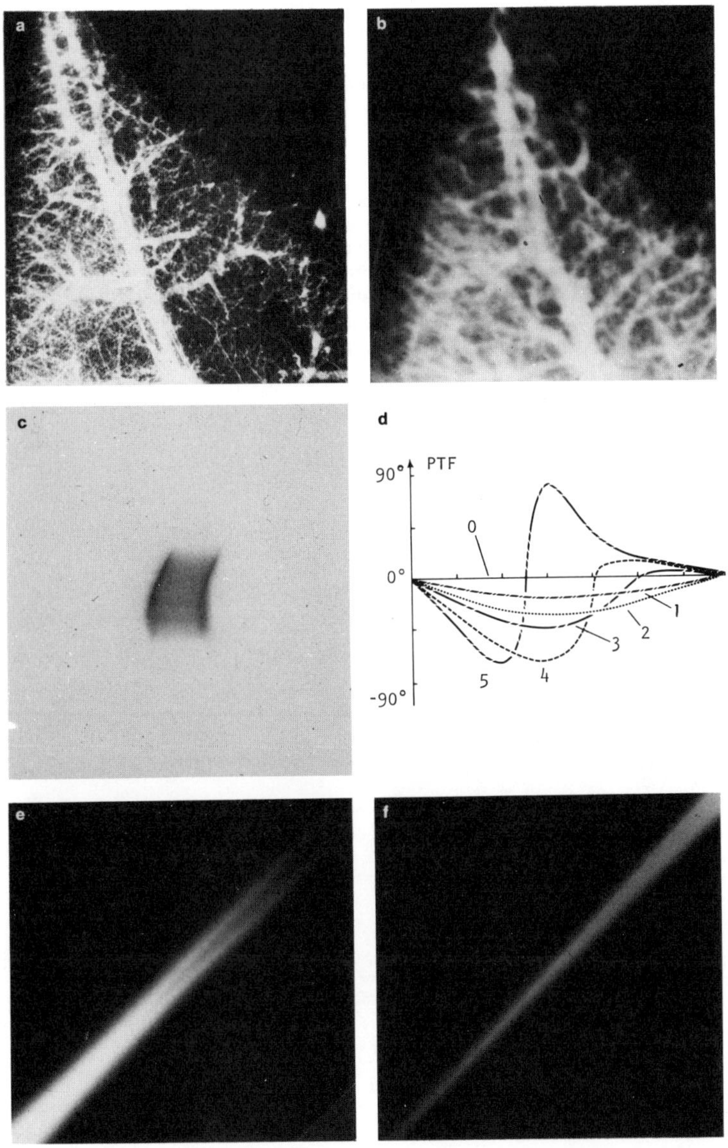

Figure 1. (a) High-resolution radiograph of peripheral vessels in the lung. (b) 2 × magnification of the radiograph in (a). (c) Pinhole photograph of 0.3-mm focal spot. (d) PTF (in degrees) as a function of relative spatial frequency for increasing (0–5) focal spot asymmetry. (e) Image of a single tapering opaque object aligned parallel to the anode–cathode axis. (f) Image of same object as in (e) aligned at 45° to the anode–cathode axis.

investigator must remain cognizant of the artifacts introduced by the focal spot intensity distribution. These, as demonstrated above, consist of loss of contrast, spurious image bifurcation, and spurious bends in image contours.

References

Gray, J. E., and Trefler, M., 1976, Phase effect in diagnostic radiological images, *Med. Phys.* (submitted).

Milne, E. N. C., 1971, The role and performance of minute focal spots in roentgenology with special reference to magnification, *C.R.C. Crit. Rev. Radiol. Sci.* **2**:269.

Milne, E. N. C., 1974, Electronic magnification of the X-ray image, *Radiology* **113**:521.

Takahashi, S., and Yoshida, M., 1957, Roentgenography in high magnification: Reliability and limitation of enlargement, *Acta Radiol.* **48**:281.

2.5. A New Low-Density, Nonaggregating Microsphere for Microcirculation Research

T. MORRISON and J. L. SÖDERBERG

The radioactive microsphere technique has been extensively described as a reliable and accurate method for measuring cardiac output and regional blood flow. Moreover, it would appear to be the only method of easily determining cardiac output and distribution in smaller animals (Bartrum *et al.*, 1974). With carbonized microspheres, inaccuracies due to variations in the diameter distribution and to aggregation of the microspheres have been reported (Reneman *et al.*, 1975). These disadvantages, however, are not encountered with tracer Sephadex microspheres.

Tracer Sephadex microspheres, 15 μm and 50 μm, are a new kind of microspheres for circulation studies in animals. They have a narrow size distribution (e.g., arithmetic mean 14.4 μm, standard deviation 1.9 μm, and arithmetic mean 52.0 μm, standard deviation 1.9 μm) and for convenience are designed for labeling by the user with a variety of metallic radionuclides. The microspheres are prepared from pure dextran and are highly crosslinked by epichlorohydrin to form a rigid gel structure which cannot be degraded by any known dextranase. The microspheres are extremely hydrophilic and during swelling take up 2.5 times their own weight of water. Because of the high water content, the microspheres have a low density, 1.12 g/cm^3. The hydrophilic surface prevents aggregation and the low density (sedimentation rate 2 mm/min in 10% Ficoll 70) makes for ease of handling. To permit labeling with a choice of metallic radionuclides, chelating groups have been covalently linked to the dextran matrix. Metallic radionuclides which may be used include transition metals, lanthanides and actinides with a charge of at least 2+, but not alkali metals. The microspheres may also be labeled with FITC for fluorescence microscopy.

References

Bartrum, R. J., Berkowitz, D. M., and Hollenberg, N. K., 1974, *Invest. Radiol.* **9**:126–132.

Reneman, R. S., Jageneau, A. H. M., van Gerven, W., *et al.*, 1975, *Pfluegers Arch.* **353**:337–347.

T. MORRISON and J. L. SÖDERBERG · Pharmacia Fine Chemicals AB, Uppsala, Sweden.

2.6. Development of an Index for Evaluating the Response of the Microvasculature in C3H Mice to Various Vasoactive Drugs

HAROLD W. PUFFER, NANCY E. WARNER, and WILLIAM P. BARRETT

During an investigation of the effect of vasoactive drugs on the microvasculature in experimental mammary tumors, it became apparent that a system for quantitation of the response would be useful (Warner *et al.*, 1976). Gray (1971, 1972, 1973) reported a standard technique for assessing vascular reactivity in neonatal skeletal muscle which relies on subjective evaluation of the response. We reasoned that a vasoactive index based on the response of the vasculature to uniform doses of a drug could be developed. We postulated that such an index might be characteristic of the vasculature of a particular tissue. This article reports the results of an investigation of the activity of certain vasoactive drugs in the microvascular bed of the mammary gland in C3H mice and the formulation of a vasoactive index to quantitate the results.

2.6.1. Methods

Using epi-illumination apparatus, the microvasculature of the resting and lactating mammary glands in C3H mice was prepared and observed as previously described (Warner *et al.*, 1968). The vessel diameters were measured using a Leitz filar micrometer. The diameter of the most prominent venule and arteriole was measured prior to the topical application of epinephrine hydrochloride, isoproterenol hydrochloride, levarterenol bitartrate, propranolol hydrochloride, and oxytocin. The vasoconstriction index (VI) was calculated using the formula $VI = VD_2/VD_1$, where VD_1 is the diameter of the vessel prior to application of the drug and VD_2 is the diameter of the vessel after application of the drug.

Blood flow was estimated according to the method of McCusky *et al.* (1972).

HAROLD W. PUFFER, NANCY E. WARNER, and WILLIAM P. BARRETT · University of Southern California, School of Medicine, Department of Pathology, Los Angeles, California.

TABLE 1 Observations on Vasoactive Drugs Applied Topically to Microvasculature of Mammary Glands in C3H Mice[a]

Drug	Threshold concentration	Minimum concentration to produce maximum response	Effective concentration to determine vasoactive index	Time for effective concentration to produce response	Flow rate of blood following application of effective dose[b]
Epinephrine HCl	1:1,000,000	1:10,000	1:100,000	15 s	3
Isoproterenol HCl	1:1000	1:10	1:100	1–2 min	1
Levarterenol bitartrate	1:1000	1:100	1:500	3–4 min	2–3
Propranolol HCl	1:10,000	1:1000	1:500	3–5 min	3
Oxytocin	0.2 unit/ml	20 units/ml	2 units/ml	1 min	3

[a] A volume of 0.2 ml of each drug was applied as a single dose containing the concentration indicated.

[b] Defined on a scale of 1–4 (4 = rapid flow, cells not detected, 3 = moderate flow, cells blurred, 2 = slow flow, individual cells seen, 1 = very slow flow, individual cells seen), according to the methods of McCusky *et al.* (1972).

TABLE II. Vasoactive Index (VI) for Selected Drugs

Drug	Concentration	VI of resting mammary gland of C3H mice		VI of lactating mammary gland of C3H mice	
		Arteriole	Venule	Arteriole	Venule
Epinephrine HCl	1:100,000	0.18 ± 0.07 n = 21	0.77 ± 0.09 n = 21	0.12 ± 0.06 n = 16	0.65 ± 0.15 n = 18
Isoproterenol HCl	1:100	0.33 ± 0.18 n = 13	0.83 ± 0.06 n = 12	0.28 ± 0.06 n = 12	0.80 ± 0.09 n = 12
Levarterenol bitartate	1:500	0.39 ± 0.14 n = 15	0.88 ± 0.15 n = 15	0.26 ± 0.12 n = 9	0.82 ± 0.18 n = 9
Propranolol HCl	1:500	0.32 ± 0.24 n = 9	0.81 ± 0.10 n = 9	0.53 ± 0.08 n = 14	0.90 ± 0.09 n = 14
Oxytocin	2 units/ml	0.22 ± 0.04 n = 5	0.84 ± 0.08 n = 5	0.37 ± 0.05 n = 4	1.00 ± 0.00 n = 4

2.6.2. Results and Discussion

The results are summarized in Tables I and II. In all cases, the arteriolar response was greater than that of the venules, as would be expected. Epinephrine, isoproterenol, and levarterenol had a stronger effect on the vessels of lactating glands, whereas propranolol and oxytocin had a greater effect on the vessels of resting mammary glands. The results indicate that a vasoactive index may be useful in evaluating the response of microvasculature to drugs.

References

Gray, S. D., 1971, Responsiveness of the terminal vascular bed in fast and slow skeletal muscles to α-adrenergic stimulation, *Angiologica* **8:**285.

Gray, S. D., 1972, Ontogenic development of vascular reactivity in fast and slow muscles of the neonatal rat hindlimb, *Angiologica* **9:**1.

Gray, S. D., 1973, Development changes in vascular reactivity in neonatal skeletal muscle, *Bibl. Anat.* **11:**376.

McCusky, R. S., Meineke, H. D., and Townsend, S. F., 1972, Studies of the hemopoietic microvenvironment. 1. Changes in the microvascular system and stroma during erythropoietic regeneration and suppression in the spleens of CFI mice, *Blood* **39:**697.

Warner, N. E., Reynolds, M., and Henning, C. E., 1968, A method of microscopy of the mammary gland in the living mouse, *Med. Exp.* **18:**151.

Warner, N. E., Puffer, H. W., and Schaeffer, L. D., Jr., 1976, Observations of the microcirculation in spontaneous mammary tumors in C3H mice, *Bibl. Anat.* (in press.)

2.7. A Microscope Laser Doppler Anemometry (LDA) System for Measurement of Flow Velocity and Velocity Profiles *in Vivo* in the Vessels of the Microvascular System

H. J. BERMAN, S. EINAV, R. L. FUHRO, J. D. FRIDMAN, S. FINE, and P. R. DiGIOVANNI

The system consists of a 0.5-MW He-Ne laser, microscope, LDA detector, and electronic processing equipment. The laser beam is transmitted through a side port in the microscope, down the objective lens, through a blood vessel (in the everted hamster cheek pouch) to the LDA detector. A 60× objective lens focuses the beam to a visual spot 22 μm in diameter in the blood vessel. In the detector, the unscattered beam, transmitted directly through the blood vessel, and the 4° scattered beam are focused separately by lenses and mixed on the cathode of a photomultiplier tube (RCA 8645), responsive to the velocity-dependent beat frequency. This difference signal is amplified, filtered, and displayed on a Hewlett-Packard storage spectrum analyzer. In some experiments, a Saicor autocorrelator was also used. In a 65-μm arteriole with a maximum flow velocity of 6.1 mm/s, the velocity profile was parabolic. With increasing vessel diameter and the same approximate maximum flow velocity (±5%), profiles became blunter. LDA velocity measurements, whenever checked, agreed closely with those obtained by a rotating-prism particle velocity meter (Berman and Fuhro, 1969). In all vessels measured, the Doppler signal amplitude profile was greatest, but it was markedly blunted in the center of the vessel, and decreased peripherally. Such amplitude measurements may provide information on RBC distribution in individual vessels. In conclusion, an LDA-microscope system has been developed that measures velocities and velocity profiles in microvessels. It also permits simultaneous viewing of a transilluminated microvascular bed and focusing of the laser beam to a small region within the blood vessel.

H. J. BERMAN, S. EINAV, R. L. FUHRO, J. D. FRIDMAN, S. FINE, and P. R. DIGIOVANNI · Department of Biology, Boston University, Boston, Massachusetts.

ACKNOWLEDGMENTS

This work was supported by NIH Grants HL-00902 and HL-09447, NASA Grant NGR 22-004-018, and NSF Grant Gk 40575.

Reference

Berman, H. J., and Fuhro, R. L., 1969, Effect of rate of shear on the shape of the velocity profile and orientation of red cells in arterioles, *Bibl. Anat.* **10:**32–37.

2.8. A Video System for Measuring the Blood Flow Velocity in Microvessels

S. E. FU and J. S. LEE

A new video correlating system has been developed to measure the velocity of flowing blood in microvessels. The velocity of the red blood cell in a microvessel is given by the ratio of moving distance ΔL to the incremental time Δt, $v = \Delta L/\Delta t$. In our system, we fix Δt according to the framing rate of the video system and employ the video signal to find ΔL by cross-correlation.

Our system first samples at a frequency 5 MHz the video signal of a raster which coincides with the center axis of the blood vessel. Any fluctuation in the signal corresponds to that of hematocrit in the vessel. These signals are stored in an analog memory of 128 buckets. The signals are then read out at a frequency of 20 kHz by a PDP-11 computer. As the sampling is completed over a period much shorter than Δt, the sequence of the sampled signals is directly related to the axial distance L along the vessel.

By correlating the signals from the same raster of two successful frames, we determine the sequential shift of the signal and compute the velocity. The velocity fluctuation in a venule and capillary so computed is

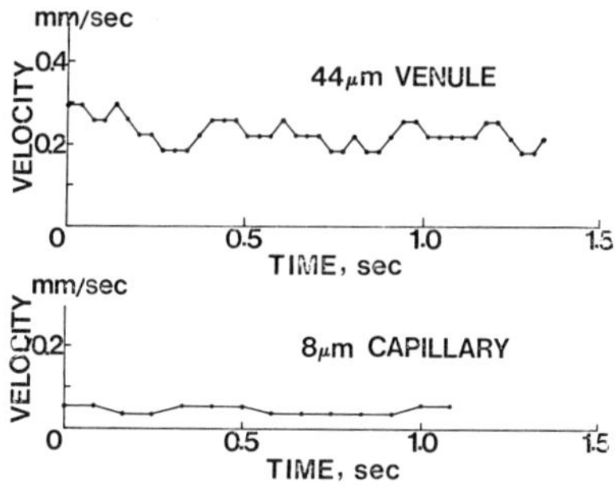

Figure 1. Computed velocity of blood flow in a venule and capillary of rat cremaster muscle. The data were obtained by cross-correlation of their video signals with appropriate averaging technique.

S. E. FU and J. S. LEE · Division of Biomedical Engineering, University of Virginia, Charlottesville, Virginia.

shown in Fig. 1. Direct visual measurement of the cell movement on the TV monitor yields comparable velocity. For the magnification used in our 9-inch TV monitor (500×), this system is capable of determining an arteriolar velocity as high as 5 mm/s.

Because of the image enhancement of a video camera, our system may not have the averaging effect inherent in a photo-optic system (Baker and Wayland, 1973). In addition, because of the minimal width of a raster, it is probable that our video method is more adaptable for computing velocity profile than the two-slit method.

Reference

Baker, M., and Wayland, H., 1973, On-line volume flow rate and velocity profile measurement for blood in microvessels, *Microvasc. Res.* **7:**131–143.

2.9. New Methods of Measuring the Different Rheological Parameters in Blood

H. CHMIEL, P. SCHWEIZER, K.-H. KRAUSE, and W. FRAMING

An increase in blood viscosity can be produced by four fundamental parameters which are in direct relationship to the blood viscosity: hematocrit, plasma viscosity, erythrocyte flexibility, and erythrocyte aggregation tendency.

These four parameters must be measured separately. To measure the aggregation tendency, a new low-shear system ($0.5\ s^{-1}$) having two concentrically arranged spheres was developed (Chmiel, 1975). Because of the viscosity, the rotation is correlated with the viscosity. A second measurement is made using an improved particle volume analyzer (PVA). A constant flow of electrolyte between two filled chambers connected by a narrow measuring orifice sweeps the sample into the center of a stream coming out of a container placed directly in front of the measuring aperture. The current generated by an electrical field between the two chambers changes impulsively because of the large difference between the conductivity of the passing particle and the surrounding fluid. This impulse is proportional to the volume of the particles (Boss *et al.,* 1973).

Plasma viscosity and erythrocyte flexibility are measured at high shear rates. For this purpose, a new type of capillary viscometer suitable for routine clinical work was developed (Chmiel, 1976).

A crossover double-blind experiment taking into consideration the circadian rhythm of human blood viscosity (Ehrly and Jung, 1973) was carried out. Thirty smokers having an increased viscosity due to smoking (Chimel *et al.*, 1973) received orally 1 g of Xantinol nicotinat. Before, after 4 h, and after 5½ h, the following parameters were determined: (1) hematocrit, measuring by Coulter counter and centrifuge; (2) plasma viscosity; (3) low and high shear viscosity of EDTA blood; and (4) particle volume distribution.

An influence of this medication on the flexibility of erythrocytes could not be observed. The aggregation tendency (low shear viscometer, PVA) showed a greater decrease from the morning values when the test group received verum (34%) instead of placebos (only 8%), because of a circadian rhythm as shown in Fig. 1.

H. CHMIEL, P. SCHWEIZER, K.-H. KRAUSE, and W. FRAMING · Helmholtz-Institut for Biomedical Engineering, Department for Internal Medicine, Clinic Aachen, West Germany.

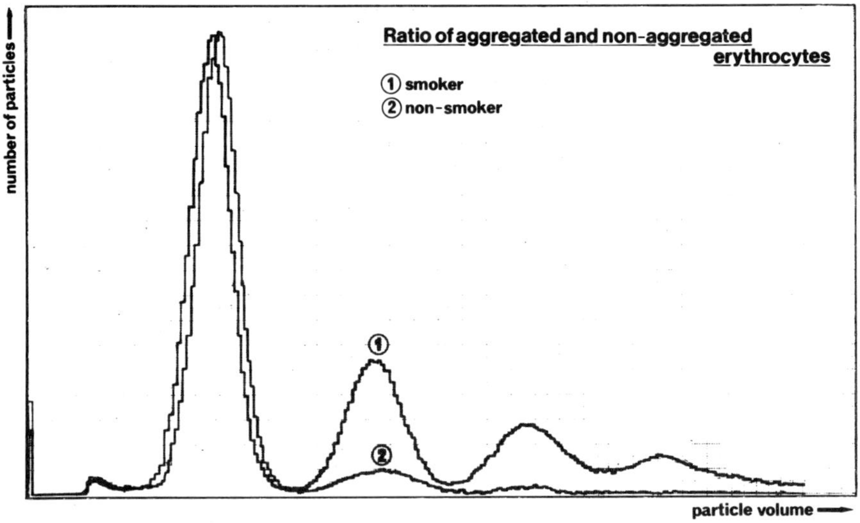

Figure 1. Ratio of aggregated to nonaggregated erythrocytes (area under the second and third peaks vs. area under the first peak before ① and 4 h after ② ingestion of 1 g Xantinol nicotinat.

References

Boss, N., Chmiel, H., Kachel, V., and Ruhenstroth-Bauer, G., 1973, Erythrozytenaggregation bei Nichtrauchern, Rauchern und Herzinfarktpatienten, *Blut* **27:**191–195.

Chmiel, H., 1976*a*, Blood rheology and its clinical application, in: *Cardiocirculatory Analysis of Aspects of Diagnosis, Assist, Therapeutic and Prosthetic Devices,* (D. N. Ghista, E. van Vollenhoven and W. J. Yang, eds.), Delft University Press, Delft, the Netherlands.

Chmiel, H., 1975, A new capillary viscometer for clinical use, *Biorheology* **12:**301.

Chmiel, H., Effert, S., and Mathey, D., 1973, Rheolgische Veränderungen des Blutes beim akuten Herzinfarkt und dessen Risikofaktoren, *Deutsch. Med. Wochenschr.* **98:**1641–1646.

Ehrly, A. M., and Jung, D., 1973, Circadian rhythm of human blood viscosity, *Biorheology* **10:**577–583.

2.10. Internal Tissue Heat during *in Vivo* Transillumination with Fused Quartz and Borosilicate Glass Rods

ROBERT ECHT, RICHARD D. DEY, and WILLIAM F. YOUNG JR.

A modified fused quartz rod transilluminator was used to quantitatively evaluate the efficacy of fused quartz and borosilicate glass as light conductors. Extremely localized internal tissue temperature readings in the optical path were effected by 40-gauge constantan–copper thermocouples. Temperatures were measured during transmission of light from each conductor with both tungsten filament and mercury vapor lamps as sources of illumination. Comparisons were made between the internal tissue temperatures produced with the fused quartz rod and with the borosilicate glass rod using the same light source, at equal light intensities, in either skeletal muscles or livers of adult rats.

With the 500-W tungsten lamp, a 4–5°C temperature difference (39.1–44.7°C) between fused quartz and borosilicate glass rods was observed at maximum light intensities during transillumination of tissue fields (Fig. 1). Increasing the light intensity (1200-W tungsten lamp) for more optimal visualization or photomicrography generated even greater tissue temperature differences. Only minimal tissue temperature increases were noted with both rods conducting light from the mercury vapor lamp. This study provides quantitative evidence favoring the use of borosilicate glass with tungsten and either fused quartz or borosilicate glass with the mercury vapor lamp for transillumination of the *in vivo* microcirculation.

ROBERT ECHT, RICHARD D. DEY, and WILLIAM F. YOUNG, JR. · Department of Anatomy, College of Human Medicine, Michigan State Unversity, East Lansing, Michigan.

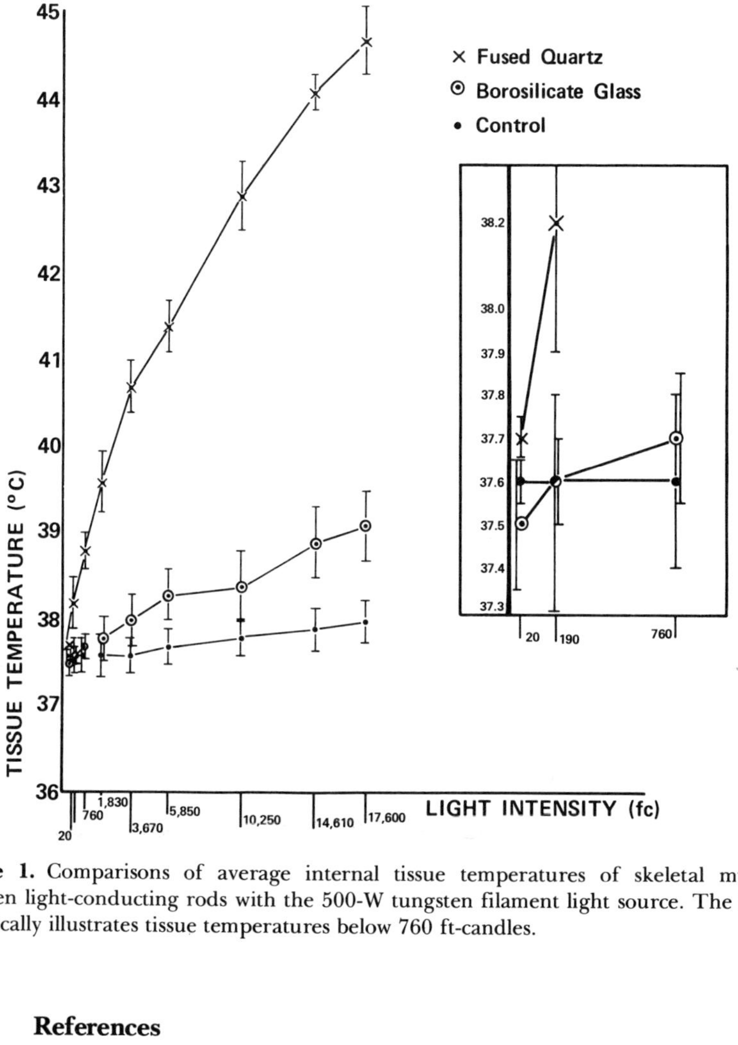

Figure 1. Comparisons of average internal tissue temperatures of skeletal muscle between light-conducting rods with the 500-W tungsten filament light source. The inset specifically illustrates tissue temperatures below 760 ft-candles.

References

Bloch, E. H., 1956, Microscopic observations of the circulating blood in the bulbar conjunctiva in man in health and disease, *Ergeb. Anat. Entwicklungsgesch.* **35:**1.

Bloch, E. H., 1973, The illumination, sensing and recording of the living microvascular system, *Bibl. Anat. Part 1,* **11:**185–210.

Holmes, K. R., 1972, Thermal conductivity of the cat (*Felis domesticus*) foot pad epidermis: Changes produced by controlled of stratum corneum, Ph.D. thesis, Michigan State University, pp. 67–69.

Knisely, M.H., 1938, Improved fused quartz living tissue illuminator, *Anat. Rec.* **71:**503.

Wilson, J. W., 1970, Borosilicate glass rod for living tissue illumination, *J. Biol. Photog. Assoc.* **38:**167.

3

Red Cell Interactions with the Microcirculation

3.1. Red Blood Cell Velocity Profiles in Arterioles and Venules of the Rabbit Omentum

GEERT W. SCHMID-SCHOENBEIN and BENJAMIN W. ZWEIFACH

We have measured RBC velocity profiles for mammalian arterioles and venules from high-speed cinematographic motion pictures. Measurements were made at 320× and 400× optical magnification over an averaging time period of 10 ms. *In vivo* profiles are uniformly nonsymmetrical, the RBCs exhibit rotation, and they frequently deviate sidewise from the overall axial direction of motion. In general, this is more pronounced on the venous side. Since all of the profiles are time variant and the average values are synchronous with the midstream velocity, individual RBC velocities will vary about the average. Profiles become more blunted in vessels with smaller diameters. In vessels below 16 μm diameter, the velocity gradients between adjacent RBCs are quite small; for large vessels, recognizable profiles develop and become fully developed in blood vessels above 30 μm in diameter. This blunting is further affected by the midstream velocity and the local hematocrit; when the velocity is reduced below 1.2 mm/s and/or an increased hematocrit is present, the profile becomes more blunted.

We have estimated the microhematocrit in these blood vessels indirectly by interpolation from systemic and capillary hematocrit distributions and have assumed it to be about 20–30%. Comparable *in vitro* profile studies indicate the same qualitative effects of hematocrit, velocity, and diameter on the RBC profiles in glass tubes (Bugliarello and Hayden, 1963; Goldsmith, 1972).

GEERT W. SCHMID-SCHOENBEIN and BENJAMIN W. ZWEIFACH · AMES-Bioengineering, School of Medicine, University of California, San Diego, La Jolla, California.

The velocity of the RBCs at the outermost edge of the bloodstream is in general higher than would be predicted for a Poiseuille profile with the same midstream velocity. Therefore, the shear rates at the endothelium cell interface can be in the range of $16{,}400^{-1}$, significantly higher than have been reported on the basis of *in vitro* experiments.

References

Bugliarello, G., and Hayden, F. W., 1963, Detailed characteristics of the flow of blood *in vitro, Trans. Soc. Rheol.* **7**:209.

Goldsmith, H., 1972, The flow of model particles and blood cells and its relation to thrombogenesis, in: *Progress in Hemostasis and Thrombosis,* Vol. I (T. H. Spaets, ed.), pp. 97–139, Grune and Stratton, New York.

3.2. Analysis of Red Blood Cell Velocity Distribution in Human Nailfold Capillaries

FELIX MAHLER, RUEDI FREY, ALFRED BOLLINGER, and MAX ANLIKER

Red blood cell velocity (V) in human nailfold capillaries was measured through the intact skin by incident light television microscopy (Bollinger *et al.,* 1974) using videodensitometric techniques (Butti *et al.,* 1976) previously developed for transilluminated tissue (Intaglietta and Tompkins, 1972). The velocity distribution in four to six different capillaries of the same field of observation and the velocity–diameter (D) relation at different sites of single loops were studied in 16 nailfolds of 14 normal subjects over periods of 2 min. While V's measured simultaneously at different sites of single capillaries were inversely related to the square of the corresponding D, there was no relation between V and D in different capillary loops. The flow pattern was continuous in 12 cases, as shown in Fig. 1, and intermittent (on–off) in two (Johnson and Wayland, 1967; Bollinger *et al.,* 1974). Even in capillaries with continuous flow, V fluctuated considerably. The variations in different loops occurred simultaneously and in the same direction in 14 nailfolds observed. The average V determined in each of the loops during a high flow phase (time 1) was 0.69 ± 0.36 mm/s (SD) and during a low flow phase (time 2) was 0.30 ± 0.23 mm/s. Although the maximal absolute differences between V's in different capillaries of the individual nailfolds ranged from 0.09 to 2.0 mm/s, the ratios between V at time 1 and V at time 2 for each of the capillaries under study were comparable in these cases with simultaneous flow variations, suggesting a common regulatory mechanism. In two selected cases, however, V variations in the opposite direction were seen. The ratios of V at time 1 and time 2 between the corresponding capillaries varied by a factor of a different order of magnitude in these two cases. The present data do not prove whether these disparities are due to different regulators or to the random distribution of blood cell size and vessel geometry (Fung, 1973), but represent a first basis for quantitative evaluation of phenomena in the human microcirculation in normal and pathological conditions.

FELIX MAHLER, RUEDI FREY, ALFRED BOLLINGER, and MAX ANLIKER
Department of Internal Medicine and Institute of Biomedical Engineering, University and ETH Zurich, Switzerland.

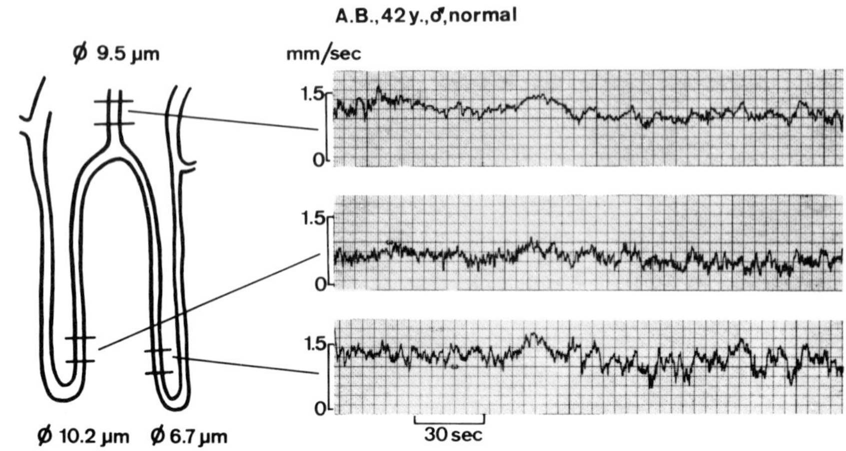

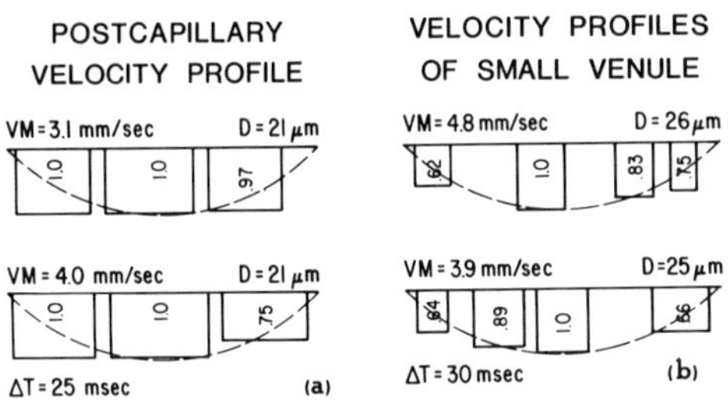

Figure 1. A branching capillary system of the nailfold capillary bed in a normal subject with the diameter (ϕ) values and original velocity tracings (cross-correlator) from the corresponding sites of measurements in the feeding vessel and two branches. The velocity changes show comparable time relations.

ACKNOWLEDGMENT

This work was supported by Grant No. 2.1160.73 from the Swiss National Fund for Scientific Research.

References

Bollinger, A., Butti, P., Barras, J. P., Trachsler, H., and Siegenthaler, W., 1974, Red blood cell velocity in nailfold capillaries of man measured by a television microscopy technique, *Microvasc. Res.* **7**:61.

Butti, P., Intaglietta, M., Reimann, H., Holliger, C., Bollinger, A., and Anliker, M., 1976, Capillary red blood cell velocity measurements in human nailfold by videodensitometric method, *Microvasc. Res.* (In press).

Fung, Y., 1973, Stochastic flow in capillary blood vessels, *Microvasc. Res.* **5**:34.

Intaglietta, M., and Tompkins, W. R., 1972, On-line microvascular blood cell flow velocity measurement by simplified correlation technique, *Microvasc. Res.* **4**:217.

Johnson, P. C., and Wayland, H., 1967, Regulation of blood flow in single capillaries, *Am. J. Physiol.* **212**:1405.

3.3. *In Vivo* Study of "Apparent Viscosity" and Vessel Wall Shear Stress in Cat Mesentery

HERBERT H. LIPOWSKY and BENJAMIN W. ZWEIFACH

The *in vivo* rheological behavior of blood in the mesenteric microcirculation of the cat was investigated by simultaneous measurement of pressure gradient and RBC velocity. Data were obtained for arterial and venous microvessels ranging in diameter from 10 to 58 μm, with length-to-diameter ratios of from 20 to 30. Intravascular pressures were measured by the electronic servonull technique developed by Wiederhielm *et al.* (1950) and modified by Intaglietta *et al.* (1970). Two servonull systems were coupled to a differential pressure transducer to facilitate measurement of the upstream-to-downstream pressure differential to within 0.05 cm H_2O. Pressure differentials ranged from 0.2 to 5.0 cm H_2O, depending on flow rate.

Vessel centerline RBC velocities were measured by a variation of the "two-slit" technique of Wayland and Johnson (1967). Velocities were computed by on-line cross-correlation of the photometric signatures detected by two photodiodes, using the self-tracking correlator developed by Tompkins *et al.* (1974). The centerline velocity (V_{CL}) was related to the bulk mean velocity (V_{mean}) of both cells plus plasma by the correction factor (V_{CL}/V_{mean} = 1.6) proposed by Baker and Wayland (1974). This correction was found to be valid (within 5 %) by *in vitro* calibration experiments for tube diameters as small as 17 μm.

These data, together with vessel geometry from high-magnification photographs, made it possible to compute "apparent viscosity" and vessel wall shear stress as a function of mean velocity. Mean velocities were varied in individual vessels by means of a pressure-actuated cuff around the superior mesenteric artery and/or microocclusion needle.

"Apparent viscosity" followed the trends associated with *in vitro* data and ranged from 20 cP, at a mean velocity of 0.3 mm/s, to 1.5 cP at 30 mm/s. For velocities associated with normal flow in mesenteric preparations, vessel wall shear stresses as high as 200 dyn/cm^2 were measured, primarily in arterioles ranging from 20 to 25 μm in diameter.

HERBERT H. LIPOWSKY and BENJAMIN W. ZWEIFACH · AMES-Bioengineering, University of California, San Diego, La Jolla, California.

ACKNOWLEDGMENT

This work was supported by United States Public Health Service Grant HL 10881.

References

Baker, M., and Wayland, H., 1974, On-line volumetric flow rate and velocity profile measurement for blood in microvessels, *Microvasc. Res.* **7**:131.

Intaglietta, M., Pawula, R. F., and Tompkins, W. R., 1970, Pressure measurements in the mammalian microvasculature, *Microvasc. Res.* **2**:212.

Tompkins, W. R., Monti, R., and Intaglietta, M., 1974, Velocity measurements by self-tracking correlator, *Rev. Sci. Instrum.* **45**:647.

Wayland, H., and Johnson, P. C., 1967, Erythrocyte velocity measurement in microvessels by a two-slit photometric method, *J. Appl. Physiol.* **22**:333.

Wiederhielm, C. A., Woodbury, J. W., Kirk, S., and Rushmer, R. F., 1950, Pulsatile pressures in the microcirculation of the frog's mesentery, *Am. J. Med.* **23**:684.

3.4. Flow Velocities of Red Blood Cells and Their Suspending Medium Measured in Glass Capillaries Using the Photometric Dual-Slit Method

P. GAEHTGENS, K. U. BENNER, and S. SCHICKENDANTZ

Suspensions of human RBCs in saline were made to flow through glass capillaries (ID 9–12 μm) at various flow rates. The image of the capillaries was projected onto a screen (magnification 90×). Signals obtained from a dual-slit arrangement of photosensors (effective separation 4 μm) were recorded to determine RBC velocities (v_{RBC}). Two additional photosensors were mounted upstream and downstream of the dual slit. Suspending

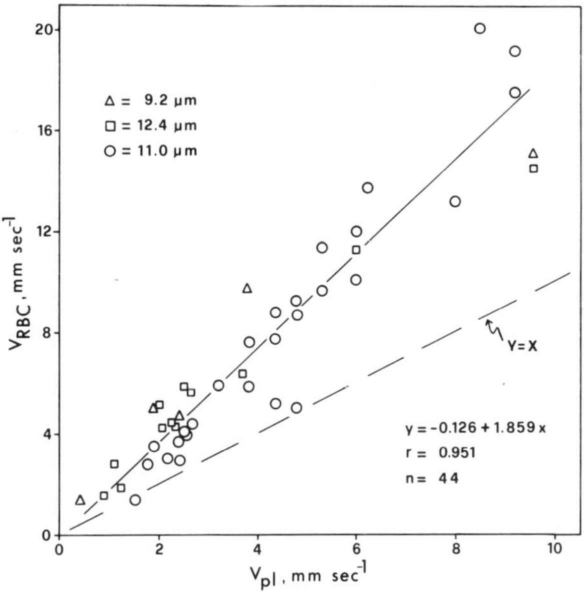

Figure 1. Red cell and suspending medium flow velocities as determined in three different glass capillaries at various flow rates. Dashed line indicates identity of both parameters.

P. GAEHTGENS, K. U. BENNER, and S. SCHICKENDANTZ · Institute for Normal and Pathological Physiology, University of Köln, West Germany.

medium flow velocity (v_{pl}) was determined from the delay between signals caused by the passage of a dye (Evans blue, 5 g%) bolus across these additional photosensors (effective separation 950 μm). All signals were recorded on tape and played back at reduced speed for visual analysis. At the flow rates used, v_{RBC} ranged between 1 and 20 mm/s, v_{pl} between 1 and 10 mm/s. In all experiments, v_{RBC} exceeded v_{pl} substantially. A linear relationship between v_{RBC} and v_{pl} was found with an average ratio v_{RBC}/v_{pl} of 1.84 ± 0.43 (Fig. 1). No effect of absolute flow rate on this ratio was observed. Similar experiments carried out in larger capillaries (ID up to 42 μm) indicated a decrease of the velocity ratios down to values below 1.0. These values, however, are in part affected by the averaging effect across several cell layers introduced by the dual-slit technique. It is concluded that the average passage time of RBCs and that of their suspending medium in the smallest capillaries are significantly different. The absence of any significant effect of the flow rate on velocity ratios may be indicative of maximum cell deformation in the high flow rate range (corresponding to $\bar{u} > 100$ tube diameters per second) used in this study.

References

Baker, M., and Wayland, H., 1974, On-line flow rate and velocity profile measurement for blood in microvessels, *Microvasc. Res.* **7**:131.

Wayland, H., and Johnson, P. C., 1967, Erythrocyte velocity measurement in microvessels by a two-slit photometric method, *J. Appl. Physiol.* **22**:333.

3.5. A New On-Line Method of Measuring High Flow Speeds in Microscopic Vessels by a Dual Video Camera Technique

M. ANLIKER and R. KUBLI

In analyzing the speed of RBCs in the capillaries of the human nailfold, it was observed that in some subjects the speed was too high even during resting flow conditions to be quantified by videodensitometry at conventional frame rates of 50 or 60 frames per second. Also, frame-to-frame analysis and videodensitometry may yield differing results when the two-slit video technique is employed (Holliger *et al.,* 1975; Butti *et al.,* 1975). This technique is based on a temporal as well as a spatial sampling process and thus discards too much of the video information available in

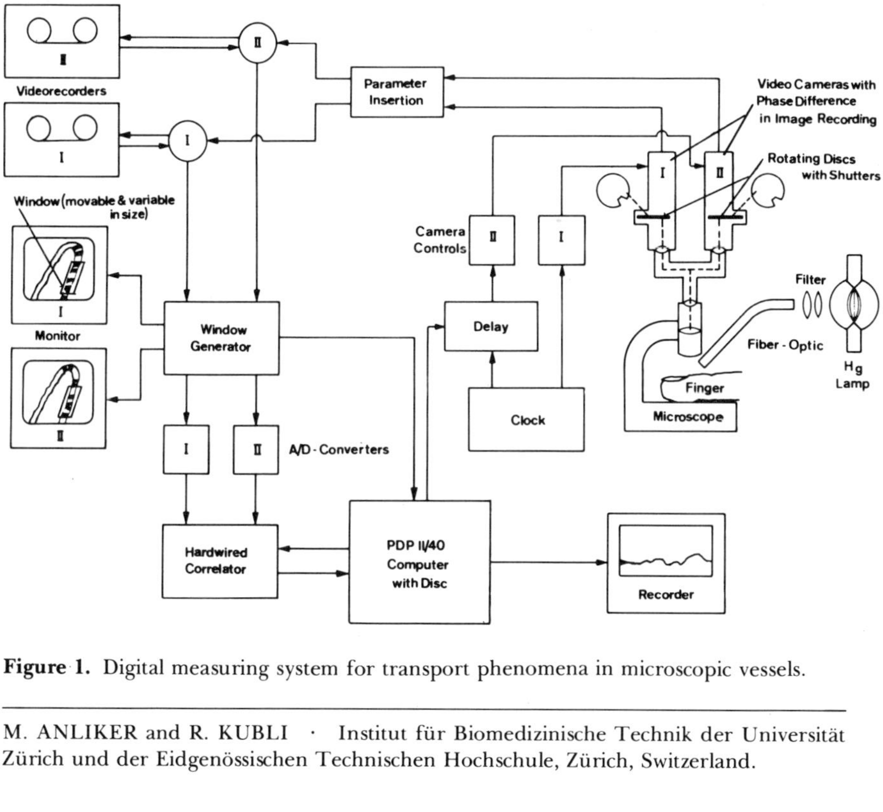

Figure 1. Digital measuring system for transport phenomena in microscopic vessels.

M. ANLIKER and R. KUBLI · Institut für Biomedizinische Technik der Universität Zürich und der Eidgenössischen Technischen Hochschule, Zürich, Switzerland.

successive frames with regard to the sequence of RBCs and plasma spaces between the two slits. Therefore, an alternate approach in the methodology appeared warranted.

A new system has been developed in which a microscopic image of the capillary bed is viewed with two video cameras whose recording cycles have a precisely controlled phase difference, as shown in Fig. 1. The cameras are modified to record all half-frames with identical line positions. The vessel of interest is surrounded by a parallelogram which forms a window. Within this window, the video signal is integrated for each line to provide a video density distribution along the vessel. The spatial correlation of the density distributions corresponding to two frames recorded within a given time interval yields a measure of the flow velocity. A custom-made digital correlator permits the evaluation of the correlograms for forward or backward flow and therefore the on-line determination of the flow speed during either recording or playback. The time delay between the two frames is chosen such that the video density distributions overlap at least 50%. With a time delay of 1 ms, the flow speed may be as high as 20–50 mm/s depending on vessel length and magnification.

References

Butti, P., Intaglietta, M., Reimann, H., Holliger, C., Bollinger, A., and Anliker, M., 1975, Capillary red blood cell velocity measurements in human nailfold by videodensitometric method, *Microvasc. Res.* **10:** in press.

Holliger, C., Anliker, M., Klingler, D., and Bollinger, A., 1975, Evaluation of an on-line videodensitometric measurement of the red blood cells speed in the capillaries of the human nailfold, *Biomed. Tech.* **20:** in press.

3.6. Blood Cells in an Annular Vortex

TAKESHI KARINO and HARRY L. GOLDSMITH

Deposits of platelet aggregates have been found on artery walls at certain sites where flow is disturbed and vortices may form. Hence we have studied the flow behavior of erythrocytes and platelets in a model of a vortex formed distal to the sudden concentric expansion of a 150-μm glass tube into a 500-μm tube, as shown in Fig. 1.

Although theory (Macagno and Hung, 1967) predicts closed vortex streamlines, single blood cells in dilute suspensions in steady flow migrated outward across the streamlines and left the vortex. Aggregates of cells, however, remained and even accumulated in the vortex, traveling on equilibrium orbits or staying in the vortex center, depending on particle

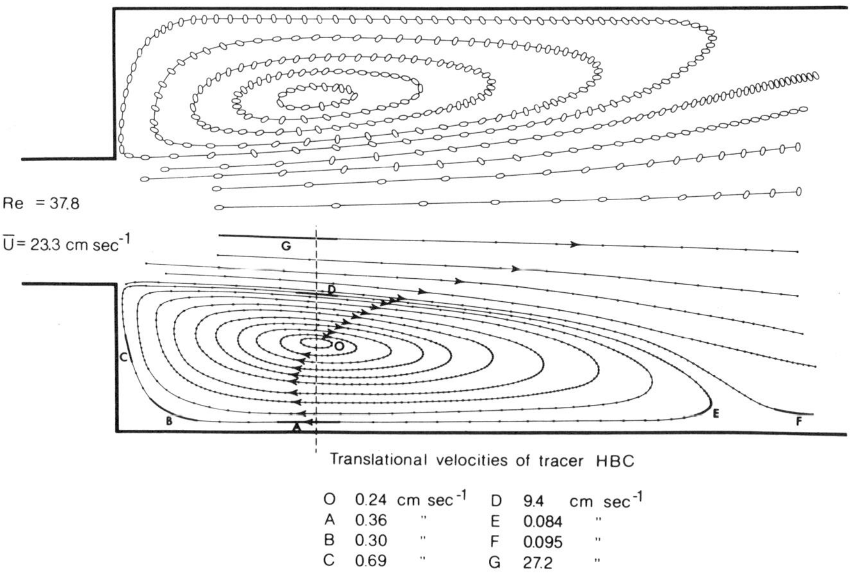

Figure 1. Annular vortex formed downstream of a sudden concentric expansion of a 150-μm tube into a 500-μm tube, showing the paths, translational velocities, and orientations of tracer-hardened red cells in the median plane of the tube. In the lower part, the velocity profile along the dashed line is given by the position of the arrows (Re and $\bar{U}$ are the upstream tube Reynolds number and mean flow rate, respectively).

TAKESHI KARINO and HARRY L. GOLDSMITH · University Medical Clinic, Montreal General Hospital, Montreal, Quebec, Canada.

size and flow rate. The rate of migration depended on the flow rate, and experiments with model rigid spheres showed that particles above 30 μm diameter remained in the vortex at all flow rates.

In pulsatile flow, the vortex varied periodically in shape and intensity. The oscillatory component of the flow enhanced the migration effects observed in steady flow. The above-described behavior also occurred with red cells in whole blood at hematocrits from 15 to 45%. Cell-free vortices developed at low steady flow rates, while in pulsatile flow the hematocrit in the vortex varied periodically but was much lower than that in the mainstream.

The observations may be relevant to the *in vivo* situation at poststenotic dilations, at obstructions, and with respect to prosthetic devices having sudden changes in vessel diameter. If aggregates of red cells or platelets are trapped in the downstream vortex where shear rates are relatively low, they may grow in size and interact with the vessel wall, causing further obstruction to the flow.

ACKNOWLEDGMENT

This work was supported by MRC Grant MT 1835 and the Quebec Heart Foundation.

Reference

Macagno, E. O., and Hung, T.-K., 1967, Computational and experimental study of a captive annular eddy, *J. Fluid Mech.* **28**:43.

3.7. Geometry of the Fetal Erythrocyte and Its Relation to Osmotic Fragility

A. W. L. JAY and J. M. WHAUN

The red cell of the newborn infant differs from that of the adult in many respects. The differences reported include cell metabolism (Oski and Smith, 1968; Whaun and Oski, 1969; Zipursky *et al.*, 1960), cell morphology (Holroyde *et al.*, 1969), and membrane structure (Haberman *et al.*, 1967). Sjölin (1954) has noted that while cord cells have a normal osmotic fragility at birth, cells obtained during the first week of life have decreased osmotic fragility; more recent studies (Gross and Hathaway, 1972) suggest that fetal cells are less deformable.

The present study investigates the relation between cell geometry and osmotic fragility. Cord blood at birth and capillary samples taken by heelprick at 1–6 h and at 2–4 days were collected from ten normal, full-term babies. The cells were suspended in Ringer solution containing 3 g/liter serum albumin. The geometry of individual cells was analyzed using photomicrographic and computer techniques. The details of the techniques have been described elsewhere (Jay, 1975). Results show that compared to adult erythrocytes, which have a mean volume of 98.1 ± 0.6 (SEM) μm^3 and a mean surface area of 133.4 ± 0.5 (SEM) μm^2, fetal cells are much larger, with mean values of about 127 μm^3 and 160 μm^2, respectively. While the mean surface area of the red cells remains unchanged during the first week of life, the mean cell volume decreases by 3.3% to 122.7 ± 1.0 (SEM) μm^3. This results in an increase in swelling index and suggests a decrease in osmotic fragility.

Studies of osmotic fragility of cells from blood samples collected from 16 babies show a progressive decrease of fragility during the first few days of life. The osmolalities at which 50% hemolysis occurs are well correlated with the swelling index from the cell geometry study, suggesting that the decreased fragility observed during the first few days of life is probably due to a reduction in cell volume.

A. W. L. JAY and J. M. WHAUN · Division of Medical Biophysics and Division of Paediatrics, Faculty of Medicine, The University of Calgary, Calgary, Alberta, Canada.

ACKNOWLEDGMENTS

This work was supported by the Alberta Heart Foundation and the Medical Research Council of Canada. Dr. Jay is a Research Fellow of the Canadian Heart Foundation.

References

Gross, G. P., and Hathaway, W. E., 1972, Fetal erythrocyte deformability, *Pediatr. Res.* **6:**593.

Haberman, S., Blanton, P., and Martin, J., 1967, Some observations on the ABO antigen sites of the erythrocyte membranes of adults and newborn infants, *J. Immunol.* **98:**150.

Holroyde, C. P., Oski, F. A., and Gardner, F. H., 1969, The "pocked" erythrocyte, *N. Engl. J. Med.* **281:**516.

Jay, A. W. L., 1975, Geometry of the human erythrocyte. I. Effect of albumin on cell geometry, *Biophys. J.* **15:**205.

Oski, F. A., and Smith, C., 1968, Red cell metabolism in the premature infant. III. Apparent inappropriate glucose consumption for cell age, *Pediatrics* **43:**473.

Sjölin, S., 1954, The resistance of red cells *in vitro*: A study of the osmotic properties, the mechanical resistance and the storage behaviour of red cells of fetuses, children and adults, *Acta Paediatr.* **43:**1.

Whaun, J. M., and Oski, F. A., 1969, Red cell stromal adenosine triophosphatase (ATPase) of newborn infants, *Pediatr. Res.* **3:**105

Zipursky, A., LaRue, T., and Israels, L. G., 1960, The *in vitro* metabolism of erythrocytes from newborn infants, *Can. J. Biochem.* **38:**727.

3.8. Electrochemical and Mechanical Factors in Red Cell Interactions

S. CHIEN, S. USAMI, and K. M. JAN

Aggregation of RBCs into rouleaux was induced by dextrans of various molecular weights and concentrations. Some of the studies were performed on RBCs with their surface charge removed by neuraminidase treatment. The degree of cell aggregation was estimated by light reflection technique in a coaxial cylinder system (Usami and Chien, 1973). Aggregation of neuraminidase-treated RBCs showed a sigmoidal relation with dextran concentrations, with plateau levels reached at concentrations above 8 g%. Aggregation of normal RBCs was similar to that of neuraminidase-treated RBCs up to dextran concentration of 4 g%, but aggregation decreased at higher concentrations, with complete disaggregation at 9 g%.

The ζ potential of RBCs was determined by electrophoresis (Seaman, 1975). The electrostatic repulsive force (F_e) between adjacent cell surfaces in the rouleaux was calculated from the ζ potential, the intercellular distance (Chien and Jan, 1973*a*), and the dielectric constant (Jan and Chien, 1973) and ionic composition of the suspending medium. In this calculation, the formula of Overbeek (1952) was used, with corrections made for the reduction of effective ionic strength by dextrans (Brooks, 1973; Chien and Jan, 1973*b*). At dextran concentrations above 4 g%, F_e increased sharply for normal RBCs, together with progressive disaggregation.

Application of moderate shear rates (0.1–1 s^{-1}) caused an enhancement of RBC aggregation, probably due to an increase in cell-to-cell encounter. With large increases in shear rate (higher than 10 s^{-1}), the resultant high shear stresses caused progressive RBC disaggregation.

The findings indicate that RBC aggregation and disaggregation represent the results of a balance of macromolecular bridging force vs. the electrostatic repulsive force and mechanical shearing force at the cell surface.

S. CHIEN, S. USAMI, and K. M. JAN · Laboratory of Hemorheology, Department of Physiology, Columbia University College of Physicians and Surgeons, New York, N.Y.

ACKNOWLEDGMENTS

This work was supported by United States Public Health Service Grants HL-06139 and HL-16851 and by U.S. Army Contract DADA-17-72-C-2115.

References

Brooks, D. E., 1973, The effect of neutral polymers on the electrokinetic potential of cells and other charged particles. II. A model for the effect of adsorbed polymer on the diffuse double layer, *J. Colloid Interface Sci.* **43:**687.

Chien, S., and Jan, K.-M., 1973*a*, Ultrastructural basis of the mechanism of rouleaux formation, *Microvasc. Res.* **5:**155.

Chien, S., and Jan, K.-M., 1973*b*, Red cell aggregation by macromolecules: Roles of surface adsorption and electrostatic repulsion, *J. Supramol. Struct.* **1:**385.

Jan, K.-M., and Chien, S., 1973, Role of surface electric charge in red blood cell interactions, *J. Gen. Physiol.* **61:**638.

Overbeek, T. T. G., 1952, Electrochemistry of the double layer, in: *Colloid Science,* Vol. I (H. R. Kruyt, ed.), pp. 115–193, Elsevier Press, Amsterdam.

Seaman, G. V. F., 1975, Electrokinetic behavior of red cells, in: *The Red Blood Cell,* 2nd ed. (D. M. Surgenor, ed.), pp. 1135–1229, Academic Press, New York.

Usami, S., and Chien, S., 1973, Shear deformation of red cell ghosts, *Biorheology* **10:**425.

3.9. Role of the Erythrocyte Surface Charge in the Microcirculation

VICTOR A. HANSON, JR., STENNIS D. WAX, and WATTS R. WEBB

This study explores a functional aspect of red cell surface charge and its influence on capillary flow. Alteration of this charge may have clinical implications in acute and chronic thromboembolic processes.

The surface charge of the erythrocyte is negative and has been attributed to the presence of carboxyl groups of sialic acid. The charge magnitude is measured *ex vivo* in an electrophoretic cell and is expressed as electrophoretic mobility (E.M.) in micrometers/second/volt/centimeter.

In anesthetized dogs, the administration of a desialylating enzyme (*Vibrio cholerae* neuraminidase) was followed by red cell clumping, rouleaux formation, and decrease of flow in the alveolar capillaries which was observed through the microscope and filmed. These flow alterations were associated with decrease in E.M. from 2.7 to 2.0 ($p < 0.001$) and decrease in arterial Po_2 from 80 to 50 mm Hg ($p < 0.001$). Similar events occurred following autotransfusion to splenectomized dogs of aged stored blood with an E.M. of less than 2.2. Low molecular weight dextran infusion, which enhances the cellular negative charge, reversed the E.M. and oxygen curves and was followed by a return to a control flow patterns in the alveolar capillaries.

We concluded that negative charge on RBCs influences the function of the microcirculation and this influence is proportional to charge magnitude.

References

Eylar, E., and Madoff, M., 1962, Contribution of sialic acid to surface charge of erythrocyte, *J. Biochem.* **237(6):**1992.

Knisely, M. H., 1951, Annotated bibliography of sludged blood, *Postgrad. Med.*, pp. 10–15.

Wells, R. E., Jr., 1964, Rheology of blood in the microvasculature, *N. Engl. J. Med.* **270(17):**832.

VICTOR A. HANSON, Jr., STENNIS D. WAX, and WATTS R. WEBB · State University of New York, Upstate Medical Center, Syracuse, New York.

3.10. Velocity-Dependent Resistance Behavior of Erythrocytes in Capillary Pores and Membrane Elasticity

P. S. LINGARD

Lingard (1974) reported pressure drop–velocity data for erythrocytes in 7-μm capillary pores (Fig. 1a) showing a constant maximum resistance below a critical velocity (K), with decreasing resistance beyond. Such resistance changes were tentatively attributed to erythrocyte distortion effects such as predicted by Lighthill (1968) and Fitz-Gerald (1969). More recent data for narrower-filter pores confirm the original findings (Lingard, 1976). The following is a simplified analysis of important features of the cell behavior.

At each velocity, we represent the cell by an equivalent, rigid, cylindrical pellet which has equal hydrodynamic resistance. The drag equation for the pellet is solved for the width (h) of the surrounding fluid film. The computed solutions for the data in Fig. 1a appear in Fig. 1b. An extended discussion reveals that the minimum film width for the original cell need not be underestimated by this approach. The narrowness of the film (yet narrower for 5-μm pores) is consistent with occupation by the cells of a substantial proportion of the capillary lumen and effectively axisymmetrical cell orientation.

Figure 1c shows the dependence of the computed film width on the pressure drop per cell. This relation agrees with Fitz-Gerald's model for large-scale cell distortion, provided that the arc lengths of the membrane faces do not vary. Fitz-Gerald (1969) assumed a Laplace law dependence of membrane curvature on deforming pressure. Better quantitative agreement is obtained, however, using a model for circular plate distortion for which the mean curvature is shown to be $4r_0^2p/Et^3$, where E is Young's modulus, t is membrane thickness, r_0 is plate radius, and p is pressure drop. E, obtained by graphical analysis from Fig. 1c, is in the range of 10^6–10^7 Pa, in agreement with estimates by Katchalsky *et al.* (1960) and Rand (1964). These findings apparently confirm the prediction of Lighthill and Fitz-Gerald of elastohydrodynamic resistance changes with velocity.

P. S. LINGARD · Research Unit for the Newborn, Children's Medical Research Foundation, Royal Alexandra Hospital for Children and The Women's Hospital, Sydney, Australia.

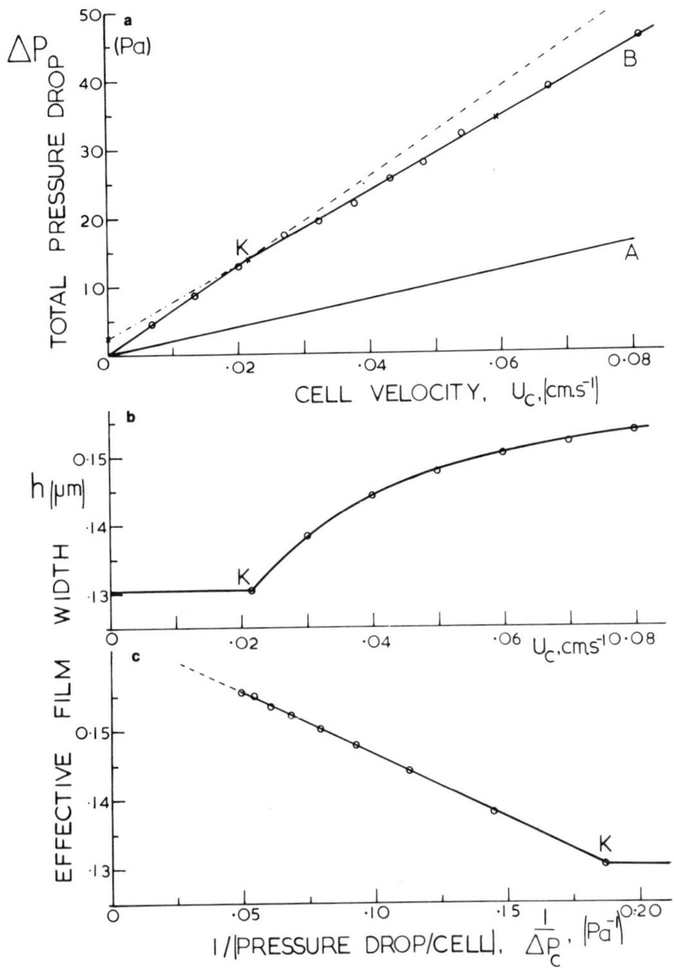

Figure 1. (a) Typical pressure drop–velocity characteristic for a suspension of human erythrocytes at hematocrit value 40%, in the 6.9-μm pores of a Nuclepore filter. Curve 0–*A* shows data for the suspending medium, a 20% (wt/vol) bovine albumin solution (pH 7.35, 290 mosM·kg^{-1}, viscosity 2.14 cP). Curve 0–*K*–*B* shows data for the erythrocyte suspension at 37°C, with change of slope at *K* ($P < 0.0005$ for difference between slopes 0–*K* and *K*–*B*, by *t* test). Leukocytes had been removed from this suspension. (b) Relation between computed film width (*h*) and cell velocity, corresponding to the data in (a). (c) Relation between computed film width and pressure drop per cell, corresponding to the data in (a) and (b).

References

Fitz-Gerald, J. M., 1969, Mechanics of red-cell motion through very narrow capillaries, *Proc. R. Soc. London Ser. B* **174:**193.

Katchalsky, A., Kedem, O., Klibansky, C., and De Vries, A., 1960, Rheological considerations of the haemolysing red blood cell, in: *Flow Properties of Blood and Other Biological Systems* (A. L., Copley and G. Stainsby, eds.), pp. 155–171, Pergamon Press, New York.

Lighthill, M. J., 1968, Pressure-forcing of tightly fitting pellets along fluid-filled elastic tubes, *J. Fluid Mech.* **34:**113.

Lingard, P. S., 1974, Capillary pore rheology of erythrocytes. I. Hydroelastic behaviour of human erythrocytes, *Microvasc. Res.* **8:**53.

Lingard, P. S., 1976, Erythrocyte motion in narrow capillaries—Effect of capillary diameter and haematocrit, *Proc. Aust. Physiol. Pharmacol. Soc.* (in press).

Rand, R. P., 1964, Mechanical properties of the red cell membrane. II. Viscoelastic breakdown of the membrane, *Biophys. J.* **4:**303.

3.11. Effects of Altered Red Cell Deformability on Capillary Flow Resistance

S. ROWLANDS, P. M. GUNTON, and A. W. L. JAY

Earlier studies have demonstrated the low resistance to flow of blood and normal erythrocytes in capillaries (Jay, *et al.*, 1972). Variation in RBC deformability as a result of changes in cell geometry, flexibility, and/or membrane viscoelasticity (Jay, 1973) will cause alterations in the pressure–flow relationships. An electronic sensing technique has been developed to measure the mean velocities of individual RBCs as they traverse glass capillaries 3–6 μm in diameter and 200–1000 μm in length. An increase in electrical resistance across the length of the glass capillary when it is partially blocked by a cell provides a pulse, the width of which is a measure of the time taken for the cell to go through the length of the capillary. The driving pressure and the time measurement are recorded simultaneously. A Wang 600 programmable calculator is used for data collection and analysis. A comparison between the slopes of the pressure–flow velocity relations for control and treated samples provides a measure of relative changes in flow resistance and cell deformability. Hypotonicity, causing swelling of erythrocytes, results in decreased cell deformability (Jay, 1973). In the present system, this is associated with a decrease in flow velocity. Flow velocity varies as the osmolality of the suspending medium. Decreased flow velocity has also been recorded for incubation of cells at 49.5°C. This is associated with a decrease in cell deformability due to membrane area decrease and cell shape change. The presence of serum albumin also decreases flow velocity. Albumin decreases cell volume (Jay, 1975); the effect is probably a result of decreased cell flexibility. The effects of some hormones are also being investigated.

ACKNOWLEDGMENTS

This work was supported by the Alberta Heart Foundation and the Medical Research Council of Canada. Dr. Jay is a Research Fellow of the Canadian Heart Foundation.

S. ROWLANDS, P. M. GUNTON, and A. W. L. JAY · Division of Medical Biophysics, Faculty of Medicine, The University of Calgary, Calgary, Alberta, Canada.

References

Jay, A. W. L., 1973, Viscoelastic properties of the human red blood cell membrane. I. Deformation, volume loss and rupture of red cells in micropipettes, *Biophys. J.* **13:**1166.

Jay, A. W. L., 1975, Geometry of the human erythrocyte. I. Effect of albumin on cell geometry, *Biophys. J.* **15:**205.

Jay, A. W. L., Rowlands, S., and Skibo, L., 1972, The resistance to blood flow in the capillaries, *Can. J. Physiol. Pharmacol.* **50:**1007.

3.12. Effect of Heat-Traumatized Blood on Microcirculatory Dynamics

M. MASON GUEST and TED P. BOND

High temperature modifies blood in tissue at the time of burning. This study was designed to evaluate effects of previously heated blood on circulation in a region of the body not heat stressed.

Blood was withdrawn from dogs, heparinized, heated, and reinfused, after cooling, into a mesenteric artery of the donor animal (Bond and Guest, 1971). Heating was performed in polyethylene tubing submerged for 1 min in a 65°C water bath. The temperature of the blood in the tubing reached 55°C and remained at this temperature, or slightly above, for no more than 2 s.

The mesenteric microcirculation was cinephotographed prior to, during, and following infusion of the previously heated blood. Cinefilm was exposed at 24 frames per second and up to 400 frames per second (Bond and Guest, 1971). Control blood (heparinized and placed in polyethylene tubing but not heated) traversed the microvessels without evidence of abnormality. In contrast, flow of blood which had been heated was abnormal; most erythrocytes were sphered and relatively rigid: flow in true capillaries was absent. Following perfusion of the previously heated blood, while the dog's nonheparinized, nonheated blood perfused the microcirculatory field, blood flow was abnormal for more than 1 h.

From observations that leukocytes tend to adhere abnormally to walls of venules and that blood flow fails to resume in some microvessels, it appears that, once heated, blood causes an alteration in endothelial surfaces. Previously heated plasma, including platelet-rich plasma containing leukocytes, did not cause discernible endothelial cell surface alteration. Hence the alteration appears to be causally related to heat-damaged RBCs.

In the plasma from the heated blood, fibrinogen and factors V and VIII were absent. The heated plasma did not inhibit coagulation.

M. MASON GUEST and TED P. BOND · Shriners Burns Institute, University of Texas Medical Branch, Galveston, Texas.

ACKNOWLEDGMENT

This work was supported by DHEW HL-16449 and the Shriners Burns institute.

Reference

Bond, T. P., and Guest, M. M., 1971, High speed cinematography of the microcirculation, in: *Cinematographic Techniques in Biology and Medicine* (A. L. Burton, ed.), pp. 151–172, Academic Press, New York.

3.13. Effect of Heat-Induced Spherocytes on Intrahepatic Microcirculation

H. HUTTEN, P. VAUPEL, I.-E. RICHTER, and P. WENDLING

In 18 rabbits anesthetized with ketamine i.p. and breathing spontaneously, regional hepatic blood flow was measured by means of the $^{85}Kr(\beta)$ clearance technique. The liver was exposed by an abdominal incision. Application of the dissolved indicator was performed through a catheter into the thoracic aorta using a slug injection. Evaluation of the clearance curves was accomplished by means of a modification of the height-over-area method (Zierler, 1965) in order to reduce the error due to the nonideal input function. Mean arterial blood pressure (MABP) was measured continuously utilizing another catheter in the femoral artery by means of a Statham pressure transducer. In each animal, repeated measurements were performed before (rHBF) and at least 30 min after injection of 2.5–3.0 ml of heat-induced spherocytes ($rHBF_0$).

3.13.1. Results

1. The correlation achieved by comparison of corresponding rHBF–$rHBF_0$ values (i.e., for the same animal and with $\Delta MABP \leq 10$ mm Hg) is described by $rHBF_0 = 0.31\ rHBF + 0.32$ and $rHBF = 0.83\ rHBF_0 + 0.63$, respectively ($p < 0.001$).
2. Mean rHBF amounts to 1.21 ml/g/min ($n = 52$, MABP = 82 mm Hg) and mean $rHBF_0$ to 0.69 ml/g/min ($n = 47$, MABP = 82 mm Hg), respectively.
3. In the range of 70–95 mm Hg for MABP, rHBF depends on MABP, whereas $rHBF_0$ is independent of MABP (Fig. 1).

3.13.2. Discussion

1. Taking into account the mass relation (in rabbits, spleen: liver = 1:80), the reduction in rHBF after injection of spherocytes cannot

H. HUTTEN, P. VAUPEL, I.-E. RICHTER, and P. WENDLING, · Department of Physiology, University of Mainz, West Germany.

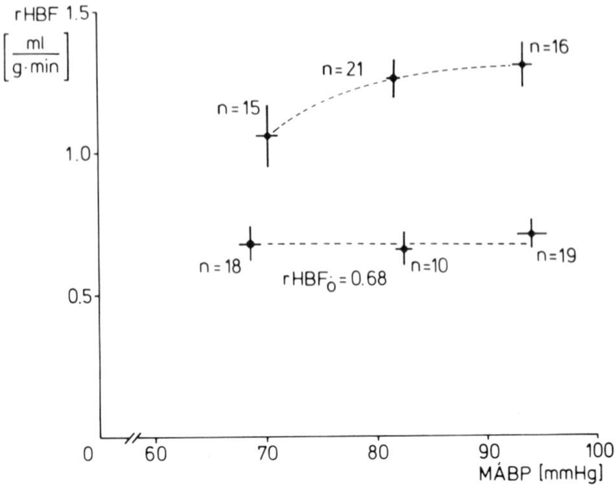

MABP	≤75	80–85	≥90	mmHg
rHBF	1.06 ± 0.11	1.26 ± 0.07	1.30 ± 0.08	ml/g/min
MABP	70.3 ± 1.1	81.7 ± 0.5	93.4 ± 1.1	mmHg
$rHBF_0$	0.68 ± 0.06	0.66 ± 0.06	0.71 ± 0.05	ml/g/min
MABP	68.6 ± 1.1	82.5 ± 0.8	94.0 ± 1.5	mmHg

Figure 1. Regional hepatic blood flow before (upper curve) and after (lower curve) application of spherocytes vs. mean arterial blood pressure (MABP). Values are means ± SEM (*n* = number of measurements).

sufficiently be explained by the obstruction of the open circulation in the spleen and thereby reduced splenic outflow to the liver.

2. According to Wagner *et al.* (1962), it can be assumed that in the spleen as well as in the liver the same volume of spherocytes (about 1 ml) is accumulated. However, total splenic blood flow is reduced only for 1.0 ml/min (Vaupel *et al.,* 1974), whereas total hepatic blood flow is diminished for 47 ml/min.
3. Scanning electron microscopic pictures reveal the different mechanisms. In the spleen, spherocytes occlude the open circulation in the perisinal meshwork of the red pulp. In the liver, single spherocytes are trapped primarily at branching points of small vessels, thereby forming microaggregates of normal erythrocytes.

References

Vaupel, P., Hutten, H., Wendling, P., and Braunbeck, W., 1974, Experimental and theoretical investigations on intrasplenic microcirculation in rabbits, *Res. Exp. Med.* **164:**223.

Wagner, H. N., Razzak, M. A., Gaertner, R. A., Caine, W. P., and Feagin, O. T., 1962, Removal of erythrocytes from the circulation, *Arch. Intern. Med.* **110:**128.

Zierler, K. L., 1965, Equations for measuring blood flow by external monitoring of radioisotopes, *Circ. Res.* **16:**309.

3.14. Locomotion and Chemotaxis of Human Neutrophils

V. G. VETHAMANY, S. K. VETHAMANY, and M. BESSIS

The apparatus used to determine locomotion and chemotaxis by easy direct observation has been described earlier (Bessis and Burté, 1964). Figure 1 shows the leukocytes and the chemotactic target at the beginning of the experiment, and Fig. 2 shows the same preparation at 9 min. The polymorphonuclear cells (PMNs) in a field of 17,600 μm^2 are counted at the time of irradiation (time 0) and at 9 min after irradiation. The PMNs forming a rosette at 9 min around the target are also counted. The ratio of PMNs in the rosette to PMNs in the field at 9 min after irradiation is defined as the chemotactic index (CI). When the velocity of the PMNs seems to depart from normal values, we also measure the velocity of individual PMNs. When cytochalasin B dissolved in DMSO is added to

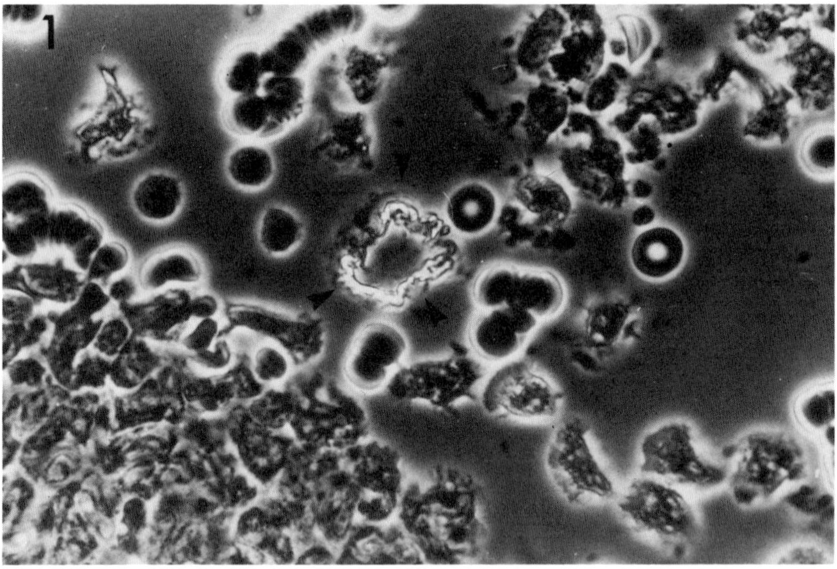

Figure 1. Leukocytes and chemotactic target (arrows) at beginning of experiment (×560; reduced for reproduction).

V. G. VETHAMANY, S. K. VETHAMANY and M. BESSIS · Department of Anatomy, Dalhousie University, Halifax, Canada, and Institute of Pathology, Paris, France.

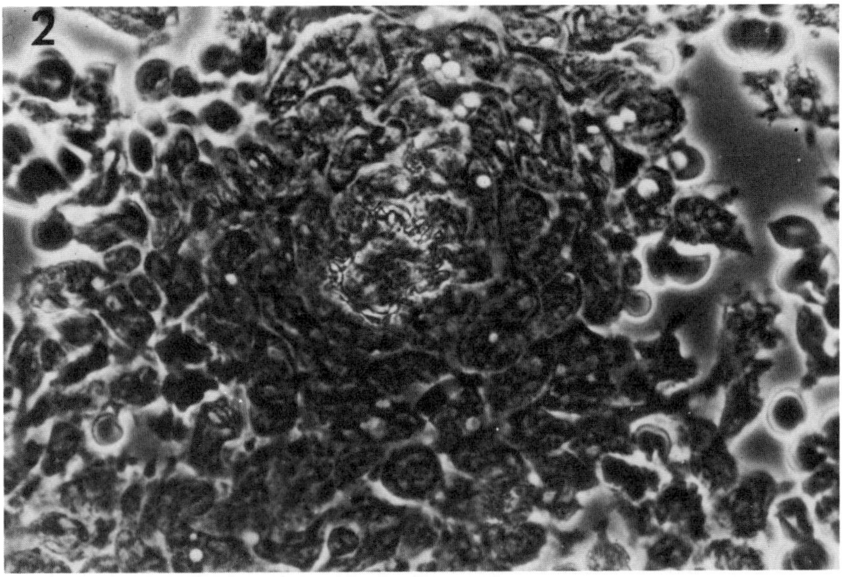

Figure 2. Same preparation as in Fig. 1 at 9 min.

leukocyte suspension at a concentration of 0.5 μg/ml and incubated for 20 min at 37°C prior to the experiment, it significantly lowered the CI (0.292 ± 0.03, t = 6.6, df = 3) as compared to DMSO control without the drug: (0.507 ± 0.09, t = 0.7, df = 3). The mean velocity of the moving leukocytes in the presence of cytochalasin B (10.25 ± 0.72 μm/min) is significantly lower than that of controls (22.55 ± 1.6 μm/min). At higher concentrations (5 and 20 μg/ml), cytochalasin B totally inhibits locomotion in this system. The lectins PHA and Con A did not have any effect on the CI. Patients with infections are found to have increased CI (0.785 ± 0.024, t = 8.6, df = 4). Such patients on antibiotics have decreased CI (0.363 ± 0.02, t = 5.8, df = 3). The leukocytes forming rosettes have normal ultrastructural morphology and contain an abundance of glycogen. Scanning electron microscopy has revealed the nature of various pseudopods classified as metapods, uropods, and rhizopods.

ACKNOWLEDGMENT

This work was supported by the MRC of Canada visiting scientist's award to Dr. V. G. Vethamany.

Reference

Bessis, M., and Burté, B., 1964, *Tex. Rep. Biol. Med.* **23:**204 (Suppl. I).

3.15. Leukocyte Adhesiveness as Influenced by Blood Velocity

HARVEY N. MAYROVITZ and MARY P. WIEDEMAN

Emigration of leukocytes is dependent on their initial adherence to vessel walls (Clark and Clark, 1935). Although many stimuli produce increases in local leukocyte adhesiveness in microvessels *in vivo* (Grant, 1973), the basic mechanisms are unknown. Atherton and Born (1973) demonstrated a linear relationship between leukocyte rolling velocity and mean blood velocity. Mayrovitz and Wiedeman (1975) showed that extravascular tissue injury increases intravascular leukocyte–wall interaction in arterial microvessels.

Based on these findings and physical considerations (Schmid-Schoenbein *et al.,* 1975), one would predict that for a given stimulus the propensity of leukocytes to become and remain adherent to the endothelial surface would decrease with increasing RBC velocity and/or blood shear stress. To test this hypothesis, leukocyte flux and velocity were

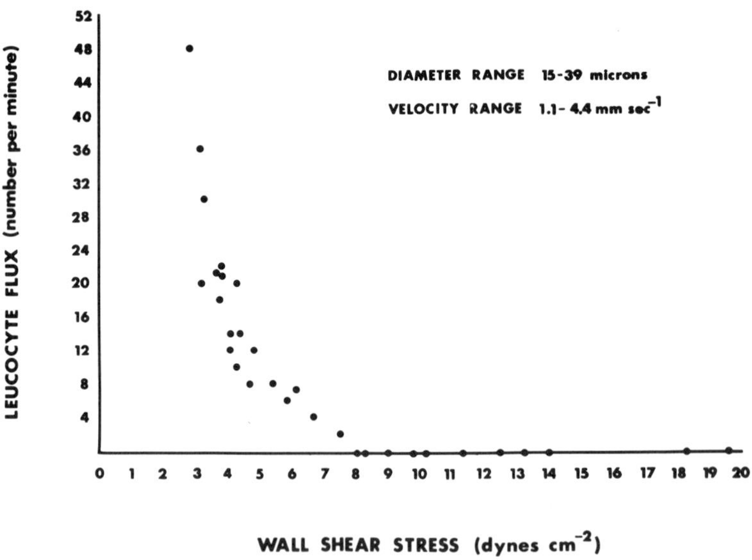

Figure 1. Leukocyte flux dependence on wall shear stress.

HARVEY N. MAYROVITZ and MARY P. WIEDEMAN · Department of Physiology, Temple University School of Medicine, Philadelphia, Pennsylvania.

measured simultaneously with blood velocity and vessel diameter in bat wing arterial vessels. Flux was determined by counting the number of leukocytes per unit time passing a fixed landmark, and leukocyte velocity was determined by timing their transit over an axial distance of 70 μm. Diameters were measured using a calibrated eyepiece micrometer. RBC velocity was measured continuously using a cross-correlation technique. Wall shear stress was calculated using the measured diameters and velocities and assuming a viscosity of 0.025 P.

The results indicate that for a given leukotactic stimulus, wall shear stress is an important parameter in determining whether leukocyte adherence occurs. As seen in Fig. 1, increasing wall shear stress is accompanied by a reduction in leukocyte flux until a threshold level is exceeded (approximately 8 dyn/cm^2) above which no leukocytes are observed. Contrastingly, leukocyte velocity data indicate that once leukocytes adhere no clear relationship is obtained between either blood velocity (range 0.5–5 mm/s) or wall shear stress (range 3–40 dyn/cm^2). These findings suggest the presence of a flow-dependent threshold mechanism for initial adherence followed by a shift in the nature and/or magnitude of the leukocyte–wall interaction process.

References

Atherton, A., and Born, G. V. R., 1973, Relationship between the velocity of rolling granulocytes and that of the blood flow in venules, *J. Physiol. (London)* **233:**157.

Clark, E. R., and Clark, E. L., 1935, Observations on changes in blood vascular endothelium in the living animal, *Am. J. Anat.* **57:**385.

Grant, L., 1973, The sticking and emigration of white blood cells in inflammation, in: *The Inflammatory Process* (B. W. Zweifach, L. Grant, and R. T. McCluskey, eds.), pp. 205–249, Academic Press, New York.

Mayrovitz, H. N., and Wiedeman, M. P., 1975, Changes in leukocyte adhesiveness accompanying laser irradiation, *Fed. Proc.* **36:**385.

Schmid-Schoenbein, G. W., Fung, Y. C., and Zweifach, B. W., 1975, Vascular endothelium–leukocyte interaction, *Circ. Res.* **36:**173.

3.16. Erythrocyte and Platelet Geometry: Comparative Quantitative Estimates by Static Microscopic and Rheo-Optical Determinations

M. M. FROJMOVIC and R. PANJWANI

The shape distributions of normal and hardened human and rabbit erythrocytes and platelets were independently obtained from static measurements of a few hundred cells in microphotographs obtained similarly as by Ponder (1930) by phase contrast microscopy at 800× magnification, as well as by a novel rheo-optical method (Frojmovic *et al.*, 1975), which allows for a direct statistical averaging for large populations ($>100 \times 10^3$ cells). In the first method, major average diameters ($\bar{d}$) and thicknesses ($\bar{t}$) were estimated for both normal and hardened cells and were used to calculate an average geometric axis ratio, $\bar{r}_p = \bar{t}/\bar{d}$, which increases to unity as cells become more spherical. Our fixation procedure (Frojmovic *et al.*, 1975) did not alter these shape parameters, for either erythrocytes or platelets: $\bar{r}_p$ was identical for both human and rabbit erythrocytes, with $\bar{d}$ and $\bar{t}$ values similar to those reported by Ponder (1930); platelets had $\bar{d} \times \bar{t} = 3.6 \pm 0.7\ \mu m \times 0.9 \pm 0.3\ \mu m$ and $3.1 \pm 0.4\ \mu m \times 0.6 \pm 0.2\ \mu m$, respectively, for human and rabbit cells; $\bar{r}_p$ values are shown in Table I. Hydrodynamic axis ratios ($\bar{r}_e$) and their standard deviations (σ_e) were obtained directly from rheo-optical measurements of fixed rabbit erythrocytes and platelets suspended in glycerol–water (3–4/1, vol/vol), where damping oscillations in transmitted light are analyzed in terms of the period of oscillation for $\bar{r}_e$ and relaxation for σ_e (Frojmovic *et al.*, 1975). Estimates of $\bar{r}_p \pm \sigma_p$ were made from the measured $\bar{r}_e \pm \sigma_e$ for the erythrocytes and platelets, using equations derived for model discs ($\bar{r} < 1$) (Frojmovic, 1975). Remarkable agreement was found for data obtained by the two methods, as well as results reported for the flow tube–microscope technique conducted by Goldsmith and Marlow (1972) for erythrocytes and privately communicated by Goldsmith for platelets.

M. M. FROJMOVIC and R. PANJWANI · Department of Physiology, McGill University, Montreal, Quebec, Canada.

Table I. Hydrodynamic and Geometric Axis Ratios of Erythrocytes and Platelets

			Hydrodynamic $\bar{r}_e \pm \sigma_e$		Geometric $\bar{r}_p \pm \sigma_p$		
	Method	Donor[a]	Erythrocytes	Platelets	Erythrocytes	Platelets	Author
A.	Static microscopy	R				0.26 ± 0.09	Forjmovic
		H/R			0.29 ± 0.04		Frojmovic
B.	Microcouette rheo-optics	R	0.43 ± 0.06		0.29 ± 0.05		Frojmovic
		H	0.44 ± 0.06		0.30 ± 0.05		Okagawa[d]
		H		0.35 ± 0.12		0.24 ± 0.10	Frojmovic
C.	Flow tube– microscope[c]						
		H	0.38 ± 0.07[b]		0.25 ± 0.07		Goldsmith
		H		0.38 ± 0.09		0.25 ± 0.08	Goldsmith[d]

[a] Rabbit (R) and human (H) donors were used as shown.
[b] All cells studied were hardened, except for this particular study.
[c] Note that 60 cells were analyzed for each of the erythrocyte and platelet studies.
[d] Personal communications.

References

Frojmovic, M. M., 1975, Rheo-optical studies of blood cells, *Biorheology* **12:**193.

Frojmovic, M. M., Okagawa, A., and Mason, S. G., 1975, Rheo-optical transients in erythrocyte suspensions, *Biochem. Biophys. Res. Commun.* **62:**17.

Goldsmith, H. L., and Marlow, J., 1972, Flow behaviour of erythrocytes. I. Rotation and deformation in dilute suspensions, *Proc. R. Soc. London Ser. B* **182:**351.

Ponder, E., 1930, The measurement of the diameter of erythrocytes. V. The relation of the diameter to the thickness, *J. Exp. Physiol.* **20:**29.

3.17. Erythrocyte Sedimentation of Human Blood at Varying Shear Rates

A. L. COPLEY, R. G. KING, and C. R. HUANG

Findings are reported on the erythrocyte sedimentation rate (ESR) of blood from four healthy human subjects. The blood, anticoagulated with EDTA at 38–44% hematocrit, was subjected to shear rates varying from 0 to 10 s^{-1}, employing a couette-type geometry fitted to a Weissenberg rheogoniometer. Recordings were made of the time taken for the plasma–erythrocytes interface to pass between two marks on the outer couette cylinder, which is made of transparent plexiglass so that this interface can be macroscopically visualized. No change in ESR was found between 0 shear and 0.01 s^{-1}. However, above 0.01 and up to 0.1 s^{-1}, the ESR increased by a factor of 3, reaching a peak at 0.1 s^{-1}. At shear rates above 0.1 s^{-1} and up to 10 s^{-1}, the ESR decreased progressively to 0. Differences

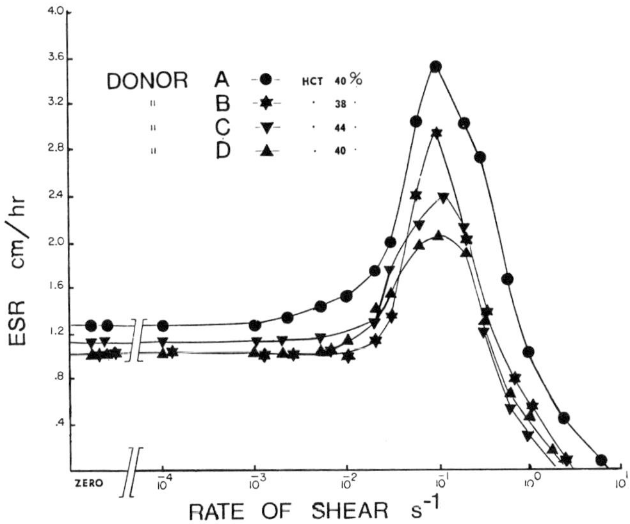

Figure 1. ESR data of EDTA-anticoagulated blood at 38–44% hematocrit, secured from four healthy adult human donors, vs. rates of shear ranging from 0 shear rate to 10 s^{-1}.

A. L. COPLEY, R. G. KING, and C. R. HUANG · Laboratory of Biorheology, Polytechnic Institute of New York, Brooklyn, New York, and New Jersey Institute of Technology, Newark, New Jersey.

were found between individual donors, but the characteristic shape of the curves remained the same, as seen in Fig. 1. Tentative explanations for the above findings are given. These include relationships between electrostatic forces and the diffusivity of erythrocytes, as well as a mathematical interpretation (Oka, 1975). The findings are a further indication that blood has a yield stress, as reported by Copley and King (1970). Our findings may mirror flow properties in certain parts of the microcirculation, since the ESR varies with changing shear rates. It is emphasized that increased ESR is not necessarily a sign of disease but can be a physiological occurrence in certain parts of the circulation (Fåhraeus, 1961; Copley, 1961, 1973) which may well be one of the prerequisites for maintaining certain functions of the blood by improving its flow characteristics.

ACKNOWLEDGMENT

This work was aided in part by Office of Naval Research Contract N00014-75-C-0222.

References

Copley, A. L., 1961, Discussion of a paper by R. Fåhraeus, 1961, *Rheol. Acta* **1**:663.
Copley, A. L., 1973, On biorheology: Joint plenary lecture, *Biorheology* **10**:87.
Copley, A. L., and King, R. G., 1970, Rheogoniometric viscosity measurements of whole human blood at minimal shear rates down to 0.0009 sec^{-1}, *Experientia* **26**:904.
Fåhraeus, R., 1961, Die intravaskuläre Erythrozytenaggregation und ihre Einwirkung auf die Rheologie des Blutes, *Rheol. Acta* **1**:656.
Oka, S., 1975, Personal communication, Tokyo.

3.18. Erythrocyte Sedimentation Rate and "a Sedimentimeter"

LAWRENCE C. CERNY, CHRISTOPHER J. PUCCINI, and DONALD M. STASIW

Every medical student, medical technologist, and nurse learns very early the technique of erythrocyte sedimentation rate (ESR). However, the frequency of its use for diagnosis appears to be quite limited. The significance of the ESR has been evaluated by Bull and Brailsford (1972). They tested the ability of three competent internists to evaluate the ESR and place results in one of five categories without previous knowledge of

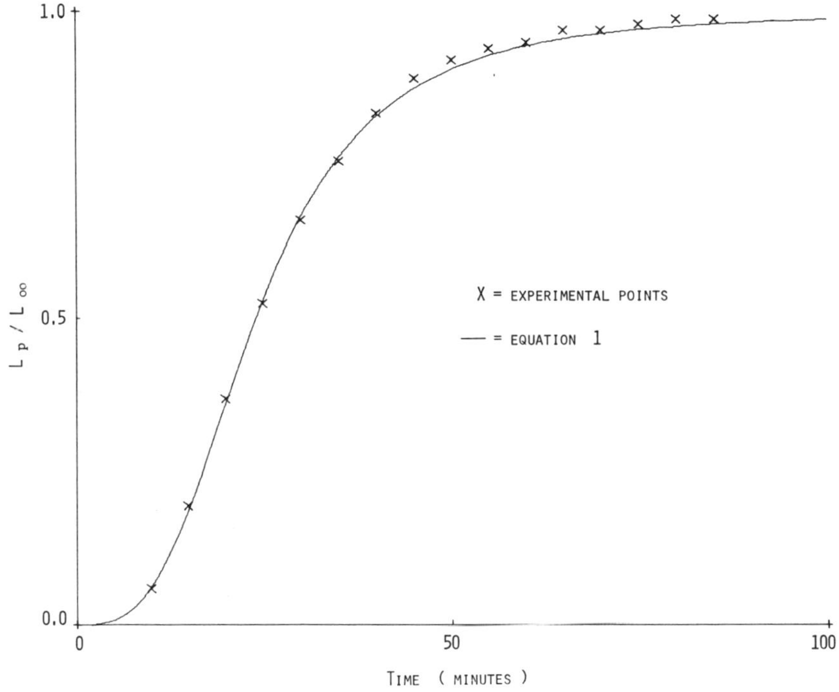

Figure 1. Typical sedimentation curve examining the validity of equation (1).

LAWRENCE C. CERNY, CHRISTOPHER J. PUCCINI, and DONALD W. STASIW · Masonic Medical Research Laboratory and Utica College of Syracuse University, Utica, New York.

the patients' condition. They state that the overall results were not reassuring and conclude that the average user of ESR data would probably not do as well.

Our approach is based on the use of the entire settling. The experience in this laboratory has been that the normal method of using just two points separated by an hour's time is extremely risky. One is actually drawing a straight line through two points and determining the slope assuming a constant rate of change, while in truth it is this part of the curve in which there is a constantly changing slope or rate of change.

At this point in our development, our approach is still semiempirical. The general shape of practically every ESR curve can be represented by a form of the logistics equation (Davis, 1960):

$$\frac{L_p}{L_\infty} = \frac{1}{1 + e^{-\beta}(\ln t - \ln t_{50})} \tag{1}$$

The advantage to this approach is the fact that this equation can be easily put into a linear form. From this linearization, the two parameters β and t_{50} can be obtained. We refer to t_{50} as the time it takes for the plasma level, L_p, to fall one-half of its final settling value.

The main difficulty in obtaining the complete sedimentation curve is the 3–5 h of technician time required to follow the settling. The basic concept of the ESR has been preserved in the design of our "sedimentimeter" (Cerny and Williams, 1975).

References

Bull, B. S., and Brailsford, J. D., 1972, The zeta sedimentation ratio, *Blood* **40:**550.

Cerny, L. C., and Williams, R., 1975, "A sedimentimeter," U.S. patent applied for.

Davis, H. T., 1960, *Introduction to Nonlinear Differential and Integral Equations,* U.S. Atomic Energy Commission, Washington, D.C.

3.19. Osmotic Fragility Curves as Frequency Distributions

JACK T. SAARI

An osmotic fragility curve may be thought of as a cumulative frequency distribution of NaCl concentrations at which erythrocytes in a given population will hemolyze. Further, this distribution may be considered a reflection of the fact that red cells within a population differ in their various properties, in particular those which determine their hemolytic concentration.

The hemolytic concentration may be represented by the relation

$$c_h = \frac{6\pi^{1/2}(c_0 - c_K)FV_0}{A^{3/2} - 6\pi^{1/2}(1 - F)V_0} - \frac{4\gamma}{RT}\left(\frac{\pi}{A}\right)^{1/2} \tag{1}$$

where c_h is the NaCl concentration causing hemolysis, c_0 the initial cell osmolarity, c_K the concentration adjustment for prelytic K^+ leak, F the osmotically active fraction, V_0 the initial cell volume, A the cell membrane area, and γ the membrane tension at hemolysis.

If the cell parameters in equation (1) are assumed normally distributed, an osmotic fragility curve may be generated by selecting random

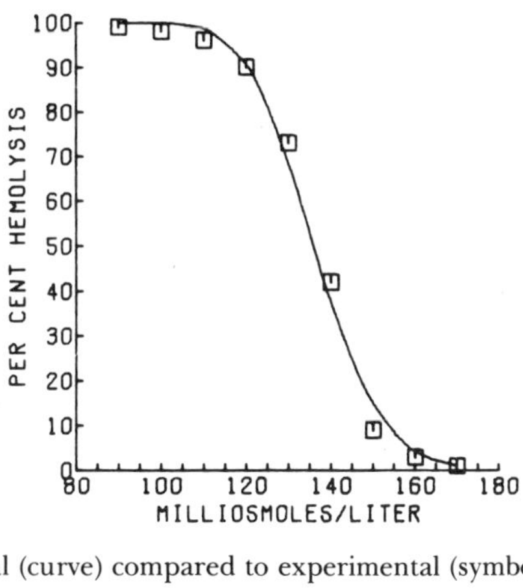

Figure 1. Theoretical (curve) compared to experimental (symbols) osmotic fragility.

JACK T. SAARI · Division of Medical Biophysics, Faculty of Medicine, The University of Calgary, Calgary, Alberta, Canada.

normal deviates in the individual distributions and solving the above equation for c_h. Progressively accumulating these randomly generated values of c_h and plotting them yields an osmotic fragility curve, which when fitted to an experimental one can give us values of unknown parameters (e.g., γ, c_K) and may indicate which parameters cause alteration of osmotic fragility in experimentally or pathologically altered erythrocytes.

Figure 1 gives an example of the fit of a theoretical osmotic fragility curve (solid line) to an experimental set of points (symbols are midpoints of the range of normal adult osmotic fragility, Dacie and Lewis, 1968). Values used in generating the theoretical curve were V_0 = 10 dyn/cm (Rand, 1964), c_K = 29.0 mosM or 10% K^+ leak (Seeman *et al.*, 1969), F = 0.58 (LeFevre, 1964)—all single valued—and V_0 = 98.1 ± 16.6 (SD) μm^3 (Jay, 1975). The value of A causing the least-squares best fit was 142.6 ± 15.8 (SD) μm^2, 6.9% in excess of the normal area given by Jay (1975).

Acknowledgments

This work was supported by the Medical Research Council (Canada) and the Alberta Heart Foundation.

References

Dacie, J. V., and Lewis, S. M., 1968, *Practical Haematology,* p. 13, J. and A. Churchill, London.

Jay, A. W. L., 1975, Geometry of the human erythrocyte. I. Effect of albumin on cell geometry, *Biophys. J.* **15:**205.

LeFevre, P. G., 1964, The osmotically functional water content of the human erythrocyte, *J. Gen. Physiol.* **47:**485.

Rand, R. P., 1964, Mechanical properties of the red cell membrane. II. Viscoelastic breakdown of the membrane, *Biophys. J.* **4:**303.

Seeman, P., Sauks, F., Argent, W., and Kwant, W. O., 1969, The effect of membrane-strain rate and of temperature on erythrocyte fragility and critical hemolytic volume, *Biochim. Biophys. Acta* **183:**476.

3.20. Psychosomatic Pain and Elevation of Blood Viscosity Factors

L. DINTENFASS and I. ZADOR

A study of patients suffering from chronic depressive or schizoid anxiety showed that blood viscosity factors (such as blood viscosity, plasma viscosity, aggregation of red cells, and apparent viscosity of artificial red/white or white thrombi) are significantly elevated compared to the normal values (Dintenfass and Zador, 1975; Zador and Dintenfass, 1975).

Subsequent continuation of this study and a division of patients into two groups, those with and without pain, showed that patients with psychosomatic pain (e.g., chest pain, abdominal pain, headache, or dermatitis) are characterized by still higher values of blood viscosity factors than chronic anxiety patients without pain.

Table I illustrates this point. Patients with psychosomatic pain have significantly higher levels of fibrinogen, a higher degree of aggregation of red cells, and a higher apparent viscosity of artificial red/white thrombi. The rheological–coagulation factors were studied using the methods of Dintenfass (1971).

Our basic finding is that psychosomatic pain is verified by the

Table I. Biophysicochemical Factors in Chronic Anxiety Patients Suffering from Psychosomatic Pain

Factor	n	$\bar{x} \pm$ SD	t	2P
Fibrinogen (mg%)				
Pain present	32	335 ± 98	1.974	<0.05
Pain absent	63	297 ± 64		
Aggregation of red cells at 37°C (mm/h)[a]				
Pain present	32	149 ± 87	2.528	<0.02
Pain absent	60	103 ± 75		
Viscosity of artificial red/white thrombus (d.u.)				
Pain present	32	5.06 ± 3.53	2.273	<0.025
Pain absent	60	3.46 ± 2.52		

[a] ESR st. pl. hc.: estimated from ESR at 37 C, corrected for plasma viscosity and adjusted to a hematocrit of 30%.

L. DINTENFASS and I. ZADOR · Haemorheology Unit and Medical Research, Sydney Hospital, and Department of Medicine, University of Sydney, Sydney, Australia.

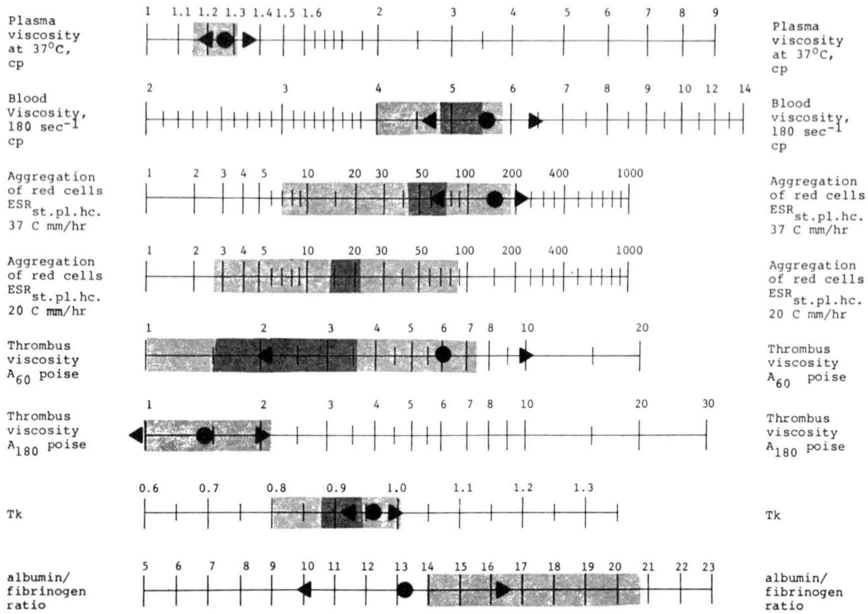

Figure 1. Novel representation of blood viscosity factors. Dots and arrows are means and range of 1 SD for patients with psychosomatic pain. Shaded areas are normal values: where the two shaded areas are superimposed, the left area is for athletes and/or females, the right area for normal males. Note that viscosity at 180 s^{-1} is particularly elevated and the albumin/fibrinogen ratio decreased in patients. "Tk" is a coefficient of rigidity/deformability in the blood viscosity equation of Dintenfass (1971). Aggregation of RBCs was estimated from the erythrocyte sedimentation rates at 60 min, corrected for plasma viscosity, and adjusted to constant hematocrit of 30%. Artificial red/white thrombi (A_{60}) and white thrombi (A_{180}) were studied by the method of Dintenfass (1971).

presence of pathological changes in blood, both the biochemical and the rheological factors being involved. One might wonder whether there is an absolute distinction between physical and psychological illness; it should be feasible to explore whether treatment of a psychological illness can include modification of hemorheological factors.

There is indeed a scope in the modification of the biochemical and blood viscosity factors, as seen from Fig. 1. Specifically, the viscosity of whole blood, which is significantly elevated, is suitable for correction.

Acknowledgment

This study was supported in part by the National Health and Medical Research Council of Australia.

References

Dintenfass, L., 1971, *Blood Microrheology, Viscosity Factors in Blood Flow, Ischaemia and Thrombosis,* Butterworths, London.

Dintenfass, L., and Zador, I., 1975, Effect of stress and anxiety on thrombus formation and blood viscosity factors, *Bibl. Haematol.* **41:**133.

Zador, I., and Dintenfass, L., 1975, Blood viscosity in chronic anxiety states, First Pacific Congress of Psychiatry, Abst. No. 174 (Melbourne, May 11–17).

3.21. Blood Viscosity Factors in Diagnostic and Preventive Medicine

L. DINTENFASS

Blood hyperviscosity syndrome (Dintenfass, 1966, 1971) is present whenever one or more of the blood viscosity factors is elevated. These include whole blood, plasma, and internal viscosity, red cell deformability and platelet aggregation, and consistency or apparent viscosity of artificial red/white and white thrombi. The syndrome might be present despite normal or decreased viscosity of whole blood.

Increased internal viscosity of red cells occurs in sickle cell and microangiopathic anemia and respiratory disorder; plasma viscosity is

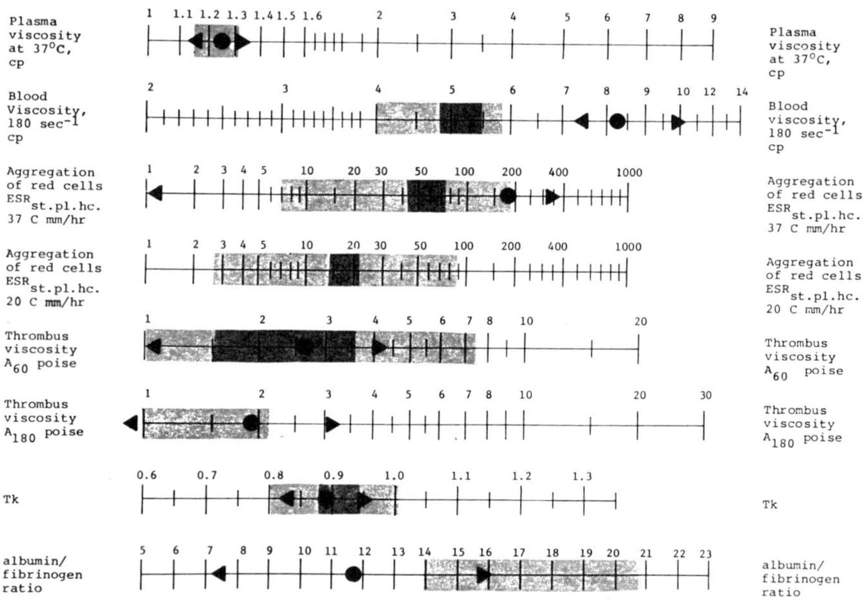

Figure 1. Blood viscosity factors. Dots are arithmetic means; arrows indicate ±1SD. Shaded areas show normal range, shaded areas to left are normal for assumed healthy men. "Tk" indicates rigidity of red cells and is a coefficient of blood viscosity equation (Dintenfass, 1971). The figure shows mean values for 12 cases of polycythemia.

L. DINTENFASS · Haemorheology Unit and Medical Research, Sydney Hospital, and Department of Medicine, University of Sydney, Sydney, Australia.

raised in macroglobulinemia or multiple myeloma, and to a lesser degree in rheumatoid arthritis and during cancer metastases; elevated apparent viscosity or the presence of red/white and/or white thrombi is characteristic of renal failure, peripheral vascular disease, and myocardial infarction; increased red cell aggregation occurs in macroglobulinemia and other paraproteinemias, as well as pulmonary embolism or cancer. Elevation of whole blood viscosity in polycythemia is due to increased hematocrit, although abnormality of other viscosity factors can be observed (Fig. 1).

The novel method of presentation of blood viscosity factors and associated biochemical factors shown in Fig. 1 allows a more rapid recognition of the disease. The prognostic value of blood viscosity factors was shown in the following studies. Dintenfass and Stewart (1971) found that with successful cadaveric kidney transplant apparent viscosity of artificial red/white and white thrombi fell to normal immediately after surgery, while rejection or complication gave sustained elevation. Dintenfass and Ibels (1975) showed that recipients of successful kidney transplants who develop occlusive arterial disease show elevation of viscosity factors even some months prior to appearance of clinical symptoms. Patients with melanoma metastases also show elevation (Dintenfass and Milton, 1973).

Population screening using blood viscosity tests would allow detection of cardiovascular and some neoplastic diseases even in their silent stage. Preventive treatment by hemodilution, plasmapheresis, drugs, etc., could counter occlusion and stasis in the microvasculature.

ACKNOWLEDGMENT

This study was supported by the National Health and Medical Research Council of Australia.

References

Dintenfass, L., 1966, A preliminary outline of the blood high viscosity syndromes, *Arch. Intern. Med.* **118**:427.

Dintenfass, L., 1971, *Blood Microrheology, Viscosity Factors in Blood Flow, Ischaemia and Thrombosis,* Butterworths, London.

Dintenfass, L., 1975, Malfunction of viscosity-receptors (viscoreceptors) as the cause of hypertension, *Am. Heart J.* (in press).

Dintenfass, L., and Ibels, L. S., 1975, Blood viscosity factors and occlusive arterial disease in renal transplant recipients, *Nephron* **11:** in press.

Dintenfass, L., and Milton, G. W., 1973, Blood viscosity factors and prognosis in malignant melanoma: Effect of ABO blood groups, *Med. J. Aust.* **1**:1091.

Dintenfass, L., and Stewart, J. H., 1971, Formation, viscosity and degradation of artificial thrombi after cadaveric-donor kidney transplantation, *Thromb. Diath. Haemorrh.* **26**:24.

3.22. Rheological Properties of Sickled Red Cells in the Microcirculation

TED P. BOND, M. MASON GUEST, and L. P. GUSTAVSON

Heparinized blood samples from sickle cell patients were sealed and stored at room temperature for 24 h. Storage in this manner resulted in sufficient O_2 depletion to cause most RBCs to assume the sickled configuration. A branch of a mesenteric artery in a dog anesthetized with pentobarbital was cannulated in the retrograde direction and distal to an arterial bifurcation (Bond and Guest, 1971).

A microscopic field of the mesenteric microcirculation supplied by the parent artery was selected by infusing Ringer solution and observing to

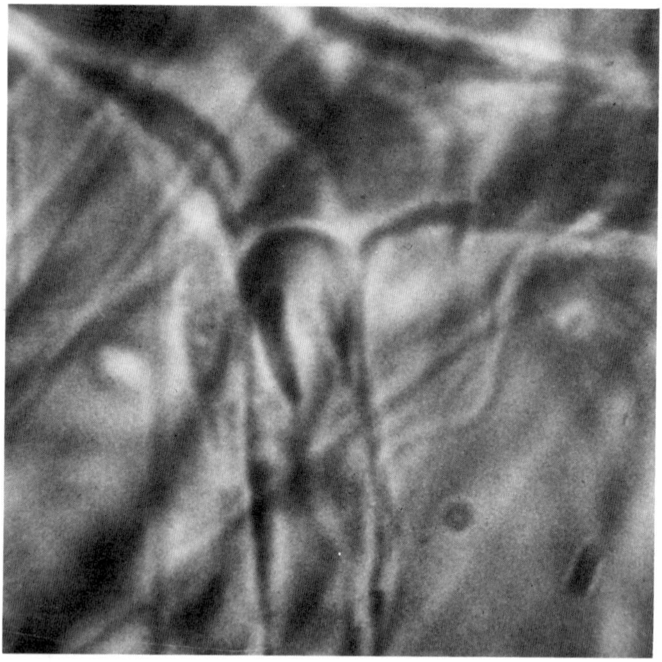

Figure 1. Sickled red blood cell blocking flow to a capillary.

TED P. BOND, M. MASON GUEST, and L. P. GUSTAVSON · Shriners Burns Institute, University of Texas Medical Branch, Galveston, Texas.

assure that the clear solution replaced the formed elements in the field under observation.

The blood containing sickled cells was then infused via the cannula. The vessels through which the sickled cells circulated were cinephotographed at conventional speeds and at up to 400 frames per second. In larger vessels, the sickled cells tended to tumble more than normal cells. The evidently rigid sickled cells frequently lodged temporarily or semipermanently at bifurcations, sharp turns in vessels, and entrances to capillaries (Fig. 1).

During perfusions of sickled cells, flow in true capillaries (<7 μm diameter) was not observed. However, flow in the smallest capillaries of dog mesentary was normal when the circulation was perfused with human nonsickled blood.

These observations are consistent with the hypothesis that the rigidity of sickled RBCs is a major factor contributing to lower life expectency of these cells. Since sickled RBCs tend to block flow to capillaries, it would appear that this could be the mechanism of the "sickle crisis."

ACKNOWLEDGMENTS

This work was supported by DHEW HL-16449 and the Shriners Burns Institute.

Reference

Bond, T. P., and Guest, M. M., 1971, High speed cinematography of the microcirculation, in: *Cinematographic Techniques in Biology and Medicine* (A. L. Burton, ed.), pp. 151–172, Academic Press, New York.

3.23. Some Effects of Tube Diameter on Oscillatory Blood Flow

G. B. THURSTON

The nonlinear viscoelastic properties of blood determine the pressure-to-volume flow relation for oscillatory tube flow (Thurston, 1975). The question considered in the present work is what are the effects of tube diameter on oscillatory flow which parallel the effects found by Fåhraeus and Lindqvist (1931) for steady flow. While the shear rates in their studies were $>100\ s^{-1}$, which tends to disrupt intercellular aggregation, in the present oscillatory flow study, the shear rates are from 0.05 to $10\ s^{-1}$. At the low shear rates, the viscoelasticity is linear and is described by a complex viscosity $(\eta' - i\eta'')$, η' being related to energy dissipation and η'' being related to elastic energy storage.

3.23.1. Methods

Measurements were made of the magnitude and phase of the oscillatory pressure, P, and volume flow, U, at 2 Hz in rigid brass tubes having radii, a, ranging from 215 to 1990 μm. Blood with CPD anticoagulant was used; the feed hematocrit was 48%, and the temperature was 24°C. From the measured components of P and U, the components of the shear stress at the tube wall, τ_w' and τ_w'', can be calculated (Thurston, 1975). τ_w' is in phase with the shear rate at the wall, $G_w(\simeq 8U/3\pi a^3)$, and τ_w'' is in quadrature. The components of the viscosity are $\eta' = \tau_w'/G_w$ and $\eta'' = \tau_w''/G_w$ (Thurston, 1972).

3.23.2. Results

First, measurements were made with increasing amplitudes of oscillation in order to determine the maximum level at which τ_w'' remains directly proportional to G_w. This maximum level, τ_{NL}'', changes vs. the tube radius, (see Fig. 1A). At this and lower levels, the apparent values of η' and η'' are seen in Fig. 1B. The decrease of η' and η'' with a is similar in appearance to the finding of Fåhraeus and Lindqvist (1931). The

G. B. THURSTON · University of Texas at Austin, Mechanical Engineering Department, Biomedical Engineering Program, Austin, Texas.

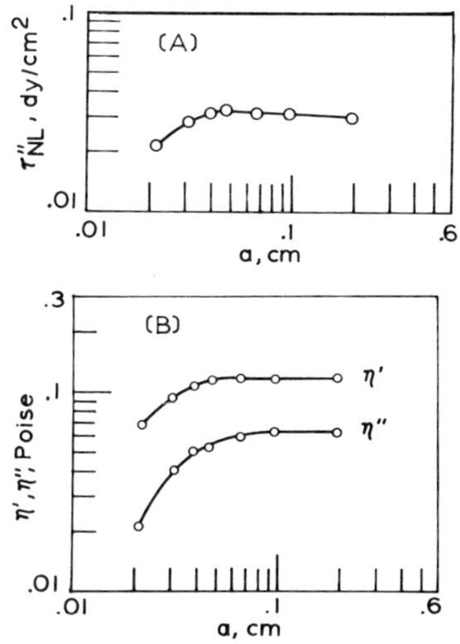

Figure 1. Elastic component of the shear stress τ''_{NL} marking onset of measurable nonlinearity in τ''_N (A), and components η' and η'' of the viscoelastic modulus (B) vs. the tube radius, a.

probable explanation of these results is that the blood near the tube wall is not in the same state of aggregation as that toward the center of the tube.

References

Fåhraeus, R., and Lindqvist, T., 1931, The viscosity of blood in narrow capillary tubes, *Am. J. Physiol.* **96:**562.

Thurston, G. B., 1972, Viscoelasticity of human blood, *Biophys. J.* **12:**1205.

Thurston, G. B., 1975, Elastic effects in pulsatile blood flow, *Microvasc. Res.* **9:**145.

4

Blood Vessel Structure

4.1. An Intracellular Tubular System in Capillary Endothelium

M. BENDAYAN, E. SANDBORN, and E. RASIO

In the current concepts of transcapillary transport by vesicular movement, many problems remain unsolved. Some of these are the synthesis of large amounts of membrane, the fusion of vesicles to the plasma membrane, its breakdown and fate, and the energy required for these processes. These difficulties may be avoided by assuming the existence of an intracellular tubular system which could be responsible for bulk transport across the cell by peristaltic action.

When fixed rapidly by perfusion with aldehyde–dimethylsulfoxide solutions, the capillary endothelial cells of the red body of the eel swimbladder reveal a series of tubules which intrude deeply into the cytoplasm from the cell membrane (Fig. 1). Frequently the channels have alternating dilatations and constrictions, giving the appearance of peristaltic waves. The circular or oval profiles, which, in thin sections, appear as isolated vesicles within the cytoplasm, can readily be accounted for as transverse or oblique sections of the tubular system. These tubules interconnect the plasma membrane with the endoplasmic reticulum (Bendayan *et al.,* 1974, 1975). Some channels lead from the cell surface to the nuclear envelope, and there is evidence of continuity between the mitochondrial outer membrane and the endoplasmic reticulum (Bendayan *et al.,* 1974; Sandborn *et al.,* 1975). When the tissue is fixed by immersion, many of the tubules present a dense content identical to that seen in the lumen of the capillary. Carbon particles and myoglobin, used as tracers, are found within some tubules, most commonly in the venular capillary cytoplasm of the organ. These findings demonstrate that the

M. BENDAYAN, E. SANDBORN, and E. RASIO · Department of Anatomy and Department of Medicine, School of Medicine, University of Montreal, Montreal, Quebec, Canada.

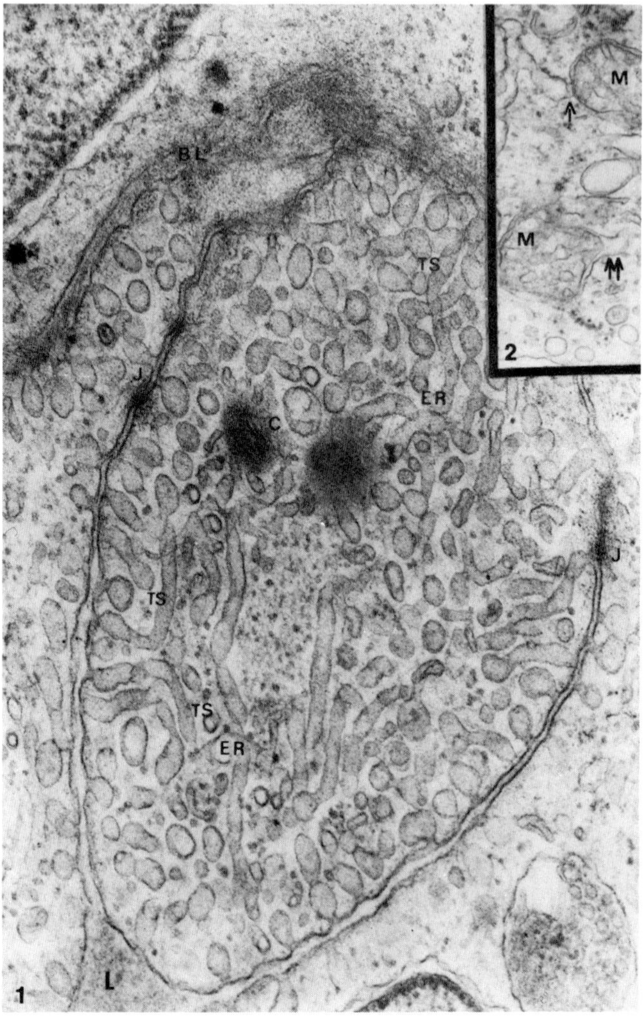

Figure 1. Electron micrograph (×50,000) of an arterial endothelial cell from the red body of the eel swimbladder. The tubular system (TS) intrudes into the cytoplasm from the lumen (L) and the base of the cell; some tubules open at the level of the intercellular junctions (J) and others seem to be in continuity with the endoplasmic reticulum (ER). (C) Centriole; (BL) basal lamina. Inset: High magnification (×30,000) of an endothelial cell showing two mitochondria (M). One of the mitochondria is in continuity with the endoplasmic reticulum (double arrow); the other mitochondrion is in close relation with the rough endoplasmic reticulum (arrow), which in turn is continuous with the smooth endoplasmic reticulum.

content of the tubular system, while being intracellular, is in fact extracytoplasmic.

The leukocyte and, in the mammal, the endothelium, mesothelium, and intestinal epithelium demonstrate similar systems (Sandborn, 1970).

It is concluded that, in most cells, a membrane-bound microcirculatory system connecting the organelles with the extracellular milieu provides an important pathway of intracellular and transcellular transport, and increases by many times the surface of the cell.

ACKNOWLEDGMENTS

This work was supported by grants from the Banting Research Foundation and the Medical Research Council.

References

Bendayan, M., Sandborn, E. B., and Rasio, E., 1974, The capillary endothelium in the rete mirabile of the swimbladder of the eel (*Anguilla anguilla*): Functional and ultrastructural aspects, *Can. J. Physiol. Pharmacol.* **52:**613.

Bendayan, M., Sandborn, E. B., and Rasio, E., 1975, Studies of capillary basal lamina. I. Ultrastructure of the rete mirabile of the eel swimbladder, *Lab. Invest.* **32:**757.

Sandborn, E. B., 1970, *Cells and Tissues by Light and Electron Microscopy,* Vols. I and II, Academic Press, New York.

Sandborn, E. B., Stephens, H., and Bendayan, M., 1975, The influence of dimethyl sulfoxide on cellular ultrastructure and cytochemistry, *Ann. N.Y. Acad. Sci.* **243:**122.

4.2. Observations of Pulmonary Capillary Endothelial Junctions Studied by the Freeze-Fracture/Etch Technique

SADAYUKI INOUE, RENE P. MICHEL, and JAMES C. HOGG

Intercellular junctions in the capillary endothelium as well as alveolar epithelium of the alveolocapillary wall of dog lungs were observed in the electron microscope with the technique of freeze-fracture and etching. The lungs of three mongrel dogs were perfused with glutaraldehyde and small pieces of lung were taken from the right upper lobe of each animal. These specimens were frozen in liquid Freon (−150°C) or liquid nitrogen, fractured in FFE accessory on an Edwards 306 vacuum coater, and etched for 2 min at −100°C followed by platinum shadowing and carbon replication. Layers of capillary endothelium, basement membrane, and alveolar epithelium were identified in the alveolocapillary wall by successive fractures of these layers along cell membranes (Fig. 1A). Fracture faces were characterized by the presence of numerous pinocytotic vesicles. Winding lines of contact between endothelial cells were observed, and occasionally a portion of cells along these lines was fractured off, revealing a surface-facing intercellular space (Fig. 1B, S). On such faces in fractured endothelium, the structure (arrow) characteristic of zonulae occludentes (tight junctions) was observed. They were made up of a parallel array of two or three strands in a narrow band of a depth of about 0.1 μm (lower inset), or, occasionally, of a less ordered, loose arrangement of these strands (upper inset). Zonulae occludentes were also observed between cells of alveolar epithelium. They were a lacelike meshwork of an assembly of closed compartments. The ultrastructure of these junctions indicates that zonulae occludentes in the epithelium are "tight" (Claude and Goodenough, 1973), while those in pulmonary capillary endothelium are of the "medium" to "leaky" type, which may be the morphological counterpart of the "small pore system" established by the physiological measurements (Landis and Pappenheimer, 1963).

SADAYUKI INOUE, RENE P. MICHEL, and JAMES C. HOGG · Department of Pathology, McGill University, Montreal, Quebec, Canada.

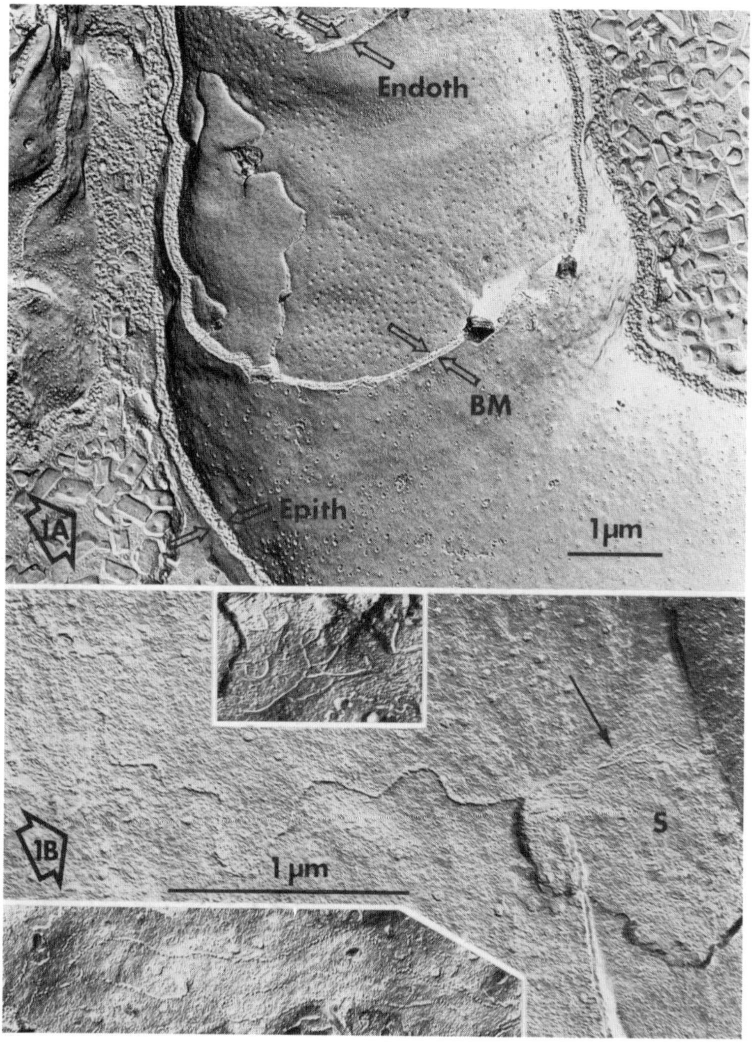

Figure 1. Freeze-fractured alveolocapillary wall of dog lung and zonulae occludentes in pulmonary capillary endothelium.

References

Claude, P., and Goodenough, D. A., 1973, Fracture faces of zonulae occludentes from "tight" and "leaky" epithelia, *J. Cell Biol.* **58:**390.

Landis, E. M., and Pappenheimer, J. R., 1963, Exchange of substances through the capillary walls, in: *Handbook of Physiology* (W. F. Hamilton and P. Dow, eds.), Section 2: Circulation, Vol. II, Chap. 29, p. 961, American Physiological Society, Washington, D.C.

4.3. On the Fine Structure of the Arteriovenous Anastomoses of the Rabbit Ear

FRITHJOF HAMMERSEN

Because the arteriovenous anastomoses (AVA) of the rabbit's ear offer the unique chance of *in vivo* study with the ear chamber technique, far-reaching conclusions were drawn from such experiments (for references, see Clara, 1956; Tischendorf and Curri, 1956; Sherman, 1963; Abramson, 1965). If these should be valid for the functional meaning of AVAs in general, then the rabbit's AVA should exhibit at least some similarities with other AVAs, particularly those of man. A fine structural study of these specialized vascular channels gave the following results:

1. Most the AVAs investigated so far showed at least one tight coil of their arterial segment that from there on gradually changed into a thin-walled venous vessel.
2. Contrary to earlier suggestions, the endothelium of the AVA forms a continuous lining of high electron density (Fig. 1) because of the large amounts of cytoplasmic filaments.
3. Sometimes a basal membrane but never an elastic lamina serves as a border toward the medium that is penetrated by numerous cytoplasmic processes establishing many myoendothelial junctions (Fig. 1).
4. The medium, particularly that of the coiled segment, consists of plumpish irregularly shaped cells that differ from typical vascular smooth muscle by (a) a looser arrangement of their myofilaments that, moreover, are oriented in different directions and (b) a more randomly distributed but higher content of organelles, especially of small mitochondria (Fig. 1).
5. The interstices are much smaller than usually found in glomus anastomoses (for references, see Hammersen, 1971). They contain delicate fibrils and a basement-membrane-like material together with many small myelin figures that seem to originate from degenerating mitochondria.
6. The relatively poor innervation contrasts to that found in other glomus anastomoses including those of man. The rabbit's AVAs show only a few small nerve bundles at the medioadventitia border

FRITHJOF HAMMERSEN · Institute for Experimental Morphology, Deutsche Sporthochschule, Cologne, FRG.

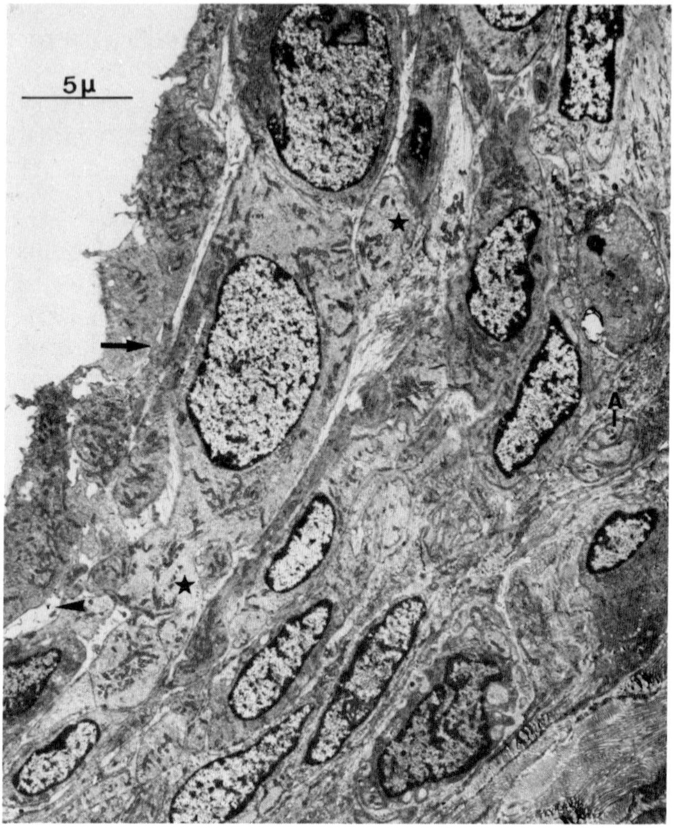

Figure 1. Low-power (×4000) electron micrograph of the arterial (coiled) segment of an AVA from the rabbit's ear. Its rather high endothelium shows the same electron density as the underlying media cells between which lighter-staining cytoplasmic profiles (★) containing clusters of mitochondria may be visualized. The broader and more translucent interstices of the media exhibit dark and spotlike corpuscles (▶) that correspond to myelin figures at higher magnifications. Note myoendothelial junctions at → and the small bundles of unmyelinated axons (A) located at the medioadventitia border.

(Fig. 1) that never penetrate any deeper into the wall and hence never achieve synaptic contacts any closer than usually found in small arteries.

References

Abramson, D. I., 1965, Pathophysiology of arteriovenous shunts in the extremities, *J. Cardiovasc. Surg.*, Suppl. 217.

Clara, M., 1956, *Die arterio-venösen Anastomosen: Anatomie–Biologie–Pathologie*, Vol. 2, Springer, Vienna.

Hammersen, F., 1971, The fine structure of epitheloid vascular cells: A comparative electron microscopic study, in: *Sixth European Conference on Microcirculation* (J. Ditzel and D. H. Lewis, eds.), pp. 406–410, Karger, Basel.

Sherman, J. I., 1963, Normal arteriovenous anastomoses, *Medicine (Baltimore)* **42**:247.

Tischendorf, F., and Curri, S. B., 1956, Experimentelle Untersuchungen zur Histophysiologie und -pathologie der arterio-venösen Anastomosen (nach Lebendbeobachtungen am Kaninchenohr). III. Morphologische und mikrooszillographische Analyse des Öffnungs- und Schliessungsmechanismus, *Z. Mikrosk. Anat. Forsch.* **62**:326.

4.4. Scanning Electron Microscopic Evaluation of Rat Femoral Artery Endothelium Following Microvascular Surgery

CARROLL P. OSGOOD, MANUEL DUJOVNY, PEDRO J. BARRIONUEVO, and RICHARD MATTA

Scanning electron microscopy (SEM) of normal arterial endothelium has shown a constant picture of fine longitudinal ridges or folds. These folds are about 14 μm across, and their smooth undulations comprise a "normal" pattern which permits assessment of various types of early endothelial damage (Hassler, 1972). SEM affords rapid, stereoscopic study of relatively large areas of endothelium with ultrafine detail. Some microvascular maneuvers may mechanically distort or obliterate normal endothelial ridging (Acland, 1973; Cobbett, 1967). In addition, fibrin–platelet–RBC cell deposits may cover damaged endothelium. One hundred and fifty rat femoral arteries, 0.6 mm in diameter, were studied with SEM following (1) microtourniquet and microclip occlusion, (2) pinching with jeweler's forceps, (3) arteriotomy and suture, (4) bipolar coagulation of a side branch 1 mm from the parent artery, 20 mV for 20 s, and (5) end-to-side microanastomosis. Arteriotomy and suture proved the most thrombogenic. Gentle pinching (jeweler's forceps) was innocuous, but hard pinching was visibly traumatic on SEM. Bipolar coagulation caused extensive endothelial distortion and platelet–fibrin deposition. Scoville-Lewis clips caused an unusual type of endothelial distortion but relatively few endothelial breaks. Small Heifetz clips caused even fewer areas of overt endothelial disruption or distortion. Khodadad clips (Fig. 1) and Mayfield MMI clips caused numerous endothelial lacerations. Several microsurgical clips now in use are characterized not only by an excessive closing force but also by a surface configuration that creates excessive tangential arterial stress along the clip edges. Serrations on the clip surfaces also cause excessive pressures on the areas of endothelium directly beneath the ridges.

CARROLL P. OSGOOD, MANUEL DUJOVNY, PEDRO J. BARRIONUEVO, and RICHARD MATTA · Department of Neurosurgery, Veterans Administration Hospital, and the University of Pittsburgh School of Medicine, Pittsburgh, Pennsylvania.

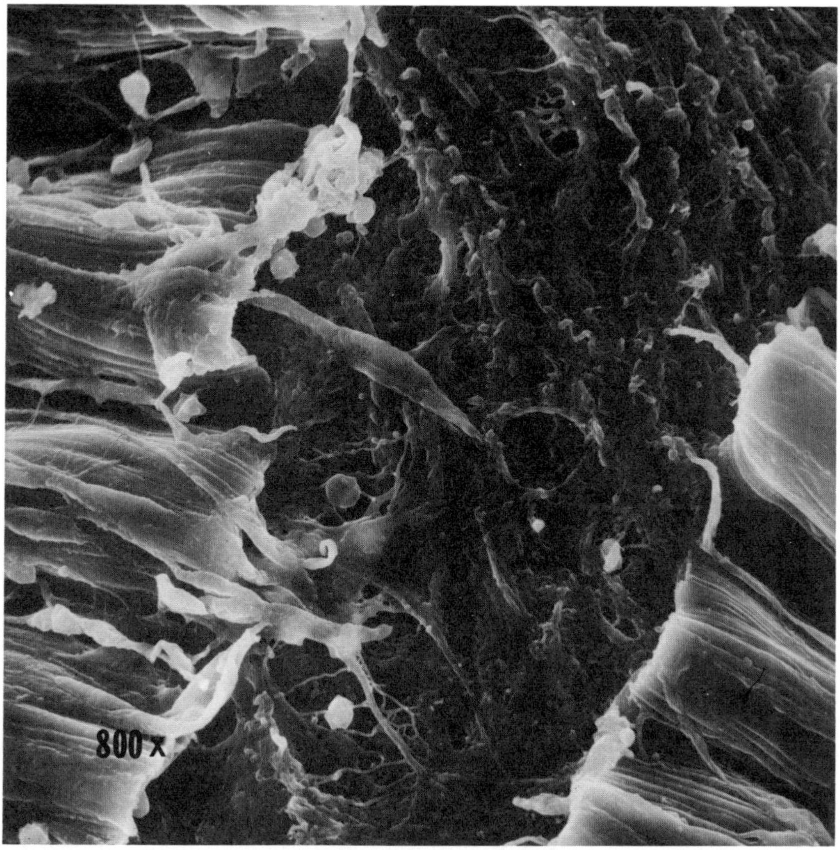

Figure 1. Endothelial lacerations caused by a Khodadad clip (×800; reduced for reproduction).

References

Acland, R., 1973, Thrombus formation in microvascular surgery: An experimental study of the effects of surgical trauma, *Surgery* **31**:766.

Cobbett, J., 1967, Microvascular surgery, *Surg. Clin. North Am.* **47**:521.

Hassler, O., 1972, Scanning electron microscopy of saccular intracranial aneurysms, *Am. J. Pathol.* **68**:51.

4.5. On the Organ Specificity of Microvessels: Heterogeneity of Arteriolar Metabolism

B. H. COOK, H. J. GRANGER, and A. E. TAYLOR

Advancements in detailed knowledge of the metabolism of microvascular smooth muscle have been severely limited by our inability to isolate microvessels without adherent parenchyma and, subsequently, to quantitate the biochemical capabilities of these vessels. *In vivo* physiological studies have suggested a marked heterogeneity between vascular beds of various organs (Norman *et al.,* 1974; Duke, 1957; Skinner and Powell, 1966; Schmid *et al.,* 1974). *In vitro* studies have, on the other hand, utilized strips of large vessels with the tacit assumption that this is a reflection of the behavior of the smooth muscle of the arteriolar wall (Coe *et al.,* 1968; Detar and Bohr, 1968). In order to explore this paradoxical problem, we have employed the semiquantitative techniques of topohistochemistry.

Four microvascular beds, heart, kidney, skeletal muscle, and intestine, were studied histochemically in order to delineate the major metabolic pathways subserving anabolic and catabolic functions of the vessels therein. Seventeen histochemical reactions on biopsies from 20 mongrel dogs were performed and the results were evaluated semiquantitatively. Enzyme reactions were performed on rapidly frozen biopsies. Samples for glycogen determination were fixed at 0°C for 16 h, then routinely processed through paraffin.

1. Myocardium: Arterioles of the myocardium were found to be rich in oxidative and, in particular, fat-catabolizing enzymes. Conversely, there were much lower levels of glycogen and anaerobic enzymes.
2. Skeletal muscle: Arterioles of this bed were found to be quite rich in both aerobic and anaerobic anzymes, suggesting a greater potential for utilization of a variety of substrates, both aerobically and anaerobically.
3. Intestine: Arterioles, primarily submucosal in distribution, were found to contain moderate levels of all enzymes and substrates studied. These activities were, however, observed to be of lesser intensity than those of vessels of similar size in skeletal muscle.

B. H. COOK, H. J. GRANGER, and A. E. TAYLOR · Department of Physiology and Biophysics, University of Mississippi School of Medicine, Jackson, Mississippi.

TABLE I. Comparative Enzymatic Activities of Four Canine Vascular Beds[a]

Enzyme or substrate	Myocardium	Kidney	Intestine	Skeletal muscle
α-Glycerophosphate dehydrogenase	+	+	++	+++
Lactate dehydrogenase	+	+	++	++++
Glycogen	+	±	+++	++
Isocitrate dehydrogenase	+++	+++	++	+++
Succinate dehydrogenase	++	++	++	++
Malate dehydrogenase	+++	++	++	++++
Glucose-6-phosphate dehydrogenase	+++	++	+++	++
DPN diaphorase	+++	+++	+++	+++
Neutral fat (nonglobular)	+	+	+	+
Lipase	++	+++	++	++
Free fatty acids	+++	+++	+++	+++
β-Hydroxybutyrate dehydrogenase	++++	+++	++	+++
Ubiquinone	++	++	++	++
Cytochrome oxidase	++	++	+	++
Wachstein-Meisel ATPase	+++	+++	+++	++++
Myosin ATPase	++++	++++	++++	++++
Alkaline phosphatase	++	0	0	0

[a] Symbols: 0, no discernible activity; ±, very weak activity; +, slight activity; ++, moderate activity; +++, strong activity; ++++, very strong activity.

4. Kidney: Renal arterioles were found to be quite rich in oxidative enzyme activity with a moderate activity of anaerobic enzymes.

Anabolic enzymes (Herman–Padykula and Wachstein–Meisel ATPases) were found to be quite rich in the microvessels of all organs studied. Alkaline phosphatase, a nonspecific phosphoesterase, was found to be patchily distributed in coronary arterioles but absent from those of kidney, skeletal muscle, and intestine.

Results for the enzymes and substrates studied are summarized in Table I. It may be noted from the table that certain enzymes deviate from the general patterns described in the text. However, the general patterns do seem to hold up quite well.

The significance of these observations may well lie in both physiological and pathological behavior of these vessels. Physiologically, as discussed in the opening paragraph, a great deal of heterogeneity has been uncovered. In addition, there appears to be a propensity for the development of arteriosclerosis within certain vascular beds, a propensity which may well depend on metabolic peculiarities of the arteriolar wall within that bed.

ACKNOWLEDGMENTS

This work was supported by NIH Grants HL 11477 and HL 11678 and by a grant from the American Heart Association.

References

Coe, J., Detar, R., and Bohr, D. F., 1968, Substrate and vascular smooth muscle contraction, *Am. J. Physiol.* **214**:245.

Detar, R., and Bohr, D. J., 1968, Oxygen and vascular smooth muscle contraction, *Am. J. Physiol.* **214**:241.

Duke, H. N., 1957, Observations on the effects of hypoxia on the pulmonary vascular bed, *J. Physiol. (London)* **135**:45.

Norman, J. N., Shearer, J. R., Napper, A. J., Robertson, I. M., and Smith, G., 1974, Action of oxygen on the renal circulation, *Am. J. Physiol.* **227**:740.

Schmid, P G., Abboud, F. M., Wendling, M. G., Ramberg, E. S., Mark, A. L., Heistad, D. D., and Echstein, J. W., 1974, Regional vascular effects of vasopressin: Plasma levels and circulatory responses, *Am. J. Physiol.* **227**:998.

Skinner, N. S., and Powell, W. J., 1966, Action of oxygen and potassium on vascular resistance of dog skeletal muscle, *Am. J. Physiol.* **212**:533.

5

Microcirculatory Flow Patterns

5.1. The Natural History of Microcirculation

W. REDISCH, E. N. TERRY, and L. R. ROUEN

Old descriptive studies of microcirculation must be reexamined. Many studies (Holland and Meyer, 1919; Jaensch, 1929) concerned with the normal, as contrasted with abnormal, development of the nailfold capillaries in infants showed that the pattern of hairpinlike loops developed at a basic rate, the loops arising from a subpapillary arteriolar plexus and reentering a venular subpapillary plexus. The mature capillary pattern is usually completed between 6 and 12 months after birth. Development of surface capillary loops in man has been fairly well documented for half a century. Heat regulation is the main function of surface vessels; its demands start early (Redisch *et al.,* 1957). Whether other beds follow similar patterns of response to changing metabolic needs during growth remains conjectural. The emergence of known architectural peculiarities in some adult beds makes such assumption plausible; however, documentation is lacking.

5.1.1. Development of Autoregulation

The development of autoregulation has been explored rather widely. Skin, kidney, brain, skeletal muscle, and intestine have been studied in excellent work, and dependence of autoregulation of perfusion on microvessel architecture and function has been established by reliable investigations (Redisch *et al.*, 1968). Heart muscle (Krulin *et al.,* 1974) is now under intensified study. It appears that the architecture of a given microcirculatory bed develops in direct response to the function of the organ it serves and that this development seems designed to facilitate the autoregulation for maintaining that particular function.

W. REDISCH, E. N. TERRY, and L. R. ROUEN · Departments of Medicine and Surgery, New York Medical College Metropolitan Hospital Center, New York, N.Y.

5.1.2. Aging of Microvessels

Changes in the microcirculation with aging are described only in relation to a control group within the scope of a study in which pathological changes are being investigated (DeNicola *et al.,* 1965; Pietrzukowoka 1966). This is unsatisfactory, because only the pathological condition under investigation in a given study is carefully excluded in the control group (Redisch *et al.,* 1970), and not the broad range of disorders which may affect the microcirculation. Utmost attention to selection of normal, healthy subjects should finally document the behavior of microcirculation with aging.

References

DeNicola, P., Maggi, G., and Tammoro, A. G., 1965, The small vessels of the skin and mucous membranes in presenile and senile age, *Bibl. Anat.* **7:**498.

Holland, M., and Meyer, L., 1919, Beobachtungen and den Hautkapillaren bei kindern mit exudativer, Diathese, *Muench. Med. Wochenschr.* **66:**1191.

Jaensch, W., 1929, *Die Hautkapillarmikroskopie,* Carl Marhold, Halle A.S.

Krulin, T. H., Kirk, E. S., Gorlin, R., Cohn, L. H., and Collins, J. J., 1974, Coronary artery bypass surgery: Assessment of revascularization by determination of blood flow and myocardial mass, *Am. J. Cardiol.* **34:**129.

Pietrzukowoka, A., 1966, Investigation of the vascular system of the senile skin, *Pol. Med. J.* **5:**44.

Redisch, W., Tangeo, F. T., and Saunders, R. H., 1957, *Peripheral Circulation in Health and Disease,* Grune and Stratton, New York.

Redisch, W., Messina, E. J., Schwartz, N. S., and Clauss, R. H., 1968, Microcirculation, in: *Cardiovascular Disorders* (A. N. Brest and J. M. Moyer, eds.), F. A. Davis Co., Philadelphia.

Redisch, W., Messina, E. J., Hughes, G., and McEwen, C., 1970, Capillaroscopic observations in rheumatic disease, *Ann. Rheum. Dis.* **29:**244.

5.2. Increased Capillary Flow Rate of Erythrocytes in Hyperosmolar Human Blood by the Addition of Pentoxifylline

A. M. EHRLY and K. SAEGER-LORENZ

In hyperosmolar blood samples *in vitro*, RBCs were found to be less deformable, thereby impairing blood flow through narrow capillaries (Braasch, 1963). In man, local hyperosmolarity of blood was found in the exercising muscle (Gray *et al.,* 1968). Recently, we presented a new pathophysiological concept of intermittent claudication (Ehrly, 1975). It showed that, besides a reduced blood flow due to occlusions or stenosis in the larger arteries, muscular microcirculation is impaired by rigid hyperosmolar RBCs.

The deformability of rigid RBCs suspended in hyperosmolar plasma can be improved by increasing their ATP content (Ehrly and Scheinpflug, 1975). Since it is known that pentoxifylline, a vasoactive drug, elicits an increase in erythrocytic ATP (Stefanovich, 1975), the following experiments were performed *in vitro* in order to establish whether it is possible to improve the flow properties of hyperosmolar blood by adding pentoxifylline and by subsequent incubation.

5.2.1. Materials and Methods

Blood was obtained from healthy volunteers, anticoagulated with heparin, and adjusted to a hematocrit of 10%. Three groups of samples were investigated: (A) normoosmolar blood, (B) hyperosmolar blood (400 mosmol) by the addition of sodium chloride, and (C) hyperosmolar blood containing pentoxifylline in a final concentration of 20 mg/100 ml blood. All samples were incubated for $2\frac{1}{2}$ h at 37°C. The number of RBCs flowing through a standardized 8-μm Millipore filter system over a period of 5 min is a measure for cell deformability (Ehrly and Rossbach, 1973).

5.2.2. Results and Conclusion

The number of normoosmolar erythrocytes (A) passing through the filters was $1.06 \pm 0.30 \times 10^8$ (mean ± SD). The filtration of hyperosmolar

A. M. EHRLY and K. SAEGER-LORENZ · Department of Internal Medicine, Division of Angiology, University of Frankfurt/Main, West Germany.

blood (B) was drastically reduced ($0.21 \pm 0.23 \times 10^8$). In hyperosmolar blood containing pentoxifylline (C), $0.54 \pm 0.35 \times 10^8$ erythrocytes passed the filters within the given time (t test B/C $p < 0.0005$). Capillary flow of hyperosmolar blood can be increased by pentoxifylline. This can be explained by an increase in the ATP content of the RBCs leading to an improved deformability.

References

Braasch, D., 1963, Verminderte Erythrozytenflexibilität (hervorgerufen durch Barbiturate, Verbrennung, Hypoxämien) und ihre Wirkungen auf den Kapillarkreislauf, *Pfluegers Arch. Gesamte Physiol.* **278:**130.

Ehrly, A. M., 1975, Rheologically induced impairment of the muscular microcirculation: A new pathophysiological concept of intermittent claudication, in: *Proceedings of the Ninth International Congress for Angiology,* Florence, 1974 (F. Pratesi, ed.).

Ehrly, A. M., and Rossbach, P., 1973, Microrheology: Studies with an 8 μm-filter system, *Bibl. Anat.* **11:**55.

Ehrly, A. M., and Scheinpflug, W., 1975, Improved deformability of crenated red cells in hyperosmolar human blood by adenosine, in: *Proceedings of the Eighth Conference of the European Society of Microcirculation,* Le Touquest, France, July 1974, in press.

Gray, S. D., Lundvall, J., and Mellander, S., 1968, Regional hyperosmolality in relation to exercise hyperemia, *Acta Physiol. Scand.* **73:**11.

Stefanovich, V., 1975, Effect of pentoxifylline on erythrocyte adenosine nucleotide levels in rats, *IRCS (Biochem. Hematol. Pharmacol.)* **3:**91.

5.3. Measurement of Arteriovenous Circulation Time and Volume Flow in the Human Retina

C. E. RIVA, I. BEN-SIRA, and W. ROBERTS

The volume of blood flowing through a closed vascular bed of the retina can be determined using the indicator dilution technique of Bulpitt and Dollery (1971). This rate of flow, F, is defined as $F = V/\bar{t}$, where V is the volume of blood in the vascular bed and $\bar{t}$ is the mean circulation time from the arterial inflow to the venous outflow. Sodium fluorescein is used as the indicator. The time course of its concentration in the artery and the vein is obtained from measurements of the fluorescence intensity, I_f, which is proportional to fluorescein concentration (Wessing, 1969).

Conventionally, I_f is detected photographically and its time variation is obtained through densitometric measurements of serial fundus photographs. This photographic technique is too time consuming for routine clinical work.

We have modified a standard fundus camera to do on-line recording of fluorescein dilution curves from human retinal vessels. The camera body housing the film has been replaced by a scanning ocular containing two optical fibers with a circular input aperture. The tips of the fibers are located in the image plane of the retina, where they collect the fluorescent light from an artery and a vein and transmit it to a photodetector. The output from the photodetector is plotted against time on a two-channel

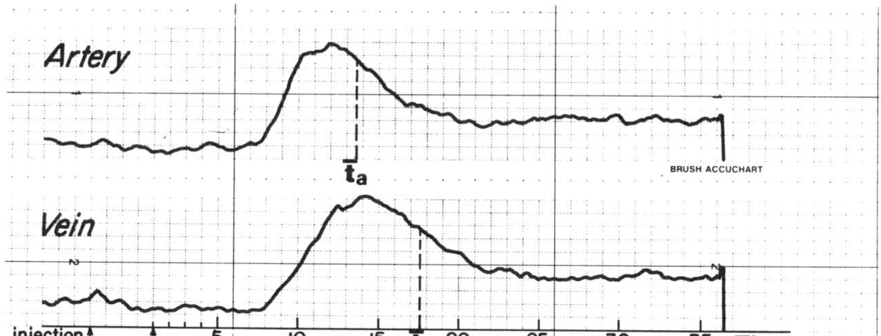

Figure 1. Fluorescein dilution curves from artery and vein in the fundus of a normal subject.

C. E. RIVA, I. BEN-SIRA, and W. ROBERTS · Eye Research Institute of Retina Foundation, Boston, Massachusetts.

recorder to give the fluorescein dilution curves. Adequate stabilization of the subject's eye is achieved by fixation on a punctual target (Riva and Ben-Sira, 1973). Figure 1 shows typical dilution curves from an artery and the corresponding vein of a normal subject after an injection of only 30 mg fluorescein. These curves are processed by a desk computer to obtain $\bar{t}$ From the diameter of the vessels, measured on color fundus slides, V is estimated.

ACKNOWLEDGMENTS

This work was supported by United States Public Health Service Grants EY-00227 and 1-R01-EY-01242-01 from the National Eye Institute, National Institutes of Health, and by the Research to Prevent Blindness William Friedkin Scholar for 1974.

References

Bulpitt, C. J., and Dollery, C. T., 1971, Estimation of retinal blood flow by measurement of the mean circulation time, *Cardiovasc. Res.* **5**:406.

Riva, C. E., and Ben-Sira, I., 1973, Reflectometry of individual blood vessels in the human ocular fundus, *J. Opt. Soc. Am.* **63**:1050.

Wessing, A., 1969, *Fluorescein Angiography of the Regina* (G. K. Noorden, trans.), p. 13, Mosby, St. Louis.

5.4. Microcirculation of the Terminal Gill Lamellae in the Freshwater Goldfish (*Carassius auratus*) and the Marine Gobie (*Lythrypnus dalli*)

M. LAURIE PHILLIPS, HAROLD W. PUFFER, and NANCY E. WARNER

It is common knowledge that certain pollutants have an adverse effect on animal life in a variety of aquatic environments (Mearns and Sherwood, 1973). In many cases, details of the mechanisms involved in causing the adverse effects are unknown. Before these mechanisms can be understood, it is necessary to establish the normal morphology and physiology of the species of animals under investigation. Therefore, we undertook this study to compare the cellular morphology and microcirculation in the gills of a marine and a freshwater teleost.

5.4.1. Methods

Fish were anesthetized with quinaldine, approximately 0.25 ml/liter, and the microcirculation in the gill was examined. Knisely's quartz rod transillumination described by Warner *et al.* (1965) was used, except that distilled water at room temperature was substituted for Ringer solution during examination of the goldfish and seawater at room temperature was substituted for Ringer solution during examination of the marine gobie. In some instances, epi-illumination also was used.

Sections of the gill in both species were prepared for scanning electron microscopy (SEM) and transmission electron microscopy (TEM) by fixation in 3% glutaraldehyde in buffered phosphate solution.

5.4.2. Results and Discussion

Several cell types are seen to be common to the surface of the gills of both species (Fig. 1). Microcirculation varies in both pattern and quantity of vascularization in the two species, particularly in the terminal division of the gill filament. The capillary system in the terminal lamella of the marine gobie, *Lythrypnus dalli*, appears to be more complex than does the capillary system in the terminal lamella of the freshwater goldfish,

M. LAURIE PHILLIPS, HAROLD W. PUFFER, and NANCY E. WARNER · Department of Pathology, University of Southern California, School of Medicine, Los Angeles, California.

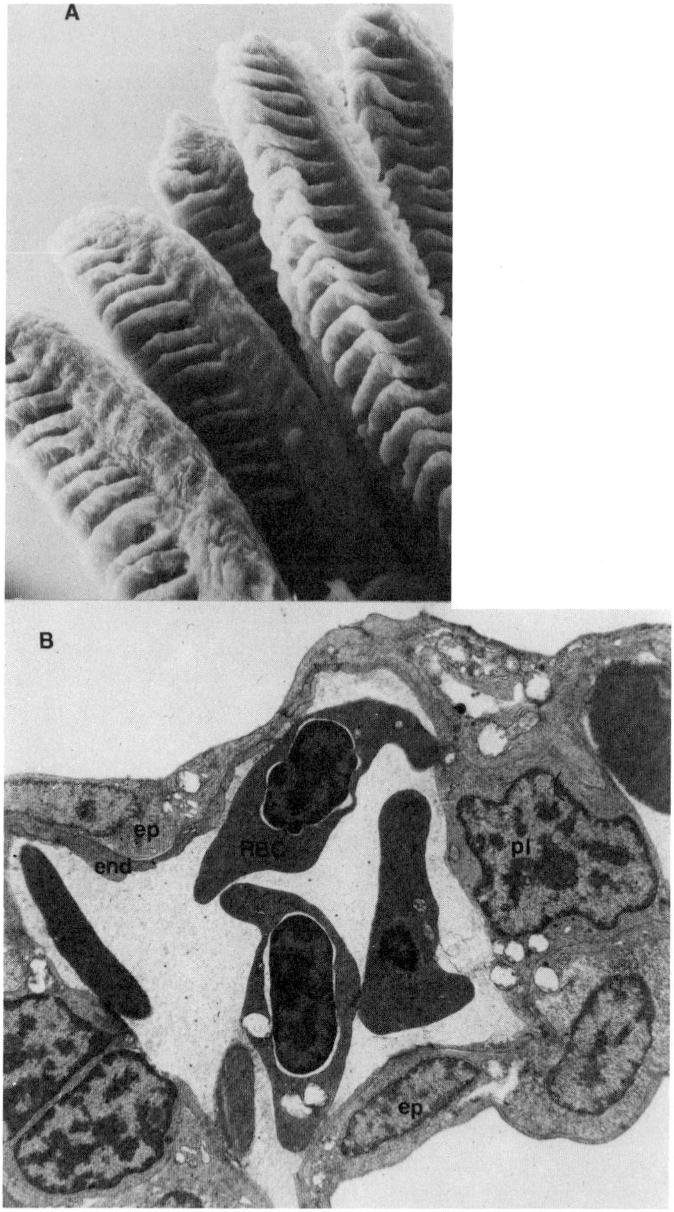

Figure 1. (A) Scanning electron micrograph of the gill filaments and terminal lamellae in the freshwater goldfish *Carassius auratus.* (B) Transmission electron micrograph of the capillary exchange surface in terminal lamellae in the same species showing capillary endothelial cell (end), pillar cell (pl), epithelial cell (ep), and red blood cell (RBC).

Carassius auratus. Basically the oxygen exchange surface in both these teleost fishes appears to be comparable to the minimal blood–air barrier in the human lung. The major difference between these two species appears to be an increase in vascularity and exhange surface in the gobie in comparison to the goldfish.

DEDICATION

This work is dedicated to the memory of Dr. Melvin H. Knisley, whose teachings inspired this work.

References

Mearns, A. J., and Sherwood, M., 1973, Coastal fish populations. The ecology of the Southern California Bight: Implications for water quality management, Southern California Coastal Water Research Project Report TR 104, El Segundo, Calif.

Warner, N. E., Bunnag, S., Bunnag, S. C., and Bennington, J. L., 1965, Microcirculation in the islets of Langerhans in experimental endotoxemia in mice, *Bibl. Anat.* **7**:449.

5.5. Flow Patterns in the Capillary Bed of Rat Skeletal Muscle at Rest and after Repetitive Tetanic Stimulation

RAYMOND J. CONNOLLY

A technique is described which can be used in skeletal muscle to mark capillaries undergoing active perfusion. Shortly after the intravenous injection of fluorescein, the selected muscle is rapidly frozen. Frozen sections are cut and are freeze-dried according to the methods of Stumpf and Roth (1967) which fix water-soluble, diffusible substances *in situ*. When the sections are examined by fluorescence microscopy, the dye is located in the lumen and walls of vessels which are being perfused at the moment of freezing. Because of the regular anatomy of skeletal muscle and its microvasculature, it is possible in a cross section to count the number of muscle fibers in a given area and the number of capillaries undergoing perfusion. These values can then be expressed as a vessel/fiber ratio (*V/F*). Capillary lumen diameters can also be measured from sections prepared this way.

To induce hyperemia, muscles were subjected to increasing durations of repetitive, brief, tetanic stimulations (train rate 0.5/s, train duration 0.5 s, stimulus rate 50/s). The contralateral muscles served as controls. Both muscles were frozen 30 s after the end of stimulation. The results are shown in Table I.

At rest, *V/F* is only a fraction of the maximum values reported (Hammersen, 1968; Eriksson and Myrhage, 1972), indicating that large numbers of capillaries are not being perfused. As the duration of stimulation increases from 4 min to 12 min, *V/F* increases, indicating a greater number of capillaries undergoing active perfusion. Both at rest and after stimulation, open capillaries are not distributed equally throughout the muscle. It is possible that this is due to the presence of different fiber types within the muscle. The capillary lumen diameters observed are similar to those previously reported (Baez, 1969; Eriksson and Myrhage, 1972). There is a 42% increase in the mean capillary diameter after 12 min of stimulation. The most probably cause of this is an increase in the transmural pressure. These results are similar to those previously reported

RAYMOND J. CONNOLLY · Tufts-New England Medical Center, Medford, Massachusetts.

Table I. Effect of Repetitive Tetanic Stimulation on the Vessel-to-Fiber Ratio and Diameters of Capillaries in the Gracilis Anticus Muscle of the Rat

Duration of stimulation (min)	Mean vessel/fiber ratio	Mean capillary diameter (μm)
Control	0.573	3.6
4	0.688	4.2
8	0.765	4.17
12	0.941	5.1

(Webb and Myers, 1973) for skeletal muscles in the reactive hyperemic state.

References

Baez, S., 1969, Simultaneous measurements of radii and wall thickness of microvessels in the anesthetized rat, *Circ. Res.* **25:**315.

Eriksson, E., and Myrhage, R., 1972, Microvascular dimensions and blood flow in skeletal muscle, *Acta Physiol. Scand.* **86:**211.

Hammersen, F., 1968, The pattern of the terminal vascular bed and the ultrastructural of capillaries in skeletal muscle, in: *Oxygen Transport in Blood and Tissue* (D. W. Lübbers, U.C. Luft, G. Thews, and E. Witzleb, eds.), pp. 184–197, Georg Thieme Verlag, Stuttgart.

Stumpf, M., and Roth, L., 1967, Freeze drying of small tissue samples and thin frozen sections below −60°C. *J. Histochem. Cytochem.* **15:**243.

Webb, C., and Myers, J., 1973, Capillary densities and luminal diameters in mixed skeletal muscle during reactive hyperemia (abst.), *Physiologist* **16:**483.

5.6. Transcapillary Pressure Gradients and Coefficients during Isotonic Mannitol Loads: Evidence for Capillary Intermittency

MURRAY A. KATZ

Mechanisms responsible for maintaining normal partition of extracellular fluid between vascular and interstitial spaces are poorly understood. Relevant information may come from study of transcapillary pressures and capillary filtration coefficients (CFC) during mannitol-induced filtration. Mannitol was infused up to 30 ml/min into ten intact dogs with chronically implanted capsules for measurement of interstitial fluid hydrostatic pressure (Pi) (Guyton, 1963). Plasma colloid oncotic pressure (πc) was determined from plasma protein, and estimates of interstitial oncotic pressure (πi) were made from assessment of mannitol-induced dilution and depletion of extravascular protein by isotopic measurement of interstitial space. Ten other dogs underwent mannitol infusion while an isolated hindlimb was being autoperfused. Capillary pressure (Pc) was determined by modification of the isogravimetric technique (Pappenheimer and Soto-Rivera, 1948). CFC was determined by strain gauge venous occlusion plethysmography, a technique which in our hands agrees closely with gravimetric techniques (Katz, 1976). Pc remained unchanged from hydropenic control values of 14.5 ± 0.9 (SEM) mm Hg, as did Pi at about -2.2 ± 1.2. πc fell from 19.4 ± 0.9 to 13.0 ± 0.5 ($p < 0.005$), while πi fell only from 4.2 to 2.5 mm Hg. CFC rose from 0.0037 ± 0.0006 to 0.0065 ± 0.0008 ml/min/mm Hg/100 mg hindlimb ($p < 0.01$). These results indicate that the driving force for mannitol-induced filtration is plasma protein dilution and a 75% increase in CFC. Since Pc is constant, capillary recruitment rather than stretch probably accounts for the rise in CFC. This supports a significant role for capillary intermittency in the regulation of extracellular fluid partition.

References

Guyton, A. C., 1963, A concept of negative interstitial pressure based on pressures in implanted perforated capsules, *Circ. Res.* **12**:399.

MURRAY A. KATZ · Renal Section, Department of Medicine, University of Arizona College of Medicine, and VA Hospital, Tucson, Arizona.

Katz, M. A., 1976, Capillary filtration measurement by strain gauge: I. Analysis of methods. *Am. J. Physiol.*, in press.

Pappenheimer, J. R., and Soto-Rivera, A., 1948, Effective osmotic pressure of the plasma proteins and other quantities associated with the capillary circulation in the hindlimbs of cats and dogs, *Am. J. Physiol.* **152**:471.

5.7. Segmental Resistances in the Microcirculation of the Mesentery and Omentum

BENJAMIN W. ZWEIFACH and HERBERT H. LIPOWSKY

The distribution of pressure and flow within the microvascular network under steady-state conditions depends on the actual driving force (net hydrostatic pressure) and the geometric makeup of the vascular segments (including length, diameter, and branching configuration), together with the flow properties of the blood (dependent on local hematocrit and velocity or shear rate). Experiments were designed to measure these parameters in the exteriorized mesentery and omentum with a view toward defining the factors concerned with the local distribution and adjustment of blood flow. The greatest drop in pressure was found to occur in the region of precapillaries 15–25 μm wide, especially across branchings. The volumetric flow rate of the blood falls off most rapidly in the larger terminal arterioles (25–35 μm wide) which feed the bed. On the basis of distribution plots for pressure and for flow, the resistance between any two points in the microcirculation could be calculated. Such average resistance values were then compared with discrete segmental resistances obtained by measuring the pressure drop directly with two micropipettes and flow at both points by a two-diode cross-correlation procedure. Considerable variance from mean resistance values was seen in the precapillary region, where individual resistances ranged from 1.5 up to 11.5 mm Hg/10^{-3} mm^3/s, reflecting the spontaneous vasomotion which is characteristic of these vessels. When the flow in a given branch was compared to that in a feeding large vessel, it was possible to use the ratio of the two flow rates to calculate the net resistance encountered at a given, horizontal cross-section of the microvascular network.

When pressure and flow were studied continuously in a given arteriole for periods of 5–10 min, it was found that the average pressure level remained reasonably constant despite changes in flow rate of over 100–200%. In contrast, in the precapillaries (<20 μm in diameter), the volumetric flow rate remained in a narrow range despite changes in pressure of as much as 10–15 μm Hg, indicating separate homeostatic adjustments in these two discrete segments of the microcirculation.

The above methods also permitted calculations of the relative value of

BENJAMIN W. ZWEIFACH and HERBERT H. LIPOWSKY · AMES-Bioengineering, University of California, San Diego, California.

pre- and postcapillary resistances. In the mesentery, these ratios varied from 3.3:1 to 1.8:1, depending on the structural level at which the two measurements were made. Because of the asymmetrical nature of the flow distribution curve for the mesentery, the principal sites for adjusting pre- and postcapillary resistances reside in different-sized vessels—in the 30–40 μm category for the arterioles and the 50–60 μm category for venules.

ACKNOWLEDGMENT

This work was supported by United States Public Health Service HL-10881.

6

Formed Elements of the Blood Platelets, and Thrombosis

6.1. Platelets in Response to the Injury in the Microcirculation—A Review

K.-E. ARFORS and D. BERGQVIST

The effects of injury in the microcirculation have been studied for about 100 years, initially more or less accidentally. The English ophthalmic surgeon Wharton-Jones (1851) described arteriolar thromboembolism in the frog's web, and the German physiologist Zahn (1872) observed the process of hemostasis in the frog's mesentery. He described the arrest of bleeding by the formation of *"ein weisslicher, nach Innen und Aussen kolbenförmig verdickter Thrombus. Genauere Untersuchung desselben erwiess, dass er, mit Ausnahme einiger wenigen eingeklemmten roter Blutkörperchen, lediglich aus farblosen Zellen bestand."* In this description, the presence of platelets in the hemostatic plug was noted for the first time.

Since these observations, several methods for studying the platelet response to the microvascular injury have been developed, and for more precise definition of thrombotic and hemostatic processes techniques have been developed in an attempt to quantitate platelet behavior *in vivo.* In 1955, Berman *et al.* used chemical injury (topical application of thrombin) to study thromboembolism in the hamster cheek pouch. Begent and Born (1970) developed a technique using the hamster cheek pouch where venular thrombus formation was induced by iontophoretically applied ADP and the growth rate of thrombi measured. Pure electrical trauma has been used by Berman and Fulton (1961). A mechanical technique for the measurement of platelet thrombosis in pial vessels of the rabbit was devised by Honour and Ross Russell (1962). Injuries caused by pinching

K.-E. ARFORS and D. BERGQVIST · Department of Experimental Medicine, Pharmacia AB, Uppsala, Sweden.

the vessels were classified as major or minor according to the presence or absence of external hemorrhage. This type of injury was later combined with chemical trauma when it was shown that activity at the sites of minor injury could be stimulated by the application of substances known to induce platelet aggregation *in vitro.*

In 1965, shortly after the construction of the first ruby laser, Kochen and Baez recognized the value of this energy source when focused on an extremely small area, and in a rat mesentery preparation they were able to make reproducible vessel injuries. In the same year, Grant and Becker (1965), with the rabbit ear chamber, also used the laser technique in combination with the systemic injection of carbon particles or dyes.

The laser technique for studying microthromboembolism has since been taken up and developed by Wiedeman (1974), Kovacs *et al.* (1973), and our group. Wiedeman *et al.* worked with arterial vessels in the bat wing using a single-pulse ruby laser. Kovacs *et al.* have used a continuous laser beam combined with the perfusion of carbon particles or dye to locate the site for vascular injury. In preliminary studies, Arfors *et al.* (1968) used a single-pulse laser injury in the rabbit ear chamber to work with unanesthetized animals over long periods of time. The animals were thus used as their own controls. As it is of paramount importance to know the precise nature of the injury being studied, we have further investigated and evaluated the laser injury.

When the laser beam is focused intravascularly and discharged, an aggregate of red cells stimulates platelet aggregation to form a microthrombus. Embolization of this thrombus provides a method for reproducibly quantifying the trauma by measuring the number of emboli during a 10-min period. Because this method of quantitation is open to criticism, a technique was developed for the planimetric measurement of the growth rate of filmed microthrombi, and it was found that there was a direct positive correlation between the mean growth rate constant and the number of emboli counted for each laser injury (Arfors *et al.*, unpublished).

To evaluate the type of platelet aggregation responsible for the growth of the laser-induced microthrombus, different inhibitors of platelet aggregation *in vitro* were investigated. Aspirin and heparin were without effect, whereas adenosine and dipyridamole inhibited the response. Conversely, small amounts of ADP stimulated microembolism (McKenzie *et al.*, 1974; Arfors *et al.*, 1975*b*). These results suggested that the aggregation of platelets at laser injury sites was primarily an ADP-mediated reaction, and an electron microscopic study showed that the thrombi had the morphological appearance of ADP-induced aggregates where complete destruction of the endothelium could not be seen (Hovig *et al.*, 1974) (Fig. 1). Below a

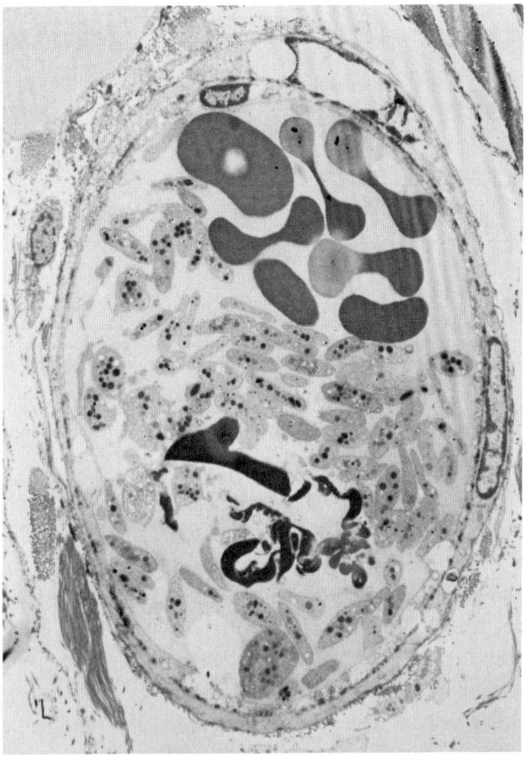

Figure 1. ADP-stimulated microembolus.

platelet count of 100,000/mm^3, a progressive reduction in platelet reactivity was seen, and this was also true for high blood flow velocities (Arfors *et al.*, 1975*a*). The method has been shown to be reliable in situations where platelet reactivity is diminshed (after dextran treatment) as well as increased (after trauma and other forms of stress) (Cockburn and Arfors, unpublished) (Fig. 2). In a statistical investigation, it was shown that in studies where platelet reactivity was supposed to be decreased, laser injury to arterioles in the rabbit mesentery could as well be used (Arfors *et al.*, 1973).

A more serious form of microvascular injury was described by Zahn (1972), who studied hemostatic plug formation after vascular transection or puncture. A number of transparent animal tissues have been used in such investigations, but most common is the microcirculatory bed of the rabbit mesentery. Different authors have studied different aspects of early hemostasis (Apitz, 1942; Zucker, 1947; French *et al.*, 1964; Marr *et al.*,

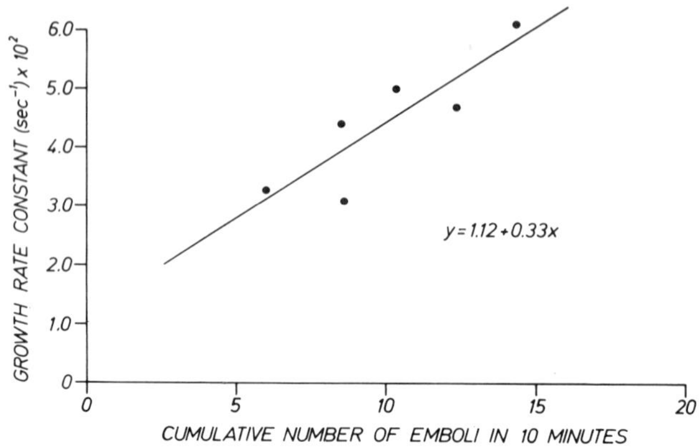

Figure 2. Number of emboli vs. growth rate constant.

1965; Packham *et al.*, 1967). Kjaerheim and Hovig (1962) established the fundamental role of platelets in initiating hemostatic plug formation by electron microscopic studies. Hugues (1953) concluded that contraction in microvessels was not a determinant in hemostatic plug formation, a view which has not been generally accepted. Several studies pointed to differences in the initial hemostatic process between arterioles and venules, although the differences were not explained and the results have been contradictory and inconclusive (Apitz, 1942; Chen and Tsai, 1948; Hugues, 1953). There is also controversy about the initiation of the hemostatic platelet aggregation, some authors favoring collagen and others ADP as the stimulus (Hugues, 1953; Kjaerheim and Hovig, 1962; Marr *et al.*, 1965; Johnson *et al.*, 1967). These different reports stimulated us in further evaluation of the technique, and our results are summarized and discussed below.

A mesenteric preparation was made for intravital microscopy in urethane-anesthetized rabbits, arterioles and venules being transected (Arfors *et al.*, 1972; Bergqvist, 1974; Bergqvist *et al.*, 1974). Bleeding stopped by the formation of a hemostatic plug, and the time until this occurred reflected primary hemostasis, which was quantitated by the primary hemostatic plug formation time (PHT). The frequency of rebleeding and the time for rebleedings were also recorded, these two measurements being combined to quantitate hemostatic plug stability. As arteriolar hemostatic plug formation time is vessel size dependent, it is important to use a well-defined vessel size range for transection in comparative studies (Bergqvist, 1974). Differences in hemostatic pattern were found between arterioles and venules, the most important being longer hemostatic plug formation time, lower plug stability, and slower plug growth rate in venules (Arfors *et al.*, 1972; Bergqvist, 1974; Bergqvist and Arfors, 1973, 1974*a,b*). It was also found that these differences could be totally abolished in animals treated with aspirin, venular hemostasis becoming similar to normal arteriolar hemostatis (Arfors *et al.*, 1972). These findings were in contrast to those of Evans *et al.* (1968) and called into question the hypothesis that hemostatic plug formation was purely collagen induced. The primary hemostatic plug formation was clearly related to the platelet count (Bergqvist and Arfors, 1973). PHT was also prolonged by dextran in high doses given 3 h before anesthesia, by heparin in high doses, by FDP, as well as by local infusion into the cranial mesenteric artery of adenosine and PGE_1 (Bergqvist and Arfors, 1974*b*). Thrombin did not influence hemostasis, whereas ADP and laser injury prior to transection shortened the PHT (Bergqvist and Arfors, unpublished). Alterations in the coagulation system did not influence primary hemostasis, but plug stability was significantly depressed, a phenomenon also seen after induction of fibrinolytic activity. Conversely, inhibition of fibrinolysis with AMCA did not influence hemostasis (Bergqvist and Arfors, 1974*b*). Using the dual-slit technique originally described by Wayland and Johnson (1967) in a modification for on-line measurements, it was possible to make continuous recordings of red cell flow velocity during the formation of a hemostatic plug (Arfors *et al.*, 1975*a*). A typical flow velocity pattern was seen during hemostasis, but none of the

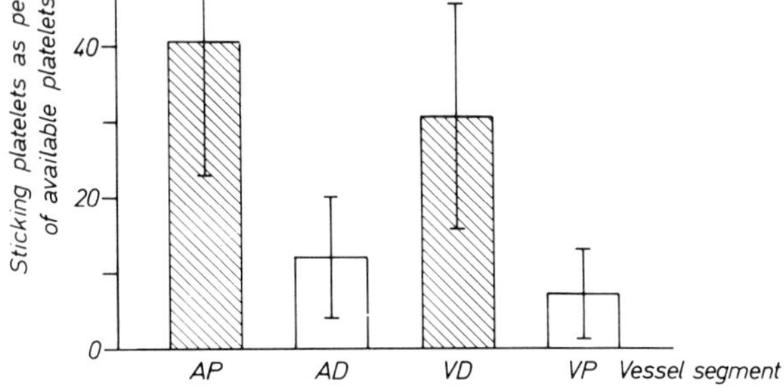

Figure 3. Platelet aggregability of vessel segments.

parameters studied was shown to be a determinant for hemostatic process. This made it possible to measure variations in vessel diameter, and, using this in combination with the flow velocity measurements and the platelet count for the rabbit under study, the total number of platelets that passed (platelet flow) before the arrest of bleeding in individual vessels could be obtained. The total number of platelets in the hemostatic plug was calculated by dividing the final plug volume obtained from the films by the volume of an individual platelet (5.5 μm^3; Arfors *et al.*, 1975). Thus individual vessel platelet aggregability as a percentage was calculated by (platelet number in final plug × 100)/(platelet flow) (Arfors and Bergqvist, 1975). Individual vessel platelet aggregability was significantly higher in plugs formed at injuries where blood flow was from the arteriolar side of the microcirculation than when it was from the venular side (Fig. 3). In injuries in the proximal arteriolar segment almost every second platelet became incorporated into the hemostatic plug, whereas in the proximal venular segment less than 10% were involved.

Different hypothetical explanations for the hemostatic difference between arterioles and venules were then tested, but none was verified: differences in fibrinolytic activity, white cell or platelet behavior, hemodynamics, vessel contraction. The conclusion made by Hugues (1953) that vascular constriction was not an important determinant of microvascular hemostasis was also firmly supported by our results.

Vascular permeability, especially in postcapillary venules, increases after trauma, a finding also true in the rabbit mesentery preparation (Arfors *et al.*, unpublished). Because the prostaglandin content of this preparation increased over time and these compounds can induce venular leakage, the equalizing effect of aspirin on the hemostatic difference between arterioles and venules was of interest. Aspirin, among other effects, inhibits prostaglandin synthesis. We therefore performed a series

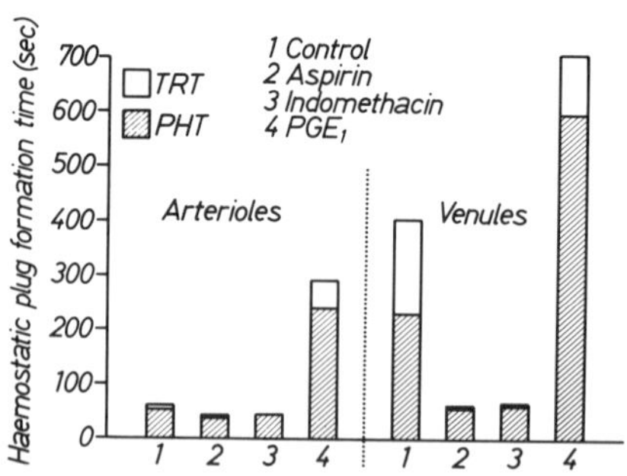

Figure 4. Arteriolar and venular hemostatic plug formation in rabbit mesentary preparation after treatment with various drugs.

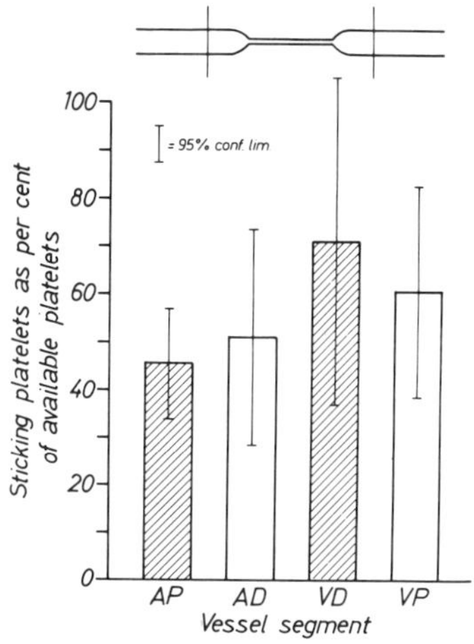

Figure 5. Platelet aggregability of vessel segments after treatment with indomethacin.

of experiments to further study this phenomenon: indomethacin totally inhibited the endogenous production of prostaglandins in the mesenteric preparation; infusion of PGE_1 into the cranial mesenteric artery significantly prolonged arteriolar as well as venular hemostatic plug formation time (Fig. 4); indomethacin (20 mg/kg given $\frac{1}{2}$ h before anesthesia and 4 mg/kg/h in continuous infusion), like aspirin, shortened the venular hemostatic plug formation time. Venular PHT did not differ from arteriolar PHT. Individual vessel platelet aggregability after indomethacin treatment was also measured, and the difference seen in untreated animals was found to be totally abolished (Arfors and Bergqvist, unpublished) (Fig. 5). It seems, therefore, that preparation of the mesentery and microvessel transection traumatized the tissue, causing prostaglandin generation. As the increased vessel permeability was localized to the postcapillary venules, the prostaglandins formed partly inhibited platelet aggregation in these vessels.

In conclusion, we suggest that primary hemostatic plug formation is mainly an ADP-induced platelet aggregation and that plug stability mainly reflects the status of the coagulation system. Prostaglandins formed locally in the mesentery preparation can explain the hemostatic differences between arterioles and venules.

References

Apitz, K., 1942, Die Bedeutung der Gerinnung und Thrombose für die Blutstillung, *Virchows Arch. Pathol. Anat.* **308:**540.

Arfors, K.-E., and Bergqvist, D., 1974, Influence of blood flow velocity on experimental haemostatic plug formation, *Thromb. Res.* **4:**447.

Arfors, K.-E., and Bergqvist, D., 1975, Platelet aggregability and vessel contraction in microvascular haemostasis, *Microvasc. Res.* **9:**22.

Arfors, K.-E., Dhall, D. P., Engeset, I., Hint, H., Matheson, N. A., and Tangen, O., 1968, Biolaser endothelial trauma as a means of quantifying platelet activity *in vivo, Nature (London)* **218:**887.

Arfors, K.-E., Bergqvist, D., Bygdeman, S., McKenzie, F. N., and Svensjö, E., 1972, The effect of inhibition of the platelet release reaction on platelet behaviour *in vitro* and *in vivo, Scand. J. Haematol.* **9:**322.

Arfors, K.-E., Bergqvist, D., McKenzie, F. N., and Nilsson, G., 1973, Platelet response to laser-induced microvascular injury in the rabbit mesentery and the rabbit ear chamber, *Thromb. Res.* **3:**75.

Arfors, K.-E., Bergqvist, D., Intaglietta, M., and Westergren, B., 1975*a*, Measurements of blood flow velocity in the microcirculation, *Uppsala J. Med. Sci.* **80:**27.

Arfors, K.-E., McKenzie, F. N., and Matheson, N. A., 1975*b*, Measurement of the platelet response to laser-induced microvascular injury: Influence of maematological and haemodynamic variables. *Thromb. Res.* (in press).

Begent, N., and Born, G. V. R., 1970, Growth rate *in vivo* of platelet thrombi, produced by iontophoresis of ADP, as a function of mean blood flow velocity, *Nature (London)* **227:**926.

Bergqvist, D., 1973, Haemostatic plug formation time and stability in the microvasculature of rabbit mesentery, *Abst. Uppsala Diss. Fac. Med.,* No. 167.

Bergqvist, D., 1974, Haemostatic plug formation in the rabbit mesentery: A methodological study, *Uppsala J. Med. Sci.* **79:**28.

Bergqvist, D., and Arfors, K.-E., 1973, The growth rate of haemostatic plug in the rabbit mesentery, *Bibl. Anat.* **12:**186.

Bergqvist, D., and Arfors, K.-E., 1974*a*, Growth rate and volume of haemostatic plugs in the mesentery of normal and thrombocytopenic rabbits, *Thromb. Res.* **4:**77.

Bergqvist, D., and Arfors, K.-E., 1974*b*, Influence of fibrinolysis and coagulation on haemostatic plug formation: An experimental study in rabbits, *Thromb. Res.* **4:**345.

Bergqvist, D., McKenzie, F. N., and Arfors, K.-E., 1974, Influence of different anaesthetic agents on the formation and stability of haemostatic plugs in the rabbit mesentery, *Uppsala J. Med. Sci.* **79:**39.

Berman, H. J., and Fulton, G. P., 1961, Platelets in the peripheral circulation, in: *Blood Platelets* (S. A. Johnson, R. W. Monto, G. W. Rebuck, and R. C. Horn, eds.), Little, Brown, Boston.

Berman, H. J., Fulton, G. P., Lutz, B. R., and Pierce, D. L., 1955, Susceptibility to thrombosis in normal young, aging, cortisone-treated, heparinised and X-irradiated hamsters as tested by topical application of thrombin, *Blood* **10:**831.

Chen, T. I., and Tsai, C., 1948, The mechanism of haemostasis in peripheral vessels, *J. Physiol. (London)* **107:**280.

Evans, G., Packham, M. A., Nishisawa, E. T., Mustard, J. F., and Murphy, E. A., 1968, The effect of acetylsalicylic acid on platelet function, *J. Exp. Med.* **128:**877.

French, J. E., Macfarlane, R. G., and Sanders, A. G., 1964, The structure of haemostatic plugs and experimental thrombi in small arteries, *Br. J. Exp. Pathol.* **45:**467.

Grant, L., and Becker, F. F., 1965, Mechanisms of inflammation. I. Laser-induced thrombosis, a morphologic analysis, *Proc. Soc. Exp. Biol. Med.* **119:**1123.

Honour, A. J., and Ross Russell, R. W., 1962, Experimental platelet embolism, *Br. J. Exp. Pathol.* **43:**350.

Hovig, T., McKenzie, F. N., and Arfors, K.-E., 1974, Measurement of the platelet response to laser-induced microvascular injury: Ultrastructural studies, *Thromb. Diath. Haemorrh.* **32**:695.

Hugues, J., 1953, Contribution a l'étude des facteurs vasculaires et sanguins dans l'hémostase spontanée, *Arch. Int. Physiol* **41**:565.

Johnson, S., Fredell, L., Shepard, J., Tebo, T., Chang, C., Pederson, H., and v. Horn, D., 1967, Red blood cells, fibrin and platelets in hemostasis, in: *Physiology of Hemostasis and Thrombosis* (S. Johnson and W. Seegers, eds.), p. 44, Thomas, Springfield, Ill.

Kjaerheim, Å., and Hovig, T., 1962, The ultrastructure of haemostatic blood platelet plugs in rabbit mesenterium, *Thromb, Diath. Haemorrh.* **7**:1.

Kochen, J. A., and Baez, S., 1965, Vascular and intravascular effects of pulsed laser micro-beam, *Bibl. Anat.* **7**:46.

Kovacs, I. B., Coalay, L., and Gorog, D., 1973, Laser-induced thrombosis in the microcirculation of the hamster cheek pouch and its inhibition by acetylsalicylic acid, *Microvasc. Res.* **6**:194.

Marr, J., Barboriak, J. J., and Johnson, S., 1965, Relationship of appearance of adenosine diphosphate, fibrin formation and platelet aggregation in the hemostatic plug *in vivo, Nature (London)* **205**:259.

McKenzie, F. N., Arfors, K.-E., and Matheson, N. A., 1974, Measurement of the platelet response to laser-induced microvascular injury: Assessment of determinants of platelet aggregation *in vivo, Thromb. Diath. Haemorrh.* **32**:704.

Packham, M. A., Warrior, E. S., Glynn, M. F., Senyi, A. S., and Mustard, J. F., 1967, Alteration of the response of platelets to surface stimuli by pyrazole compounds, *J. Exp. Med.* **126**:171.

Wayland, H., and Johnson, P., 1967, Erythrocyte velocity measurement in microvessels by a two-slit photometric method, *J. Appl. Physiol.* **22**:333.

Wharton-Jones, T., 1851, On the state of the blood and blood vessels in inflammation, ascertained by experiments, injections, and observations by the microscope, *Guy's Hosp. Rep. 2nd Ser.* **7**:1.

Wiedeman, M., 1974, Vascular reactions to laser *in vivo, Microvasc. Res.* **8**:132.

Zahn, W., 1872, Untersuchungen über Thrombose, *Centralbl. Med. Wiss.* **10**:129.

Zucker, M. B., 1947, Platelet agglutination and vasoconstriction as factors in spontaneous hemostasis in normal, thrombocytopenic, heparinized and hypoprothrombinemic rats, *Am. J. Physiol.* **148**:275.

6.2. Double Labeling of Platelets with ^{51}Cr and [^{14}C]Serotonin

K. RÅDEGRAN

A method has been devised for combined labeling of platelets with ^{51}Cr, firmly bound to the platelet particle, and [^{14}C]serotonin, readily released. Canine platelets isolated from ACD blood were labeled with ^{51}Cr (according to Aas and Gardner, 1958, modified by Abrahamsen, 1968). [^{14}C]Serotonin was added to the suspension at the same time as the chromate.

Blood samples from experimental animals were collected in ACD solution. The ^{51}Cr activity of whole blood, red cells, platelet-rich plasma (PRP), and platelet-poor plasma (PPP) was determined in a Packard liquid scintillation meter. Corrections were made for the influence of ^{51}Cr activity on the ^{14}C measurements as well as for variations in quenching.

Eleven experiments were performed on splenectomized dogs. Five experiments served as a control group. In six experiments, *in vivo* platelet aggregation was induced on the day after platelet reinjection by protamine chloride infusion (Rådegran and McAslan, 1972).

6.2.1. Results

On the day after reinjection of platelets, there was 46 ± 4% recovery in ^{51}Cr activity in whole blood (11 experiments). A relative measure of ^{14}C recovery was calculated by dividing platelet-bound ^{14}C radioactivity (PRP-PPP) per milliliter of PRP by the platelet-bound ^{14}C radioactivity per milliliter of platelet suspension injected. This calculation was also applied to ^{51}Cr label. A ratio ($^{14}C/^{51}Cr$) was obtained by dividing the relative recoveries of ^{14}C by those of ^{51}Cr. This was 2.1 ± 0.3 in the 1-h and 1.9 ± 0.3 in the 1-day sample. Taking the latter as 100%, during the following 3 days, $^{14}C/^{51}Cr$ increased in controls to 184 ± 18% (Fig. 1). There was no correlation between whole blood recovery of ^{51}Cr activity and the relative recovery ratio ($^{14}C/^{51}Cr$) in PRP at either 1 h or 1 day after reinjection. The $^{14}C/^{51}Cr$ ratio correlated well with the ^{51}Cr activity in the red cell portion obtained after centrifugation (to produce PRP).

In six experiments, *in vivo* platelet aggregation was induced on day 1 by intravenous protamine infusion. An acute but transient fall in the

K. RÅDEGRAN · Surgical Research Laboratory, Karolinska Sjukhuset, Stockholm, Sweden.

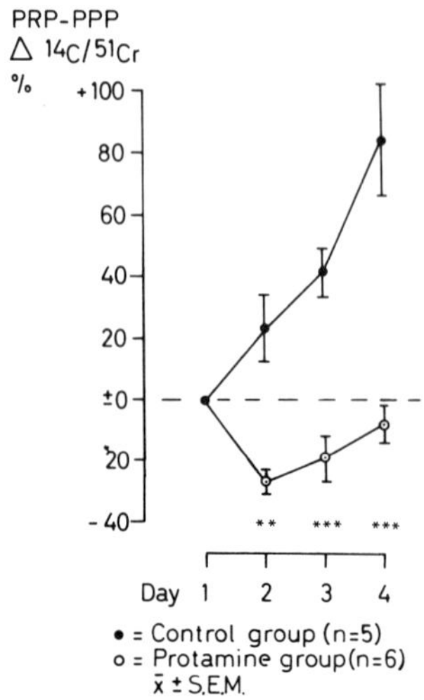

Figure 1

platelet count of blood exceeding 90% of the preinfusion values occurred in 4 min. The platelet count and the ^{51}Cr activity of blood remained below control values throughout the study. Platelet-bound ^{14}C activity of PRP was disproportionately lowered on day 2 as compared with the ^{51}Cr-activity, clearly shown by a 27% fall in the relative recovery ratio (^{14}C/^{51}Cr) for PRP, which is to be compared with a 23% rise in the control experiments (Fig. 1). Thus release of [^{14}C]serotonin from platelets had been induced. The pronounced rise in relative recovery ratio (^{14}C/^{51}Cr) observed in the control animals did not occur in those infused with protamine.

References

Aas, K. A., and Gardner, F. H., 1958, Survival of blood platelets labelled with chromium^{51}, *J. Clin. Invest.* **37**:1257.

Abrahamsen, A. F., 1968, A modification of the technique for Cr^{51}-labelled blood platelets, *Scand. J. Haematol.* **53**:5.

Rådegran, K., and McAslan, C., 1972, Circulatory and ventilatory effects of induced platelet aggregation and their inhibition by acetylsalicylic acid, *Acta Anaesthesiol. Scand.* **16**:76.

6.3. Inhibition of Platelet Function by Angiographic Contrast Media

J. GOLDSTONE and N. H. SANDOW

Angiographic procedures employing water-soluble, iodinated contrast media are of great importance in clinical medicine. Although thromboembolic complications constitute the major risk of such procedures (Judkins and Gander, 1974), we have encountered a clinically significant impairment in primary hemostasis in a few patients who were operated on shortly after extensive diagnostic angiography. Alterations in platelet adhesiveness to glass beads as well as in several coagulation proteins have been attributed to contrast agents (Jacobsson *et al.,* 1969). The purpose of this study was to determine their effects on *in vitro* platelet aggregation.

6.3.1. Methods

The contrast media selected for study were Renograffin-60, Renograffin-76, and Hypaque-50. They contain, respectively, 60%, 76%, and 50% diatrizoate, and were chosen because of the frequency with which they are used clinically. To 0.5 ml of platelet-rich plasma were added 25, 50, 75, and 100 μl of these solutions, which were incubated for periods up to 1 h and then tested for platelet aggregation using the turbidometric method of Born (1962). ADP (5 μM) and *l*-epinephrine (22.5 mM) were used to stimulate aggregation.

6.3.2. Results

Maximum percent aggregation was reduced from a normal value of 75.5% to 61.8%, 39.9%, 10.9%, and 0% by the addition of above-listed doses of contrast (Fig. 1). This marked inhibition was immediate and irreversible. It was more pronounced with the more concentrated agents. Lower concentrations of contrast media inhibit the secondary wave of aggregation, while higher concentrations inhibit even the primary wave. Addition of contrast to already aggregated platelets did not produce disaggregation.

J. GOLDSTONE and N. H. SANDOW · Surgical Service, Veterans Hospital, and Department of Surgery, University of California, San Francisco, California.

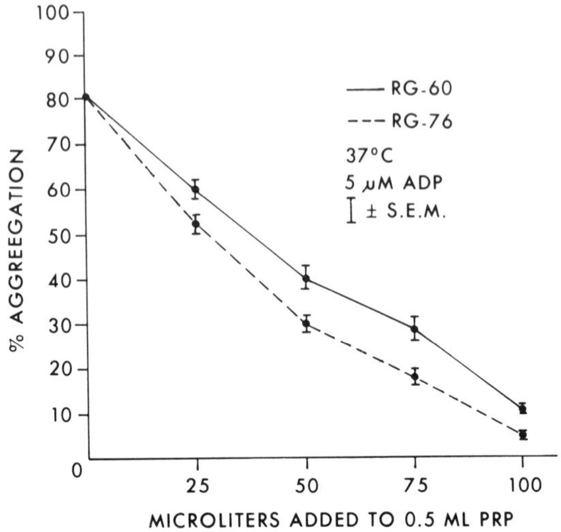

Figure 1. Effects of adding increasing quantities of Renograffin–60 and Renograffin–76 to platelet-rich plasma. The results are all statistically significant ($p < 0.01$) relative to control but not between the two contrast agents.

6.3.3. Discussion and Conclusions

There are several possible explanations for this profound inhibition of aggregation (Mustard and Packham, 1970; Sahud, 1972). The contrast agents bear no structural similarity to ADP. They are very hypertonic, but addition of similar aliquots of hypertonic mannitol or saline failed to mimic this effect. The binding of calcium by the EDTA present in the contrast agents is not the mechanism, because addition of up to 8 μM calcium to the platelet-rich plasma did not prevent the inhibition. The fact that the inhibitory action is so prompt suggests that uptake of the contrast by the platelets is not necessary, so their site of action may be at the platelet membrane.

Although the exact mechanisms have not been elucidated, marked inhibition of platelet aggregation occurred at dosage levels comparable to those used clinically. Therefore, these agents should be used with caution in patients who are about to undergo major surgery or who have hemostatic defects.

References

Born, G. V. F., 1962, Aggregation of blood platelets by adenosine disphosphate and its reversal, *Nature (London)* **194:**927.

Jacobsson, B., Bergentz, S. E., and Ljungquist, U., 1969, Platelet adhesion and thrombus formation on vascular catheters in dogs, *Acta Radiol. Diagn.* **8**:221.
Judkins, M. P., and Gander, M. P., 1974, Prevention of complications of coronary arteriography, *Circulation* **49**:599.
Mustard, J. F., and Packham, M. A., 1970, Factors influencing platelet function: Adhesion, release and aggregation, *Pharmacol. Rev.* **22**:97.
Sahud, M. A., 1972, Platelet disorders—A review of disturbances in adhesion, aggregation, and release reaction, *Calif. Med.* **116**:21.

6.4. Electronic Particle Size Measurement of Platelet Aggregates

PETER S. KENNEDY and R. THOMAS SOLIS

Numerous methods have been developed for assessing platelet function, including platelet retention tests, screen filtration of aggregates, changes in optical density, and others (Mustard and Packham, 1970). Many of these methods analyze the formation of aggregates indirectly and require the preparation of platelet-rich plasma. Several demand standardization of platelet concentration in plasma. The present study describes the use of an electronic particle analyzer to quantitate platelet aggregation in blood.

6.4.1. Methods

The use and operation of the particle size analyzer (Coulter Electronics, Hialeah, Florida) to measure the size distribution of platelet aggregates in plasma have been described (Solis *et al.*, 1974, 1975). The measurement of platelet aggregates in blood is similar to measurement in plasma except that blood is diluted 1:101 in an Eagle's solution (Isoton, Coulter Electronics) containing a lysing agent (Zap-Isoton, Coulter Electronics). Particle size analysis is completed within 20 s of dilution.

6.4.2. Results

Preliminary studies indicated that electronic measurements of platelet aggregates in platelet-rich plasma were not altered by addition of lysing agent to the diluent. As platelets began to clump after exposure to ADP (0.2 μmol), the total volume and size of aggregates increased (Fig. 1A), while there were opposite changes during platelet deaggregation (Fig. 1B). With higher concentrations of ADP, the total volume and size of aggregates formed during the initial 60 s increased (Fig. 1C); subsequently, only their size increased, and they dissociated more slowly.

When the platelet concentration in blood was increased by serial dilutions while a constant hematocrit was maintained, the mean size of the aggregates varied linearly with the total volume of aggregates that were formed (Fig. 1D) ($r = 0.94$).

PETER S. KENNEDY and R. THOMAS SOLIS · Department of Medicine, Baylor College of Medicine, Houston, Texas.

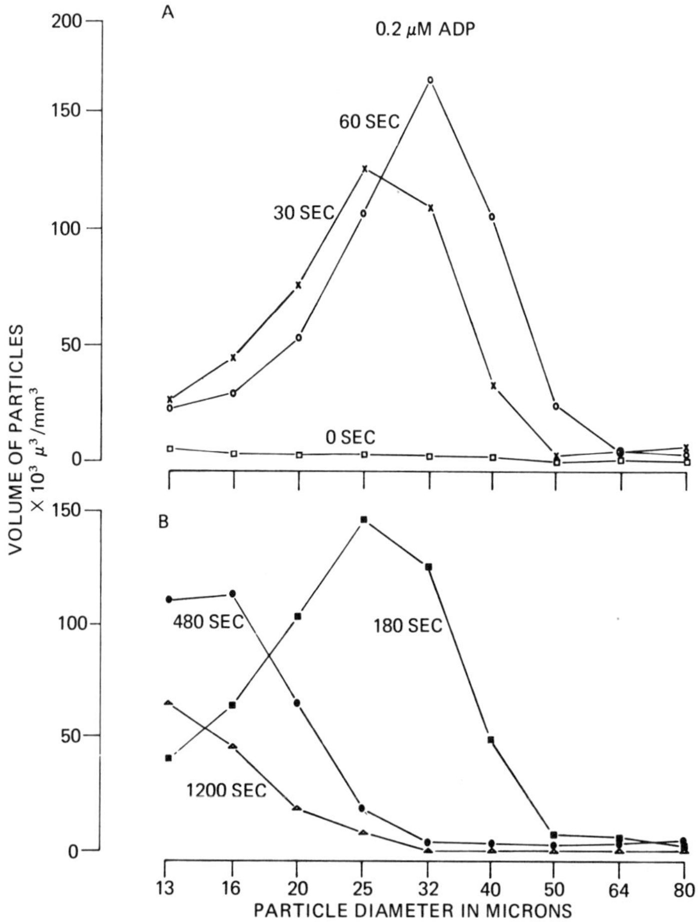

Figure 1. (A) Volume distribution of platelets during aggregation in blood after addition of ADP (0.2 μmol). (B) Volume distribution of platelets during deaggregation after ADP (0.2 μmol).

When the platelet count in blood was kept constant, the mean size of aggregates varied inversely with changes in the hematocrit ($r = 0.98$).

6.4.3. Discussion

These studies show that ADP-induced platelet aggregates in whole blood can be quantitated using the electronic particle size analyzer. Preliminary work suggests that measurement of mean aggregate size, when corrected for platelet concentration and hematocrit, can serve as an index of the functional mass of circulating platelets.

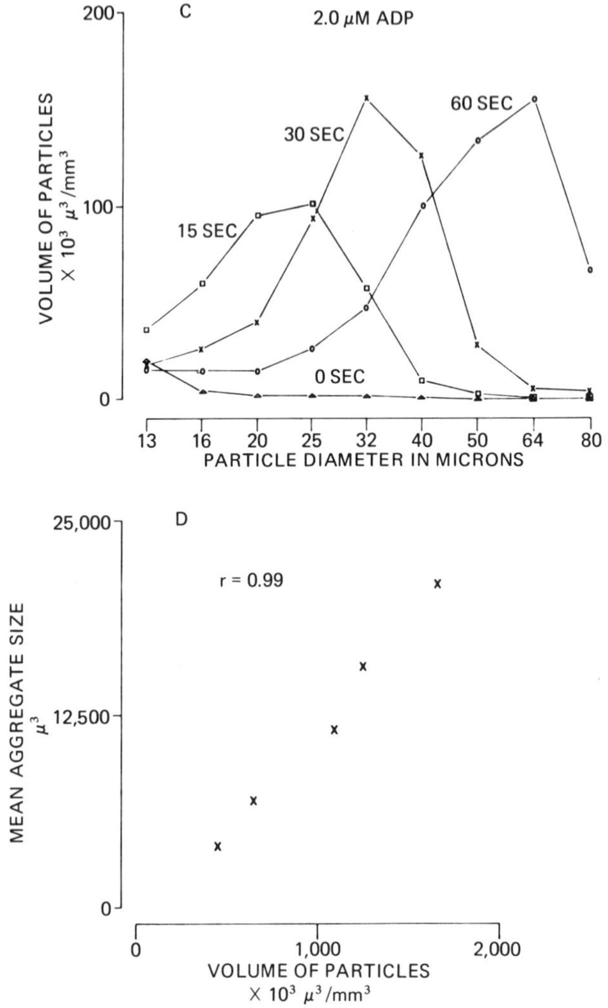

Figure 1. (C) Volume distribution of platelets during aggregation after ADP (2.0 μmol). (D) Relationship between mean aggregate size and total volume of particles measured 60 s after addition of ADP (2.0 μmol).

References

Mustard, J. F., and Packham, M. A., 1970, Factors influencing platelet function: Adhesion, release, and aggregation, *Pharmacol. Rev.* **22:**97.

Solis, R. T., Goldfinger, D., Gibbs, M. B., and Zeller, J. A., 1974, Physical characteristics of microaggregates in stored blood, *Transfusion* **14:**538.

Solis, R. T., Wright, C. B., and Gibbs, M. B., 1975, Electronic particle size measurements of platelet aggregates formed *in vitro*, *J. Appl. Physiol.* **38:**739.

6.5. Videomicroscopy and Videodensitometry of Platelet Aggregation under Controlled Conditions of Blood Flow and ADP Convective Diffusion

ERIC F. GRABOWSKI, KATHLEEN K. HERTHER, and PAUL DIDISHEIM

The overall objective of this work has been to quantify and control the effects of flow and diffusion (of ADP) on platelet adhesion and aggregation in whole blood. Toward this end, a blood flow chamber (Grabowski *et al.*, 1974; Grabowski, 1976) has been designed and constructed within which platelet aggregates form at and adhere to a specified microscopic site on a cuprophane (Bemberg PT 150) membrane (see Fig. 1a). Important chamber features include controlled ADP diffusion into the flowing blood at the microscopic site and a design permitting continuous *in situ* observation and quantification (e.g., aggregate mean thicknesses and volumetric growth rates) by means of videomicroscopy and densitometry of video recordings. Video calibration requires use of differing but known thicknesses of blood film between light source and microscope objective. Although the wavelength of the incident light is 800 ± 90 nm (mean ± half-bandwidth for 50% peak intensity), the Lambert-Beer law is applicable to the present system, as shown by separate determination of the relative constancy of the absorptivities of both whole blood (±2%) and packed platelets (±12%) over the range of 700–900 nm.

Results obtained with citrated or heparinized dog blood (or platelet-rich plasma) and ADP in micromolar concentrations at the membrane–blood interface are as follows: (1) in agreement with the *in vivo* findings of Begent and Born (1970), aggregate growth rate prior to embolization (see Fig 1b) passes through a maximum (between 200 and 400^{-1}) with respect to surface shear rate, the maximum being 2.7 ± 0.63, 6 (mean ± SE, *N*) μ/min per 200,000 platelets/mm^3; (2) adhesion but not aggregation is negligible in the absence of RBCs; and (3) aspirin inhibits aggregation but not adhesion. Therefore, aggregate growth rates appear to be limited in general by platelet convection, finite platelet–ADP interaction times, and platelet function.

ERIC F. GRABOWSKI, KATHLEEN K. HERTHER, and PAUL DIDISHEIM · Mayo Clinic, Graduate School of Medicine and Medical School, Rochester, Minnesota.

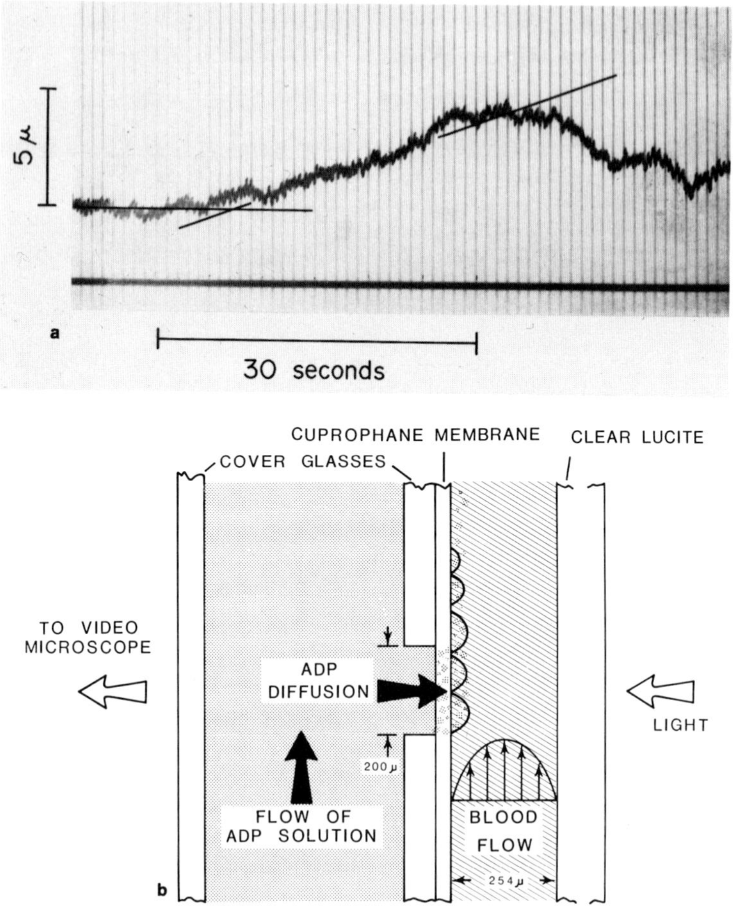

Figure 1. (a) Chamber detail showing site of ADP entry by diffusion. "Bumps" represent adherent platelet aggregates. (b) Calibrated paper recording of output from densitometer window: ordinate is mean thickness of adherent aggregates forming in whole blood with ADP in millimolar concentrations at the membrane–blood interface at a shear rate of 986^{-1}; growth rate is taken to be the maximum slope.

Acknowledgment

This research was supported by grants from the Minnesota Heart Association and NIH (HL 17443) to Dr. Grabowski.

References

Begent, N., and Born, G. V. R., 1970, Growth rate *in vivo* of platelet thrombi, produced by iontophoresis of ADP, as a function of mean flow velocity, *Nature (London)* **227**:926.

Grabowski, E., Herther, K. K., and Didisheim, P., 1974, Platelet aggregation quantified in an *ex vivo* chamber by means of videodensitometry, in: *Platelets, Thrombosis and Inhibitors* (P. Didisheim, T. Shimamoto, and H. Yamazaki, eds.), pp. 127–134, F. K. Schattauer Verlag, Stuttgart.

Grabowski, E. F., 1976, Platelet aggregation in flowing blood *in vitro*. I. Production by controlled ADP convective diffusion and quantification by videodensitometry, *Microvasc. Res.*, submitted for publication.

6.6. Effects of Agar on Platelet Aggregation

GILBERT E. HERMAN and RAYMOND L. HENRY

Two principles mediating platelet aggregation *ex vivo* were noted from investigations on extracts drawn from *Pseudomonas aeruginosa* cultures on media containing Bacto-Agar (Difco Laboratories, Detroit, Michigan). One activity was specifically related to bacterial products within the media, while the other was related to the media. These findings prompted us to investigate further the character of the media. Platelet aggregating activity was found to be due to the Bacto-Agar component of the media.

Agar gels (1.5% in distilled water) were resolubilized by the freeze–thaw method. Particulate matter was first removed by syneresis with cheesecloth, filtered through glass Gelman type E prefilter pads with syringe, and finally filtered through a 0.2-μm metrical type GA-8 membrane. Material collected was stored at 4°C and was stable for at least 3 months.

Carbohydrate content of prepared agar extract, determined by the orcinol reaction, was 2.366 mg/ml. Platelet aggregometry was performed using standard methods suggested by Mustard. Agar (100 μl) was added to citrated platelet-rich plasma (400 μl) adjusted to 200,000 platelets/mm^3. Agar irreversibly aggregated human and dog platelets. Aggregation was inhibited by increasing concentrations of EDTA, indicating a divalent cation-depending surface interaction (see Fig. 1). EDTA also inhibited ADP aggregation, as noted by Marcus and Zucker (1965); however, lag time was not increased and slope at time of one-half maximum aggregation was not significantly altered (see Fig. 1). Neither dialysis nor autoclaving interfered with aggregating ability of agar. Thus ions inherent in agar and tertiary structure could not account for aggregating effects. Partial thromboplastin times and prothrombin times were not altered by agar on either human or dog plasma. Effects of agar on platelet aggregation are not likely due to effects on blood enzymology. Caution should be exercised when evaluating platelet-aggregating effects suspected to be mediated by agents from bacteria grown on agar culture.

References

Marcus, A. J., and Zucker, M. B., 1965, *Physiology of Blood Platelets,* p. 50, Grune and Stratton, New York.

Mustard, J. F., *Chrono-Log Procedural Manual,* Chrono-Log Corp., Broomall, Pa.

GILBERT E. HERMAN and RAYMOND L. HENRY · Wayne State University School of Medicine, Detroit, Michigan.

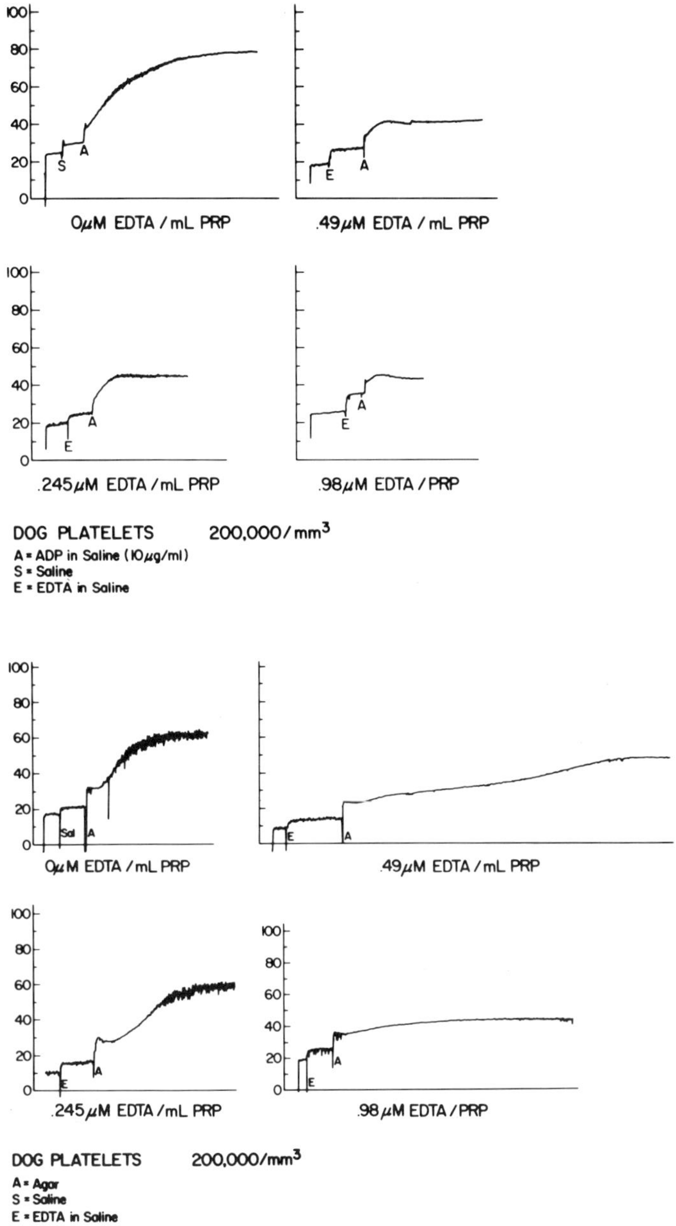

Figure 1. Effects of EDTA on platelet aggregation. Top: ADP-mediated aggregation. Bottom: Agar-mediated aggregation. Note decreased slope and increased lag phase with progressive EDTA inhibition of agar-mediated aggregation.

6.7. Effects of pH and P_{CO_2} on ADP-Induced Platelet Sphering and Aggregation for Human and Rabbit Citrated Platelet-Rich Plasma

S. S. TANG, R. PANJWANI, and M. M. FROJMOVIC

There are large changes in pH, P_{CO_2}, and P_{O_2} of human and rabbit citrated platelet-rich plasma preparations at 37°C during processing and storage of the samples in air in tightly closed tubes. These parameters were measured with the 3M5-3MK2 blood microsystem (Radiometer, Copenhagen). All these changes occurred most rapidly for samples kept in closed tubes vs. open tubes; P_{O_2} equilibrated toward atmospheric P_{O_2}, while P_{CO_2} and pH changed in parallel. The pH generally rose to 7.8 ± 0.2 between 1 and 3 h after bleeding, and the P_{CO_2} decreased in parallel to 10–20 mm Hg. In order to control these changes, we have used a simple gas incubation method (Rogers, 1972) to keep constant P_{CO_2} and pH. Physiologically normal P_{CO_2} (~35 mm Hg) and pH (~7.45) gave reduction in primary (P) and secondary (S) aggregation induced by 20 μM serotonin and in P aggregation induced by 7 μM epinephrine as compared to low P_{CO_2} (~18.3 mm Hg) and high pH (~7.74) conditions. However, ADP-induced P and S aggregation were insensitive to these pH, P_{CO_2} changes. These results indicate that the P_{CO_2} and pH do not alter the intrinsic P and S aggregation mechanisms. Moreover, ADP- and serotonin-induced sphering was unaltered. We could rule out the possibility that P_{CO_2} and pH altered the binding of drugs to the specific disced-platelet receptors (Born, 1970) or reduced the sensitivity of receptors to drugs, leading to sphering. Decreasing the plasma calcium level by increasing the concentrations of sodium citrate can lead to clear inhibition of the aggregation to ADP when normal P_{CO_2}, pH and low P_{CO_2}, high pH are compared. It is suggested that the selective action of P_{CO_2} and pH might result from an influence on the specific transmission process between the receptors and the mechanisms of P and S aggregation through changes in the level of bound calcium (Mongar and Schild, 1958). This process may have different thresholds affecting the P and S aggregations for various agents.

S. S. TANG, R. PANJWANI, and M. M. FROJMOVIC · McGill University, Montreal, Quebec, Canada.

References

Born, G. V. R., 1970, Observations on the change in shape of blood platelets brought about by adenosine diphosphate, *J. Physiol. (London)* **209:**487.

Mongar, J. L., and Schild, H. O., 1958, The effect of calcium and pH on the anaphylactic reaction, *J. Physiol. (London)* **140:**272.

Rogers, A. B., 1972, The effect of pH on human platelet aggregation induced by epinephrine and ADP, *Proc. Soc. Exp. Biol. Med.* **139:**1100.

6.8. Effect of a New Potent Inhibitor of Platelet Aggregation (BL-3459) on Experimental Thrombosis

J. S. FLEMING and J. P. BUYNISKI

The present need for a clinically useful inhibitor of arterial thrombosis is well recognized, and after many years of experience with the anticoagulants we are aware of the need for a more effective form of therapy (Weiss, 1974). A number of compounds have recently been investigated for their effects on platelet aggregation and thrombosis. However, most of these, such as aspirin, dipyridamole, and sulfinpyrazone, are agents actually on the market for other purposes and have demonstrated variable and often inconsistent activity (Vermylen *et al.,* 1973).

6-Methyl-1,2,3,5-tetrahydroimidazo[2,1-b]quinazolin-2-one hydrochloride monohydrate (BL-3459)

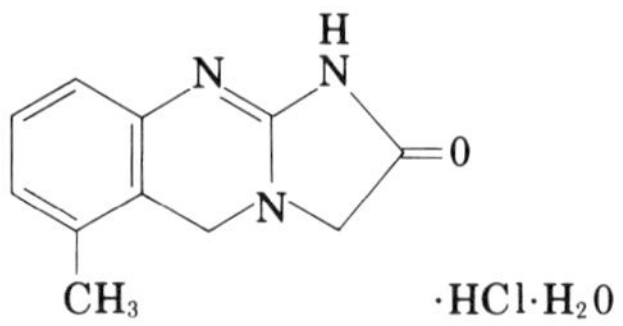

is a new potent inhibitor of platelet aggregation which has proven to be particularly effective in *in vivo* animal models of thrombosis (Fleming *et al.,* 1975). BL-3459 inhibited platelet aggregation induced *in vitro* by a variety of agents including ADP in platelet-rich plasma obtained from various species at concentrations in the range of 0.4–4 μM. This activity carried over to the *ex vivo* situation, and the compound demonstrated impressive activity in various *in vivo* animal models of thrombosis following oral dosing in the range of 0.5–10 mg/kg. *In vivo* models employed included laser-induced thrombosis in dogs, endotoxin shock in rats, hemorrhagic shock in dogs, and epinephrine-induced myocardial necrosis in dogs. BL-3459 was rapidly absorbed following oral administration and had a pharmacological half-life of 13.4 h in rats. In contrast to aspirin, BL-3459

J. S. FLEMING and J. P. BUYNISKI · Department of Pharmacology, Bristol Laboratories, Division of Bristol Myers Company, Syracuse, New York.

Table I. Comparison of BL-3459 to Aspirin, Dipyridamole, and Sulfinpyrazone in Various *in Vitro*, *ex Vivo*, and *in Vivo* Experimental Systems

	Aggregometry—rabbit PRP				*In vivo* animal model ED_{50}'s (mg/kg)		
	In vitro EC_{50} (μg/ml)		*Ex vivo* ED_{50} (mg/kg i.p.)				
Compound	ADP	Collagen	ADP	Collagen	Rabbit biolaser thrombosis	Dog electrical thrombosis	Rat endotoxin shock
Aspirin	>512	7	>100	3	>60 i.v.	50 p.o.	>256 p.o.
Dipyridamole	>512	245	>100	>100	>60 i.v.	>35 i.p.	>256 p.o.
Sulfinpyrazone	>512	62	>100	3	>60 i.v.	>100 p.o.	>128 p.o.
BL-3459	0.4	0.09	0.4	0.1	12 p.o.	1 p.o.	10 p.o.

had little effect on bleeding time in guinea pigs. In addition, the compound lowered aortic blood pressure, stroke volume, and peripheral vascular resistance and elevated cardiac rate and cardiac contractile force in dogs following oral and intraduodenal administration. Separation of platelet effects from cardiovascular effects was possible by selection of the proper dosing regimen. Although the precise mechanism of action of BL-3459 has not been determined, an agent possessing this type of pharmacological profile (Table I) may prove particularly interesting as a candidate for clinical evaluation.

References

Fleming, J. S., Buyniski, J. P., Cavanagh, R. L., and Bierwagen, M. E., 1975, Pharmacology of a potent, new antithrombotic agent, 6-methyl-1,2,3,5-tetrahydroimidazo[2,1-b]quinazolin-2-one hydrochloride monohydrate (BL-3459), *J. Pharmacol. Exp. Ther.* **194:**435.

Vermylen, J., deGaetano, G., and Verstraete, M., 1973, Platelets and thrombosis, in: *Recent Advances in Thrombosis* (L. Poller, ed.), pp. 113–150, Churchill Livingstone, London.

Weiss, J., 1974, Inhibition of platelet induced thrombus formation, *Schweiz. Med. Wochenschr.* **104:**114.

6.9. Hematological Effects of a Splenic Extract

C. R. SPILLERT, E. J. LAZARO, L. P. PARMER, and A. A. SCHNERRING

In a previous report from our laboratory (Lazaro *et al.,* 1975), we described the isolation of a bovine splenic extract that inhibits platelet aggregation *in vitro* and increases mouse mesenteric bleeding time. In this communication, the effects of this extract on platelet count, thrombin time, fibrinogen concentration, ADP-induced platelet aggregation, and disseminated intravascular coagulation (DIC) are detailed. Intravenous administration of 2 mg/kg of the extract into dogs (16) decreased platelet counts between 20 and 70% (average 25%) of preinjection values within 3 h. ADP-induced platelet aggregation was inhibited 10–60% (25% average) of preinjection values. Plasma thrombin time was increased 10–70% (20% average). Plasma fibrinogen concentrations were reduced up to 50% (15% average) after injection. DIC was produced in 60 Swiss white mice by *Escherichia coli* endotoxin. After 72 h, 70% of the saline controls were dead whereas only 27% of the extract-treated mice died.

The results of this study indicate the ability of this splenic extract to modify the factors which control the development of intravascular thrombosis. Of greatest consideration in this respect is the significant inhibition of ADP-induced platelet aggregation. Other parameters such as increased bleeding times and *in vitro* inhibition of ADP-induced platelet aggregation reported previously by us further substantiate this effect.

In extensive administration of this extract to various species of laboratory animals, no acute or chronic toxic effects have thus far been noted.

Previous investigators have demonstrated the role of blood platelets in the development of endotoxin-induced Shwartzman reactions, which are currently believed to be part of the pathological process of DIC. Since endotoxin aggregates platelets with the release of platelet constituents, it is reasonable to assume that alteration of platelet function and inhibition of aggregation should markedly reduce the mortality of this DIC state by lowering the incidence of intravascular thrombosis.

Reference

Lazaro, E. J., Spillert, C. R., Parmer, L. P., and Schnerring, A. A., 1975, Antiplatelet, antithrombotic effects of a splenic extract, *Fed. Proc.* **34(3)**:259.

C. R. SPILLERT, E. J. LAZARO, L. P. PARMER, and A. A. SCHNERRING · College of Medicine and Dentistry of New Jersey, New Jersey Medical School, Newark, New Jersey.

6.10. Inhibition of ADP-Induced Platelet Aggregation by Canine Spleen Alkaline Phosphatase

ROGER R. CALAM, GEORGE E. GRIGNOL, RAYMOND L. HENRY, and GENESIO MURANO

This study was conducted in an attempt to elucidate an aspect of spleen reservoir function, the prevention of irreversible aggregation of activated intrasplenic platelets. The spleen is known to give up its contents in response to stress, including the release of sequestered, viable, functional, but already activated platelets (Elgjo and Hovig, 1972; Ljingqvist, 1971; Koskins and Lee-Gunning, 1917; Toghill and Prichard, 1964). We propose that within the spleen there is a membrane-bound alkaline phosphatase capable of hydrolyzing ADP, thereby allowing sequestration of nonaggregated but activated platelets. Erythrocyte ADP (in this case, likely from leakage by senescent, fragile red cells during splenic phagocytosis) is well established as a mediator of platelet adhesiveness (Hellem, 1968). In addition, collagen induces platelet aggregation by contact within the splenic cordal system (Elgjo and Hovig, 1972; Hovig, 1963).

Alkaline phosphatase (AP: orthophosphoric monoester phosphohydrolase, E.C. 3.1.3.1) activity was extracted from canine spleen using the nonionic detergent, Triton X-100. Triton was removed from the extract with Bio-Bead SM-2 column chromatography to eliminate interference with platelet aggregation. Purification employing DEAE-cellulose chromatography resulted in a specific activity increase of 325%. Two bands of phosphatase activity were observed from the purified material using polyacrylamide gel electrophoresis. One band, designated as the "anodic band," demonstrated faster migration than the other, designated as the "cathodic band." Similarities to bone alkaline phosphatase were noted from thermal inactivation studies, while similarity to liver alkaline phosphatase was found from chemical inhibition procedures. Neither inactivation nor inhibition studies resulted in a differentiation of anodic from cathodic alkaline phosphatase.

Crude extracts of spleen alkaline phosphatase-like material were previously shown to inhibit ADP-induced platelet aggregation (Steiman and Henry, 1970). Our purified extract was also capable of *ex vivo*

ROGER R. CALAM · Saint John Hospital, Detroit, Michigan. GEORGE E. GRIGNOL, RAYMOND L. HENRY, and GENESIO MURANO · Wayne State University School of Medicine, Detroit, Michigan.

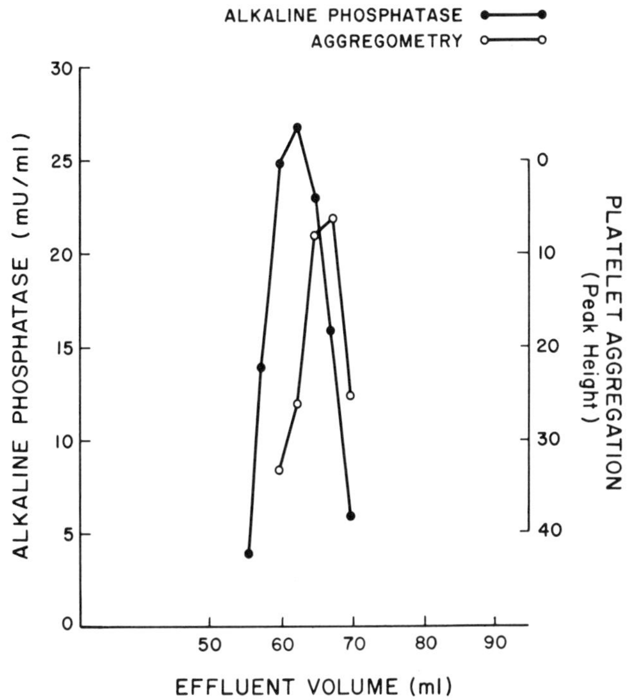

Figure 1. Graphic composite representation of alkaline phosphatase (mU/ml) and platelet aggregation (peak height) demonstrating the association between anodic phosphatase and platelet inhibitory activities.

inhibition of platelet aggregation. Both anodic and cathodic fractions had alkaline phosphatase activity, but only the anodic fraction inhibited ADP-mediated platelet aggregation (Fig. 1). These findings direct us to investigate *in vivo* actions of splenic alkaline phosphatase in relation to splenic platelet sequestration function.

ACKNOWLEDGMENT

This work was supported in part by the Michigan Heart Association.

References

Elgjo, R. F., and Hovig, T., 1972, Ultrastructural studies of platelet activation and aggregation in normal spleen from different species, *Scand. J. Haematol.* **9:**587.

Hellem, A. J., 1968, Platelet adhesiveness, *Ser. Haematol.* **1:**99.

Hoskins, R. G., and Lee-Gunning, R. E., 1917, The effects of adrenin on the distribution of the blood volume changes and venous discharge in the spleen, *Am. J. Physiol.* **43:**298.

Hovig, T., 1963, Aggregation of rabbit blood platelets produced *in vitro* by saline extract of tendon, *Thromb. Diath. Haemorrh.* **9:**248.

Ljingqvist, L., 1971, Properties of splenic vein platelets in the dog, *Acta Chir. Scand.* **137:**103.

Steiman, R. H., and Henry, R. L., 1970, Effects of splenic extracts on platelet aggregation, in: *Proceedings of the Eighteenth Annual Symposium on Blood: Platelet Adhesion and Aggregation in Thrombosis: Countermeasures* (E. F. Mammen and F. K. Schattauer, eds.), p. 365, Verlag-Stuttgart.

Toghill, P. J., and Prichard, B. N. C., 1964, A study of the action of noradrenaline on the splenic cell pool, *Clin. Sci.* **26:**203.

6.11. Effect of Diflunisal, a Novel Salicylate, on Platelet Function and Blood Coagulation

C. T. SMIT SIBINGA, K. F. TEMPERO, and G. O. BREAULT

The use of analgesic drugs is limited by bleeding tendencies. Salicylate and particularly the acetylated compounds have a definite effect on platelet function (O'Brien, 1968; Zucker and Peterson, 1970). We studied a new analgesic, diflunisal (2′4′-difluoro-4-hydroxy-1′1,-diphenyl-3-carboxylic acid), on platelet function and blood coagulation in volunteers. The drug was double-blind tested in 20 healthy males, randomly assigned to diflunisal and placebo groups.

6.11.1. Methods

Test systems were Hb, mH, blood glucose, platelet counts, bleeding time, ADP and collagen platelet aggregation (Born, 1962), PT, PTT, thrombin time, fibrinogen, antithrombin III, clot lysis, serum FDP, and diflunisal blood levels. Paired-*t* and covariance tests were computed.

The study design was as follows:

1. Acute single-dose trial: 250 mg diflunisal or placebo orally on day 1. Tests were monitored before and 4 and 8 h after administration and further in the fasting state at days 2, 4, 8, 10, and 12.
2. Chronic multiple-dose trial: 250 mg diflunisal or placebo b.i.d. orally from day 15 to day 21. The same tests were monitored before and 4 and 8 h after administration on day 15, and in the fasting state on days 16, 18, 21, 25, 29, 31, and 33.

6.11.2. Results

In both groups, age and weight ranges were equal. All plain samples for drug analysis exhibited normal background fluorescence. Diflunisal blood levels rose to a mean of 24 μg/ml after a single dose of 250 mg and reached a constant mean level of 37 μg/ml after chronic administration of 250 mg b.i.d. for 1 wk.

At day 4 in the single-dose study and day 25 in the multiple-dose

C. T. SMIT SIBINGA · Coagulation Laboratory, Department of Internal Medicine, University of Groningen, Groningen, the Netherlands. K. F. TEMPERO · Merck Sharp & Dohme Research Laboratories, Rahway, New Jersey. G. O. BREAULT · Merck Institute for Therapeutic Research, West Point, Pennsylvania.

study, diflunisal levels had decreased to background activity. Fasting blood glucose levels showed no differences between groups.

Bleeding time and platelet function as well as fibrin formation and fibrinolysis showed no significant change in either the acute or chronic trial as compared to the control.

References

Born, G. V. R., 1962, Aggregation of blood platelets by adenosine diphosphate and its reversal, *Nature (London)* **194:**927.

O'Brien, J. R., 1968, Effect of anti-inflammatory agents on platelets, *Lancet* **i:**894.

Zucker, M. B., and Peterson, J., 1970, Effect of acetylsalicylic acid, other nonsteroidal anti-inflammatory agents, and dipyridamole on human blood platelets, *J. Lab. Clin. Med.* **76:**66.

6.12. Polyphloretin Phosphate, an Inhibitor of Platelet Function

J. SWEDENBORG, H. LAGERGREN, P. OLSSON, and L. SCHALIN

Polyphloretin phosphate (PPP), a polyester of phloretin and phosphoric acid, was tested as an inhibitor of platelet function. The substance had earlier been reported to inhibit several enzymes (Diczfalusy *et al.,* 1953) and also to inhibit prostaglandins. The former effect is located among the larger molecules of the compound together with a weak heparinlike activity. The latter effect is located among the small molecules of the polymer (Eakins, 1971).

PPP inhibited the platelet aggregation and subsequent fall of platelet count induced by intravenous infusions of thrombin but did not inhibit the fall of fibrinogen (Swedenborg, 1974). This effect on the platelets was not due to the heparinlike activity since the compound was equally effective in inhibiting platelet aggregation induced by protamine. Aggregation induced by protamine *in vivo* is not inhibited by heparin.

PPP was also tested as an inhibitor of adhesion. Specially designed arteriovenous shunts were placed between the femoral artery and vein in dogs whose platelets had previously been labeled with ^{51}Cr. The dogs were defibrinogenated with defibrase in order to eliminate the influence of fibrin formation. PPP reduced the uptake of platelets on the shunts to less than 5% of the initial value (Swedenborg *et al.,* 1974). This effect was not linked to its heparinlike activity. Even in animals with a normal fibrinogen level, the effect was the same but the dosage had to be increased. PPP was also compared to dipyridamole and acetylsalicylic acid. The latter two substances reduced the platelet uptake considerably less (50–65%).

References

Diczfalusy, E., Fernö, O., Fex, H., Högberg, B., Linderot, T., and Rosenberg, T., 1953, Synthetic high molecular weight enzyme inhibitors. I. Polymeric phosphates of phloretin and related compounds, *Acta Chem. Scand.* **7**:913.

Eakins, K., 1971, Prostaglandin antagonism by polymeric phosphates of phloretin and related compounds, *Ann. N.Y. Acad. Sci.* **18**:386.

Swedenborg, J., 1974, Inhibitory effect of polyphloretinphosphate upon platelet aggregation and hemodynamic and respiratory changes caused by protamine and thrombin, *J. Pharmacol. Exp. Ther.* **188**:214.

Swedenborg, J., Olsson, P., and Lagergren, H., 1974, Polyphloretinphosphate, an antithrombogenic substance which inhibits platelet adhesion, *Thromb. Res.* **4**:687.

J. SWEDENBORG, H. LAGERGREN, P. OLSSON, and L. SCHALIN · Surgical Research Laboratory, Thoracic Clinics, Karolinska Sjukhuset, Stockholm, Sweden.

6.13. Platelet Aggregation and Particulate Microembolization during Cardiac Operations

R. THOMAS SOLIS, PETER S. KENNEDY, and MICHAEL E. DeBAKEY

Aggregation and microembolization of platelets may cause pulmonary, cerebral, and hemostatic complications after heart operations (Kendall and Lowenstein, 1962; Swank and Porter, 1963; Allardyce *et al.,* 1966). In the present study, we used an electronic particle size analyzer to compare the effects of membrane and bubble oxygenators on particulate microembolization and platelet function during cardiopulmonary bypass.

6.13.1. Method

The total volume of microemboli in venous, arterial, and cardiotomy reservoir blood and that of platelet aggregates 13–80 μm in diameter induced *in vitro* in the blood of patients undergoing cardiac operations were measured as previously described (Solis *et al.,* 1974, 1975).

6.13.2. Results

There was a small but significant ($p < 0.05$) increase in the total volume of microemboli in blood on passage through a bubble oxygenator (Travenol Laboratories, Morton Grove, Illinois) which was not noted with microporous membrane (Travenol Laboratories) oxygenation. However, the volume of microemboli in extravasated blood collected through the coronary suction system was markedly increased, did not differ in membrane and in bubble oxygenator patients, and was similar to the volume of platelet aggregates that could be induced *in vitro* in the patients' arterial blood. The percent by volume of these microemboli that remained in cardiotomy reservoir blood after passage through five different in-line blood filters was as follows: 40-μm pore mesh (Ultipore, Pall Corporation, Glencove, New York), 39 ± 5%; polyurethane foam (PF427, Bentley Laboratories, Santa Ana, California), 39 ± 5%; 25-μm pore mesh (Ultipore), 33 ± 4%; dacron wool (CA 100, Cardiotomy Blood Filter, Pioneer Laboratories, Hillsboro, Oregon), 10 ± 10%; and woven fabric

R. THOMAS SOLIS and PETER S. KENNEDY · Department of Medicine, Baylor College of Medicine, Houston, Texas. MICHAEL E. DeBAKEY · Department of Surgery, Baylor College of Medicine, Houston, Texas.

(Intersept, Johnson and Johnson, New Brunswick, New Jersey) 8 ± 5% (mean ± SD, n = 10).

A comparable degree of thrombocytopenia developed with the two oxygenators; however, the total volume and mean size of platelet aggregates induced *in vitro* by ADP (0.2 μmol) after membrane oxygenation (1.19 < 0.11 × 10^6 $\mu m^3/mm^3$ and 10.0 ± 1.7 × 10^3 μm^3, respectively) were significantly greater than after bubble oxygenation (0.65 ± 0.10 × 10^6 and 4.5 ± 0.7 × 10^3, $n = 20, p < 0.001$).

6.13.3. Discussion

This study shows that use of a membrane oxygenator reduces particulate microembolization and preserves platelet function when compared to a bubble oxygenator. However, a large volume of microemboli continue to be generated in coronary suction blood, indicating the continued need for effective blood filters within the cardiotomy system.

References

Allardyce, D. B., Yoshida, S. H., and Ashmore, P. G., 1966, The importance of microembolism in the pathogenesis of organ dysfunction caused by prolonged use of the pump oxygenator, *J. Thorac. Cardiovasc. Surg.* **52**:706.

Kendall, A. G., and Lowenstein, L., 1962, Alterations in blood coagulation and hemostasis during extracorporeal circulation (Part I), *Can. Med. Assoc. J.* **87**:786.

Solis, R. T., Noon, G. P., Beall, A. C., Jr., and DeBakey, M. E., 1974, Particulate microembolization during cardiac operation, *Ann. Throac. Surg.* **17**:332.

Solis, R. T., Beall, A. C., Jr., Noon, G. P., and DeBakey, M. E., 1975, Platelet aggregation: Effects of cardiopulmonary bypass, *Chest* **67**:558.

Swank, R. L., and Porter, G. A., 1963, Dissappearance of micro-emboli transfused into patients during cardiopulmonary bypass, *Transfusion* **3**:192.

6.14. Growth Patterns of Platelet Thrombi and Their Relationship to Microemboli

MICHAEL M. CHEN, M. B. STEMERMAN, T. H. SPAET, and RICHARD K. BLAISDELL

Theoretical analyses and *in vivo* and *in vitro* experimental evidence are presented concerning the dynamics of platelet thrombus formation. In acute thrombus formation processes, the thrombogenicity of the surface—whether it consists of an exposed connective tissue or the surface of a rapidly growing aggregate of activated platelets—is usually so high that the dominant process limiting the rate of growth of the thrombus is platelet transport. Under such circumstances, the surface of the thrombus has a natural tendency to become uneven and wavy, even leading somtimes to the formation of fingerlike projections, as shown in Fig. 1. This tendency is the consequence of a self-amplifying process, first discussed by Petschek and Weiss (1970) in a different context, which is initiated by natural nonuniformities in early platelet adhesion. Subsequent platelet aggregation on the adherent layer tends to favor the high spots at the expense of the recessed low spots, which are less accessible to the circulating platelets. This process continuously amplifies the nonuniformities, thus resulting in an uneven profile. Theoretical analyses based on the convective–diffusive equations of platelet transport (Chen, 1974) suggest that the predominant wavelength of such irregularities should be in the 30–300 μm range. Such wavy profiles can be seen distinctly on *in vivo* thrombi formed on rabbit subendothelium upon exposure to whole blood after balloon de-endotheliation, as seen in Fig. la (see Stemerman, 1973). Similar patterns are seen on *in vitro* thrombi (Fig. 1b) formed on rabbit adventitia rotated in heparinized blood (see Blaisdell *et al.*, 1974). It is suggested that as the growth of the wavy projections continues they will become fragile and will embolize under the hemodynamic forces. A study of the process might then shed light on the conditions of formation and size distribution of the resulting microemboli.

MICHAEL M. CHEN · University of Illinois at Urbana-Champaign, Urbana, Illinois. M. B. STEMERMAN and T. H. SPAET · Montefiore Hospital and Medical Center and Albert Einstein College of Medicine, Bronx, New York. RICHARD K. BLAISDELL · University of Hawaii, Honolulu, Hawaii.

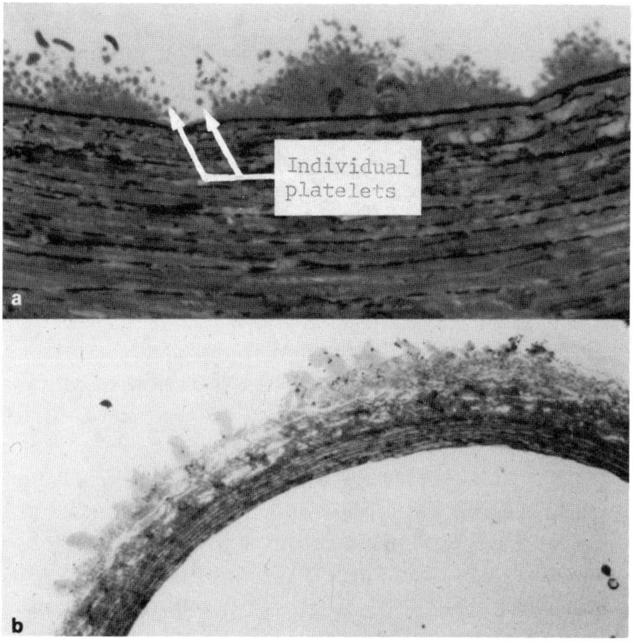

Figure 1. Growth of mural thrombi. (a) Wavy formations on *in vivo* thrombi on rabbit aorta after balloon de-endotheliation. (b) *In vitro* thrombi on rabbit adventitia rotated in heparinized blood. Note that the waves have developed into prominent projections.

References

Blaisdell, R. K., Stemerman, M. B., Chen, M. M., and Spaet, T. H., 1974, A new *in vitro* method for measuring platelet deposition on the vessel surface, *Thromb Diath. Haemorrh. Suppl.* **60:**35.

Chen, M. M., 1974, On the continuum formulation of platelet and related transport pertaining to thrombogenesis, Paper presented at the American Institute of Chemical Engineering 77th National Meeting, June 2–5, Pittsburgh, Pa.

Petschek, H. E., and Weiss, R. F., 1970, Hydrodynamic problems of blood coagulation, AIAA Aerospace Sciences Meeting, January, New York, Paper No. 70-787.

Stemerman, M. B., 1973, Thrombogenesis of the rabbit arterial plaque: An electron microscopic study, *Am. J. Pathol.* **73:**7.

6.15. Effect of Hormonal Contraceptives on Electrically Induced Thrombosis Times in Rats

GRAZYNA SCHWAN, DOUGLAS NEIMAND, NARAYANAN RAMASAMY, and PHILIP N. SAWYER

Hormonal contraceptives have been implicated in the etiology of thromboembolism and stroke in women (Dugdale and Masi, 1971; Group Study for Stroke, 1973). We have determined the *in vivo* thrombotic effects of several hormonal steroids and the protective action of vitamin C in the intact cardiovascular system of rats. The technique of current-induced occlusion times of rat mesenteric vessels was employed (Sawyer *et al.*, 1960; Aaron *et al.*, 1970). The hormones were administered orally (except Depo-Provera) for 2 wk at 10 times the human dose to a group of adult male and female rats. The following hormonal steroids were studied: (1) ethynodiol diacetate, (2) norgestrel, (3) Depo-Provera (Upjohn), medroxyprogesterone acetate, (4) Ovral (Wyeth), a combination of norgestrel and ethynyl estradiol, (5) Demulen (Searle), a combination of ethynyl estradiol and ethynodiol diacetate, (6) a combination of mestranol and norethindrone, and (7) mestranol, norethindrone, and vitamine C. The results were compared with those for controls (no drug) and rats on vitamin C. Ovral was given to a group of adult male rats, also. Depo-Provera was administered as a single intramuscular dose and occlusion times were determined at 3 and 7 days after the injection. The times for complete occlusion of the rat mesenteric vessels in all these cases are shown in Table I.

The study shows that all contraceptive hormonal steroids, irrespective of the type, whether estrogenic or progestational or combination of both, significantly accelerate current-induced thrombosis in female rats. Male rats appear to be unaffected by these agents. Depo-Provera has a marked prothrombotic effect in the cardiovascular system of rats only within the first few days of administration. The protective effect of vitamin C is clearly evident, as it reverses the pernicious thrombogenic effects induced by the steroidal hormones in rats.

GRAZYNA, SCHWAN, DOUGLAS NEIMAND, NARAYANAN RAMASAMY, and PHILIP N. SAWYER · Electrochemical and Biophysical Laboratories of the Vascular Surgical Services, Departments of Surgery and Surgical Research, State University of New York, Downstate Medical Center, Brooklyn, New York.

Table I. Effect of Hormonal Contraceptives on Thrombosis in Rats

Drug[a]	Number of rats	Duration of treatment (days)	Occlusion time (min) (mean ± DS)	p (less than)
Control[b]	7	14	47.9 ± 2.7	—
Ethynodiol diacetate	5	14	28.2 ± 7.8	0.005
Norgestrel	6	14	15.5 ± 3.0	0.005
Depo-Provera[c]	7	3	29.1 ± 11.3	0.005
	8	7	36.4 ± 9.7	0.05
Demulen	8	14	28.6 ± 7.5	0.005
Ovral	6	14	27.5 ± 4.3	0.005
Ovral[d]	5	14	47.1 ± 9.1	0.15
Mestranol (M) and norethindrone (N)	5	7	27.0 ± 7.6	0.005
M + N + vitamin C	9	7	106.7 ± 23.8	0.005
Vitamin C[b]	7	3	118.6 ± 19.9	0.005

[a] All the contraceptive steroids were given orally at 10 times the normal human dose per unit body weight. Adult female rats were used.
[b] Adult male and female rats were used.
[c] Single intramuscular injection. Determinations were carried out 3 and 7 days after the injection.
[d] Adult male rats were used.

Acknowledgments

The authors thank the National Institute of Health (Grant No. HL 15123) and the Sawyer Foundation for research support.

References

Aaron, R. K., Srinivasan, S., Burrowes, C. B., and Sawyer, P. N., 1970, Effects of chemical compounds upon current induced thrombosis in rat mesenteric vessels, *Thromb. Diath. Haemorrh.* **23:**621.

Dugdale, M., and Masi, A. T., 1971, Hormonal contraception and thromboembolic disease: Effects of oral contraceptives on hemostatic mechanisms—a review of the literature, *J. Chronic. Dis.* **23:**775.

Group Study for Stroke, 1973, Oral contraceptives and increased risk of cerebral ischemia and thrombosis, *N. Engl. J. Med.* **288:**871.

Sawyer, P. N., Suckling, E. E., and Wesolowski, S. A., 1960, Effects of small electric currents on intravascular thrombosis in the visualized rat mesentery, *Am. J. Physiol.* **198:**1006.

6.16. Interaction between Platelet Thrombi and the Vessel Wall

MARY P. WIEDEMAN and RONALD F. TUMA

The fact that platelets will adhere to the wall of a blood vessel in certain specific conditions has been well documented since it was first described over 100 years ago, but the reason for the adherence has not been discovered.

It has previously been reported that a sequence to adherence of a platelet aggregate is the appearance of platelets rolling along the vessel wall upstream, extending farther upstream with time (Wiedeman, 1974). A study was made to determine the extent of the adherence of platelets upstream and the time course. In 27 trials using bat wing vessels in eight animals, platelet aggregates were produced with a beam from a single-pulse ruby red laser. Initially, a platelet aggregate is formed by the adherence of platelets to a cluster of heat-coagulated red blood cells stuck to the vessel wall. After a delay of about 10 s, platelets become visible

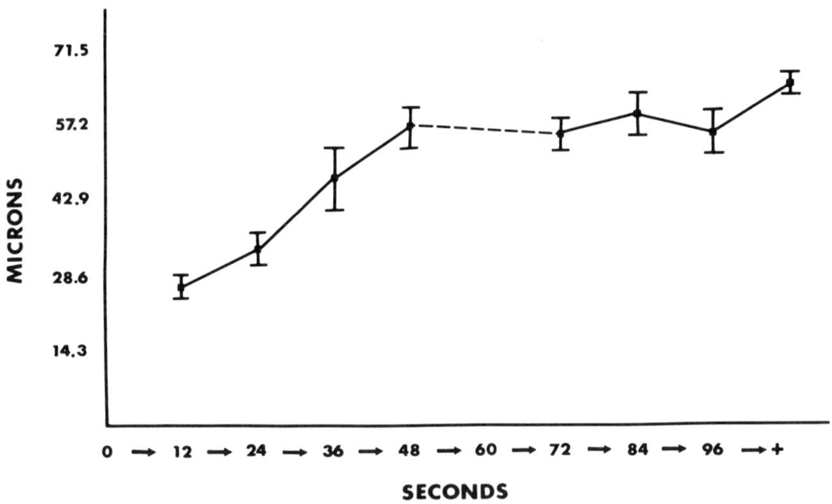

Figure 1. Relationship between appearance of upstream platelets and time after initial platelet aggregate.

MARY P. WIEDEMAN and RONALD F. TUMA · Department of Physiology, Temple University School of Medicine, Philadelphia, Pennsylvania.

rolling along the wall of the vessel approximately 26.3 μm upstream. Within the next 30 s, this distance has increased to 39.9 μm, which remains the upper limit for about 5 min. However, within the next 1 or 2 h, the distance upstream that platelets are visible on the vessel wall has increased to 57.2 μm. The data are shown in Fig. 1.

Two possible explanations can be given for the extension of upstream adherence to the vessel wall with time as well as for the attraction of platelets to a site of injury in a distal branch of the parent vessel. One, the mechanism for developing adhesiveness is dependent on stimulus strength, so a subliminal stimulus would require a longer development time. Alternately, platelet mass may generate a wall change that affects the next adjacent wall area and so progresses from the initial site.

ACKNOWLEDGMENT

This work was supported in part by SCOR. Thrombosis HL-14217-04.

Reference

Wiedeman, M. P., 1974, Vascular reactions to laser *in vivo, Microvasc. Res.* **8:**132.

6.17. Platelet and Fibrinogen Preservation in Intraoperative Autotransfusion

W. WALL, R. O. HEIMBECKER. F. N. McKENZIE, A. ROBERT, and R. BARR

Salvage and reinfusion of blood lost during vascular surgery have been used successfully (Brener *et al.,* 1973; Duncan *et al.,* 1974; Pilon *et al.,* 1973). Although the procedure has many potential advantages over homologous transfusion, a paucity of information exists on the changes occurring in blood salvaged during surgery and in the recipients after its infusion (Aaron *et al.,* 1974; Brener *et al.,* 1973).

Hematological and coagulation parameters were studied in six patients receiving an average of 17,700 ml intraoperative autotransfusion during major vascular surgery (four abdominal and two thoracic cases). The patients were systematically heparinized during operation. The autotransfusion unit was a modification of the cardiotomy suction used in open heart surgery. No patient received donor blood or blood products during operation or while the coagulation studies were carried out postoperatively. Therefore, any changes could be attributed to autotransfusion alone. Table I shows the values in samples of autotransfused blood. The hemoglobin was slightly below normal. Mean platelet counts and fibrinogen levels were normal in autotransfused blood and in the patients postoperatively. No bleeding tendencies occurred, and the coagulograms measured postoperatively were normal in all patients. No patient suffered any complication that could be attributed to autotransfusion. Donor blood transfusion was avoided in five of the six cases by salvage and reinfusion of shed blood. The average hemoglobin at the time of discharge was 11.0 g%. Using our technique and systemic anticoagulation, intraoperative autotransfusion was safe and economical, and dramatically reduced donor blood requirements in vascular operations.

ACKNOWLEDGMENTS

This work was supported in part by the Ontario Heart Foundation, the Bickell Foundations, the Nelson Hyland Foundation, and the Medical Research Council of Canada.

W. WALL, R. O. HEIMBECKER, F. N. McKENZIE, A. ROBERT, and R. BARR
Department of Cardiovascular and Thoracic Surgery, University Hospital, University of Western Ontario, London, Ontario, Canada.

Table I. Hematological and Coagulation Parameters

	Autotransfused blood		
	Mean	Range	n^a
Hb (g%)	11.5	10.3–14.2	10
WBC (mm^3)	7,400	5,100–12,700	10
Platelets (mm^3)	156.000	94–210,000	5
Plasma Hb (mg%)	256	29–840	9
Fibrinogen (mg%)	257	165–325	9
FDPs (μg/ml)	40–160	40–160	3
Euglobulin clot lysis (min)	90	90	10

[a] Number of determinations.

References

Aaron, R. K., Beazley, R. M., and Riggle, G. C., 1974, Hematologic integrity after intraoperative autotransfusion: Comparison with bank blood, *Arch. Surg.* **108:**831.

Brener, B. J., Raines, J. K., and Darling, R. C., 1973, Intraoperative autotransfusion in abdonimal aortic resections, *Arch. Surg.* **107:**78.

Duncan, S. E., Klebanoff, G., and Rogers, W., 1974, Patient experience with intraoperative autotransfusion, *Rev. Surg.* **31:**121.

Pilon, R. N., Cough, N. P., and Brown, W. J., 1973, Autotransfusion with a renal allograft: A case report, *Anesth. Analg. (Cleveland)* **53:**403.

Wall, W., Heimbecker, R. O., Robert, A., and Barr, R., 1976, Intraoperative autotransfusion in major elective vascular surgery: A clinical assessment, *Surgery* **79:**82.

6.18. Effect of Gliclazide on Irradiation-Induced Experimental Atheromatosis

C. T. SMIT SIBINGA and R. A. WIERINGA

Gliclazide (Diamicron) is a new oral antidiabetic drug (Malaisse and Leclercq-Meyer, 1972). A sulfonylurea molecule is endocyclically linked to a nitrogen-containing heterocyclic group. The drug seems to have a protective effect against diabetic angiopathy. Animal experiments disclosed a favorable preventive effect in experimentally induced obstruction of the rat mesenterical microcirculation. Barre *et al.* (1975) reported a favorable effect of gliclazide in a control retinopathy study of 261 diabetic patients: significantly more improvement and significantly less increase in retinopathy were found as compared to the controls. In this study, gliclazide, compared to glibenclamide and a control, was tested for a protective effect on X-ray-induced atheromatosis in the rabbit carotid artery (Smit Sibinga, 1973).

6.18.1. Model

Rabbits were fed a 0.5% cholesterol diet, irradiated 1 wk later on one carotid artery (2000 R single dose, the nonirradiated carotid artery being the control), kept on the diet for another 4 wk, and then killed for histological examination of the carotid arteries. Blood for cholesterol and glucose examination was drawn in a fasting state at the start, before irradiation and sacrifice. Gliclazide dosages were 25 mg/kg and 15 mg/kg body weight daily mixed with the food; the glibenclamide dosage was 0.07 mg/kg.

6.18.2. Results

1. Control: In the presence of markedly elevated serum cholesterol levels, the irradiated carotid arteries showed clear evidence of atheromatosis (Fig. 1). The nonirradiated control arteries were completely normal.
2. Glibenclamide: The irradiated carotid arteries showed intimal and medial infiltrations of lipid with foam cells. The nonirradiated

C. T. SMIT SIBINGA · Coagulation Laboratory, Department of Internal Medicine, University of Groningen, Groningen, the Netherlands. R. A. WIERINGA · Department of Radiopathology, University of Groningen, Groningen, the Netherlands.

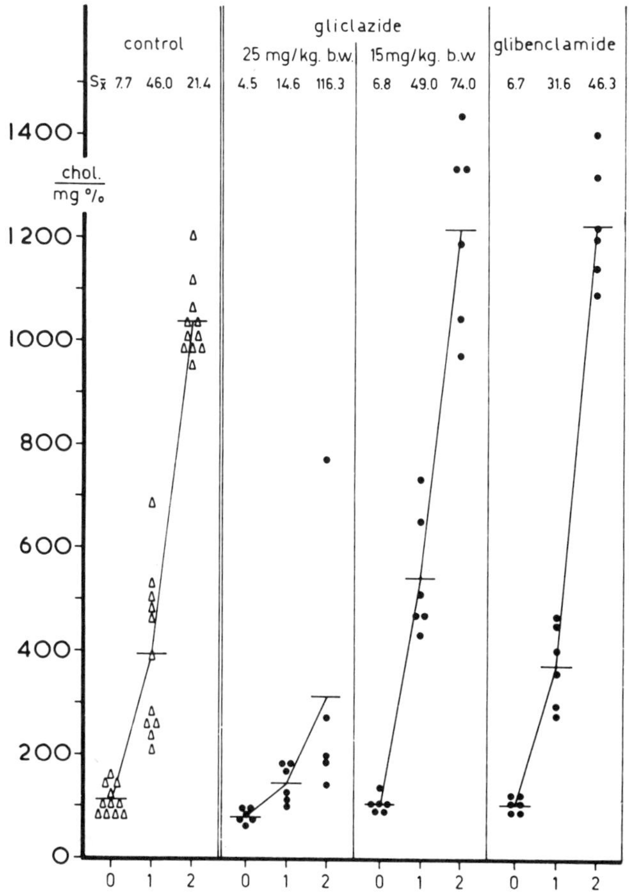

Figure 1. Individual and mean cholesterol levels in the various groups. Abscissa: 0, start; 1, irradiation; 2, sacrifice.

control arteries were normal. Serum cholesterol levels were markedly elevated.

3. Gliclazide: Both the 25 mg/kg and 15 mg/kg treated groups showed no signs of lipid infiltration or deposition, despite marked elevations in serum cholesterol in the 15 mg/kg group and slight but distinct elevations in the 25 mg/kg group.

6.18.3. Conclusion

Gliclazide, in the dosages used, has a preventive effect on infiltration and deposition of lipid in irradiation-damaged vessel walls.

References

Barre, Y., Canivet, J., Deuil, R., Foucquier, E., Molinier, A., and Zara, M., 1975, Le gliclazide dans le traitement de la rétinopathie diabétique: Résultats préliminaires portant sur 18 mois de traitement, *Gaz. Med. Fr.* **82:**167.

Malaisse, W. J., and Leclercq-Meyer, V., 1972, Insulinotropic action of a new sulfonylurea: Gliclazide, *Rev. Eur. Etud. Clin. Biol.* **17:**310.

Smit Sibinga, C. T., 1973, Prevention of vessel wall damage in experimental irradiation, *Bibl. Anat.* **12:**242.

6.19. A Diagnostic Sign in the Small Blood Vessels of the Conjunctiva in Arteriosclerosis

ELI DAVIS and LEON RAUCH

Arteriosclerosis (AS) of the conjunctival small vessels as revealed by clinical biomicroscopy has been described by Davis *et al.* (1966). In the present study, 200 patients aged 45 or over were examined. One-hundred patients presented with AS with a clinical complication such as coronary artery ischemia, cerebrovascular disease, or peripheral vascular disease, and 100 patients presented with nonvascular disease such as peptic ulcer, bronchitis, or rheumatism. All had a full clinical examination and most had electrocardiograms, chest X-ray, blood sugar tests, and blood cholesterol tests. The conjuctiva was examined by slit lamp at ×25.

The AS sign in the conjunctiva consists of very tortuous venules, accompanied by straight, narrow arterioles surrounding very thin capillaries. The arteriolar venular ratio is 1:3 or 1:4 in place of 1:2. The capillaries are 5 μm in diameter in place of 10–15 μm. The capillaries are also reduced in number (Fig. 1). Intravascular red cell aggregation is usually present.

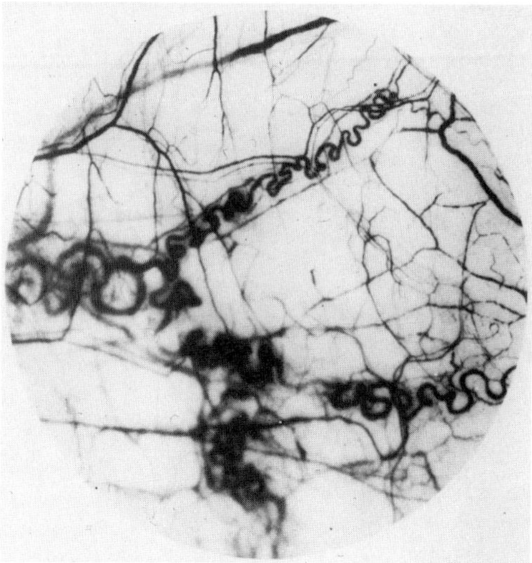

Figure 1. Small blood vessels of the conjunctiva in AS (×4 on negative).

ELI DAVIS and LEON RAUCH · Hadassah University Hospital, Jerusalem, Israel.

Table I. Prevalence of AS Sign

	Presenting disease	
Age	Vascular	Nonvascular
45–54	10 of 25	4 of 25
55–64	17 of 25	5 of 25
65–74	20 of 25	5 of 25
75+	23 of 25	15 of 25

The AS sign was present in 70% of the patients with clinical AS and in 29% of the patients with nonvascular disease. Half of the latter were found to have AS on investigation. The prevalence of the sign increased with age, but age was not the main factor in prevalence (Table I).

An AS retina can be diagnosed by an experienced ophthalmologist, and was nearly always found when the conjunctival AS sign was present. The sign in the conjunctiva is much more clear-cut and distinct than the AS fundus, which is often interpreted differently by different observers.

References

Davis, E., and Landau, J., 1960, The small blood vessels of the conjunctiva and nailbed in arteriosclerosis, *Angiology* **11:**173.

Davis, E., Landau, J., and Ivry, M., 1966, *Clinical Capillary Microscopy,* Thomas, Springfield, Ill.

6.20. Ventilatory Dysfunction after Long-Lasting Intravascular Platelet Aggregation

JARLE VAAGE

Pulmonary microembolism with platelet aggregates has been claimed to be a pathogenetic component in the development of acute respiratory distress (Blaisdell, 1974). Suddenly induced intravascular platelet aggregation will cause pulmonary vasoconstriction and airway constriction (Vaage *et al.*, 1974), and the transvascular fluid balance in the lungs will be disturbed as well (Nicolaysen *et al.*, 1975).

To evaluate whether intravascular platelet aggregation might cause respiratory insufficiency, a collagen suspension was infused intravenously over 1 h to open-chested cats given positive-pressure ventilation with air. To avoid intravascular coagulation, the animals were given large doses of heparin. Such infusions markedly reduced the number of circulating platelets, decreased dynamic lung compliance ($DynC_L$) by about 40%, and increased pulmonary vascular resistance (PVR). Systemic blood pressure and cardiac output showed smaller changes. A severe arterial hypoxemia developed (arterial Po_2 about 60 mm Hg). A linear correlation between the reduction in $DynC_L$ and in arterial Po_2 was found (r = 0.92). pH decreased to about 7.30. When the collagen infusion was ended, $DynC_L$, PVR, arterial Po_2, and pH gradually improved. Normal values could be restored in this period by deep lung inflations.

Cats breathing spontaneously were also tested. During collagen infusion, they showed similar disturbances in gas exchange, and the respiratory frequency (f) doubled. This increased f was sustained during the 2 h following the end of collagen infusion, resulting in a respiratory alkalosis. However, Po_2 returned to a normal value after the end of infusion.

In conclusion, intravascular platelet aggregation may cause a severe but mainly reversible ventilatory dysfunction. The beneficial effect of lung inflations suggests airway closure to be a key factor in the development of this dysfunction. As a fulminant, acute respiratory distress syndrome did not develop in these cats, it might be that in addition to platelet aggregation other pathogenetic components are necessary.

JARLE VAAGE · Institute of Physiology, University of Oslo, Oslo, Norway.

References

Blaisdell, F. W., 1974, Pathophysiology of the respiratory distress syndrome, *Arch. Surg.* **108**:44.

Nicolaysen, G., Vaage, J., and Waaler, B. A., 1975, Changes in the hydraulic conductivity of pulmonary capillaries after induced intravascular aggregation of blood platelets, in: *Proceedings of the VIIIth European Conference on Microcirculation,* le Touquet, 1974, Karger, Basel.

Vaage, J., Bø, G., and Hognestad, J., 1974, Pulmonary responses to intravascular platelet aggregation in the cat, *Acta Physiol. Scand.* **92**:546.

6.21. Studies on Platelet and Red Cell Survival after Cardiopulmonary Bypass (CPB) without Blood Filter

F. N. McKENZIE, A. ROBERT, and R. O. HEIMBECKER

An arterial line filter is generally considered essential for safe CPB (Ashmore *et al.*, 1968). The possibility that the filter may itself cause significant injury to the blood elements due to its inability to handle 5 liter/min blood flows was examined by comparing serial measurements of platelet count, hemoglobin (Hb), plasma Hb, and blood loss in two groups of patients who underwent hypothermic (32°C) CPB for valve replacement or coronary artery surgery. CPB was carried out with a disposable bubble oxygenator (Bentley) primed with up to 2 liters of Ringer lactate. The results in 61 consecutive patients studied are shown in Table I. In the *absence* of an arterial line filter (study group, 43 patients), the maximal decrease in platelet count and blood loss were reduced by half compared to the control group of 18 patients. All patients in the control group required blood transfusion. In the study group, 60% required no blood transfusion and none was given platelet or plasma transfusion. Scanning electron microscopy (SEM) of the arterial line filter in the control group showed gross platelet and fibrin deposition. SEM of the filter used in the cardiotomy suction line *only* in the study group showed minimal changes. We conclude that for routine CPB an arterial line filter is neither necessary nor desirable (McKenzie *et al.*, 1975), for it can cause a degree of consumptive coagulopathy.

ACKNOWLEDGMENTS

This work was supported in part by the Ontario Heart Foundation, the Bickell Foundations, the Nelson Hyland Foundation, and the Medical Research Counil of Canada.

F. N. McKENZIE, A. ROBERT, and R. O. HEIMBECKER · Department of Cardiovascular and Thoracic Surgery, University Hospital, University of Western Ontario, London, Ontario, Canada.

Table I

	Age (yr)	Perfusion time (min)	Postoperative blood loss (ml)		Blood transfusion (mean units/ patient)	Plasma/platelet (number of patients)	Bloodless CPB (OR and ICU)	Hb at discharge (g%)	Mean maximum decrease in platelet count (% of preoperative)
			0–12 h	12 h+					
Control (*n* = 18)	59	63	635	410	5.5	10	0	11.5	26
Study (*n*) = 43)	58	58	375	457	1.3	0	26	11.3	72

References

Ashmore, P. G., Svitek, V., and Ambrose, P., 1968, The incidence and effects of particulate aggregation and micro-embolism in pump oxygenator systems, *J. Thorac. Cardiovasc. Surg.* **55:**691.

McKenzie, F. N., Heimbecker, R. O., Barnicoat, K. T. N., Robert, A., Gergely, N. F., Del Maestro, R., and Wall, W., 1975, Bloodless open heart surgery with atraumatic extracorporeal circulation, *Can. Med. Assoc. J.* **112:**1073.

6.22. Osmotic Fragilities and the Kalmedic Fragiligraph Model D-3

DONALD M. STASIW, SUSAN ROSATO, and LAWRENCE C. CERNY

The Kalmedic fragiligraph permits the determination of erythrocyte osmotic fragilities on a time scale suitable for a routine clinical testing procedure (Danon *et al.*, 1965; Danon, 1967). In its delivered configuration, the fragiligraph displays the sigmoidal fragility curve and either the salt diffusion or differential hemolysis curve plotted on a time-based, two-channel strip chart recorder. Since the independent variable of interest is salt concentration and not time, the strip chart recorder was replaced with two *X-Y* recorders. This allows the plotting of both the hemolysis and differential hemolysis curves directly against effective salt concentration. Additional procedural changes made include the continuous monitoring of the hemolysis cell temperature, the direct calibration of the salt channel, and the dialysis of the sample cell membrane prior to use to remove residual salt.

The sigmoidal hemolysis curve can be fitted to an equation of the form

$$Y = T_c/T_{c=0} = \frac{1}{1 + \exp(\beta C_{50} - \beta C)} \tag{1}$$

In equation (1), Y is the ratio of transmittances at a given salt concentration, c, to that at zero salt concentration (i.e., complete hemolysis), C_{50} is the salt concentration at which half the cells have hemolyzed, and β is related to the range of salt concentrations over which hemolysis begins and reaches completion. Transforming equation (1) to a linear form

$$\ln [1/(y - 1)] = \beta C_{50} - C\beta \tag{2}$$

allows rapid calculation of band C_{50}. Goodness of fit (Fig. 1) can then be determined by comparing the fragiligraph-generated differential hemolysis curve with the curve calculated by analytically differentiating equation (1) and using the values of β and C_{50} obtained from equation (2). This procedure is in total agreement with that employed by DeTraglia *et al.* (1974) to interpret osmotic fragility data obtained by a modification of the method of Good (1971).

DONALD M. STASIW, SUSAN ROSATO, and LAWRENCE C. CERNY · Masonic Medical Research Laboratory and Utica College of Syracuse University, Utica, New York.

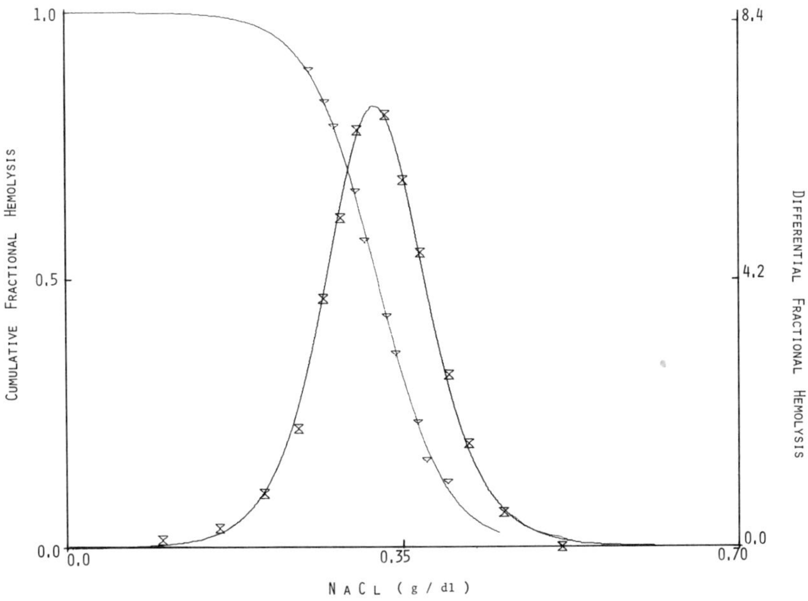

Figure 1. Typical cumulative and differential hemolysis curves obtained with the Kalmedic fragiligraph. The solid lines represent curves calculated from equation (1) and its derivative. Points are from the experimentally obtained fragility curves.

References

Danon, D., 1967, The fragiligraph and its applications, automation in hematology, *Br. J. Haematol.* **13:**273.

Danon, D., Shiffman, A., and Efrati, P., 1965, Analysis of osmotic fragility as a routine test in clinical practice, *Isr. J. Med. Sci.* **1:**4.

DeTraglia, M., Cook, F. B., Stasiw, D. M., and Cerny, L. C., 1974, Erythrocyte fragility in aging, *Biochim. Biophys. Acta* **345:**213.

Good, W., 1971, Haemolysis experiments on erythrocytes, *Exp. Physiol. Biochem.* **4:**163.

7

Lymphatics

7.1. Electron Microscopic Studies of the Lymphatic Endothelium in Lymphangiectasia of the Small Intestine

M. TSUCHIYA, H. ASAKURA, N. HIBI, Y. WATANABE, and Y. ENOMOTO

We (Tsuchiya *et al.*, 1973) have reported that the lymphangiectasia of the small intestine was revealed not only in protein-losing enteropathy but also in liver cirrhosis and Behçet's disease. Although lymphangiectasia of the small intestine does not necessarily cause enteric protein loss, what mechanism does trigger this loss?

The aim of this article is to clarify the mechanism of enteric protein loss from the dilated lymphatic vessel in primary protein-losing enteropathy.

7.1.1. Materials and Methods

Biopsy specimens were obtained under fluoroscopy by the peroral technique or at laparotomy from seven patients with primary protein-losing enteropathy. Each subject fasted overnight more than 15 h prior to biopsy. Specimens were fixed in 1% osmium tetroxide and embedded in Epon after dehydration through graded concentration of ethanol and acetone. Epon blocks were sectioned with a glass knife and stained with uranyl acetate.

M. TSUCHIYA, H. ASAKURA, and N. HIBI · Department of Internal Medicine, Keio University, Tokyo, Japan. Y. WATANABE and Y. ENOMOTO · Department of Pathology, Keio University, Tokyo, Japan.

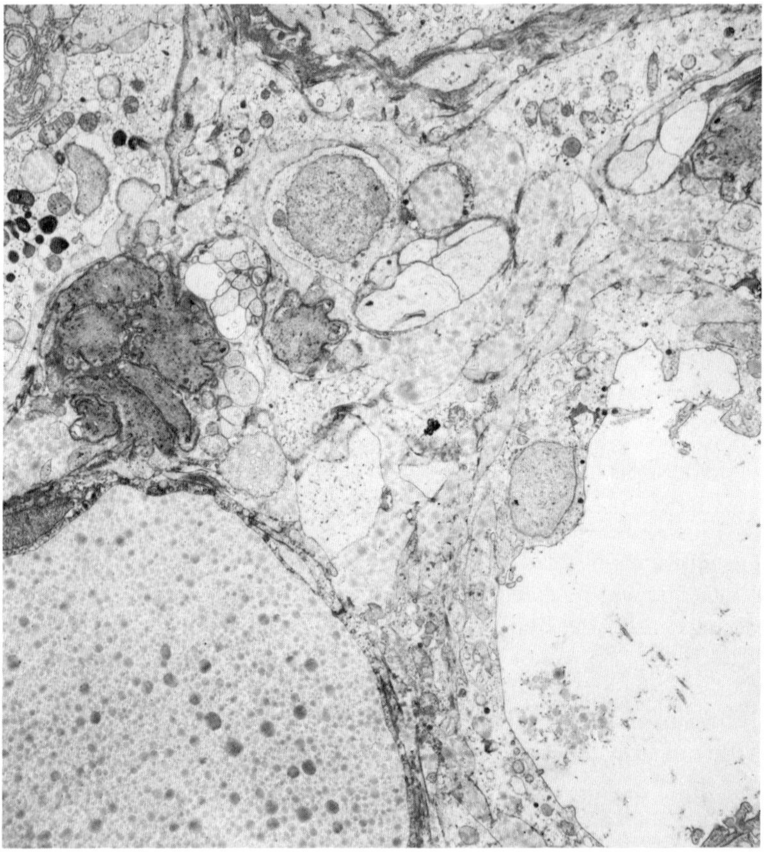

Figure 1. Electron microscopic photograph showing endothelium of lymphatic vessels in the lamina propria, which was varied in its thickness (×3000; reduced for reproduction).

7.1.2. Results

Electron microscopic study of lymphatic endothelium revealed the following:

1. An abundance of chylomicronlike substances and precipitated lymphoproteins were seen within the lumen of lymphatic vessels and in extracellular spaces of the lamina propria of the intestinal mucosa.
2. Lymphatic endothelium which contained numerous chylomicron-like substances in its cavity became thin, while the endothelial cells

of the lymphatic vessels which contained a small amount of chylomicronlike substances were normal in thickness (Fig. 1).
3. Large vesicles which contained chylomicronlike substances were observed in endothelial cells.
4. Widening of interendothelial junction was rarely seen in the specimens studied.
5. Many chylomicronlike substances were seen in the interepithelial spaces between the absorptive cells. These substances were present even within the apical portion of the interepithelial spaces as well as in the basal portion.

These findings suggested that the inverted mechanism of lymphatic endothelial pinocytosis and the transportation process of the interepithelial spaces might be related to enteric protein loss in primary protein-losing enteropathy.

Reference

Tsuchiya, M., Asakura, H., Shimabukuro, K., Morita, A., Morishita, T., Watanabe, Y., and Enomoto, Y., 1973, Lymphangiectasia of the small intestine, *Bibl. Anat.* **11**:317.

7.2. Microcirculation of the Human Lymph Node

P. G. FORKERT and J. W. DAVIDSON

In mammals, the topographies of small blood vessels and lymphatic spaces in and around follicles within the cortex of the lymph node form "microcirculatory units" (Davidson *et al.*, 1973, 1975). This arrangement of lymph-containing spaces and blood vessels may be of basic significance with respect to dynamic functions of lymph nodes.

None of the previous studies (Millikin, 1966, Fukuda, 1968; Herman *et al.*, 1972) demonstrated the unitary relationship between blood vessels and lymphatic spaces within and around the cortical follicles. The topography and relationships of both vascular and lymphatic structures may be studied in three dimensions by injection of Microfil (Canton Bio-Medical Products, Boulder, Colorado) of different colors into lymphatics and arteries afferent and efferent to lymph nodes in human cadavers. This communication describes the circulation within peripheral and visceral lymph nodes.

7.2.1. Materials and Methods

Lymph nodes from both embalmed and fresh human cadavers were examined in a sample representing a range of ages and both sexes. In 12 subjects aged 15–80 yr, including one aged 15 yr and a second 27 yr, the arterial supply to individual lymph nodes was displayed by injection of Microfil into main arteries to various regions. Lymph nodes from the groin, axilla, retroperitoneum, and mediastinum were examined.

7.2.2. Results and Discussion

Despite varying degrees of filling of both blood vessels and lymphatic spaces within lymph nodes, this approach enables more complete three-dimensional study of their topography than previous methods. In man, our studies demonstrate even better defined microcirculatory units than in animals (Fig. 1). A single arterial twig feeds a rounded network of

P. G. FORKERT · Department of Anatomy, University of Toronto, Toronto, Ontario, Canada. J. W. DAVIDSON · Associate Clinical Professor of Radiology, McMaster University Medical Center, Hamilton, Ontario, Canada.

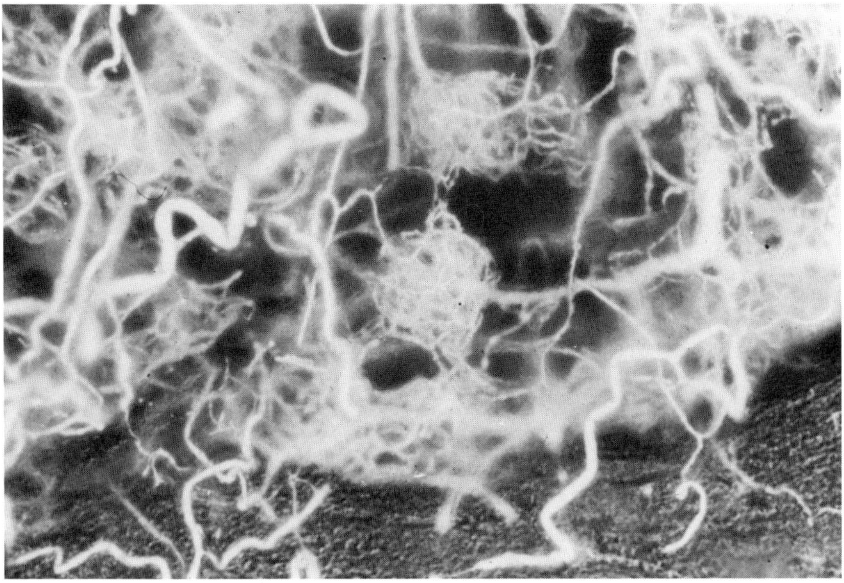

Figure 1. Cortex of cleared human inguinal lymph node (×40) following injection of Microfil into the external iliac artery. Note the microcirculatory units in the center of the specimen.

capillary-size vessels within the periphery of each follicle at the site of lymphocyte transference. From this network emerges the draining vein. Examination with higher magnification of the cut surface reveals that, within the node, peripherally located postcapillary venules join to form the draining vein, which is usually seen outside the deep pole of the germinal center. These veins join to drain small areas or segments of the parenchyma, and in turn the segmental veins lead to larger lobular veins at the corticomedullary junction of each node. Around this vascular complex is a network of intercommunicating lymphatic spaces extending from the margin of the node to the medulla.

The cortical thickness in barrier nodes appeared to decrease with age, a finding similar to that of Denz (1947). However, considerable variation in the size of lymphatic domes and vascular units is observed in different subjects. This suggests cyclical changes or responses to the antigenic background, similar to those described histologically. This difference in morphology of the basic microcirculatory unit is in keeping with its adaptation by hypertrophy, multiplication, or both during immune reactions secondary to lymph-borne antigens.

References

Davidson, J. W., Fletch, A. L., McIlmoyle, G., and Roeck W., 1973, The technique and applications of lymphography, *Can. J. Comp. Med.*.**37:(2):**130.

Davidson, J. W., Hobbs, B. B., and Fletch, A. L., 1974, The microcirculatory unit of the mammalian lymph node, in: *Proceedings of the VIIth European Congress on Microcirculation,* Karger, Basel.

Denz, F. A., 1947, Age changes in lymph nodes, *J. Pathol. Bacteriol.* **59:**575.

Fukuda, J., 1968, Studies on the vascular architecture and the fluid exchange in the rabbit popliteal lymph node, *Keio J. Med.* **17:**53.

Herman, P. G., Yamamoto, I., and Mellins, H. J., 1972, Blood microcirculation in the lymph node during the primary immune response, *J. Exp. Med.* **136:**697.

Millikin, P. D., 1966, Anatomy of germinal centres in human lymphoid tissue, *J. Arch. Pathol.* **82:**499.

7.3. Quantitation of Blood Flow to and Lymph Output from Single Lymph Nodes

BARRY B. HOBBS and JOHN B. HAY

Nuclide-labeled microspheres (15 μm diameter) were injected into the arterial system of sheep, and their distribution to a variety of single lymph nodes as well as several major organs was measured. Catheters were fluoroscopically positioned in the ascending aorta near the aortic valve. Adequate mixing occurred, and the bilateral distribution of microspheres to the kidneys, lymph nodes, and eyes was symmetrical. Blood flow to kidneys was found to be 11.9 ± 1.6%, spleen 1.8 ± 0.3%, and lymph nodes 0.012 ± 0.001% of the cardiac output, based on measurements in ten animals. Chronic lymphatic fistulas were established in the efferent vessels from one or more peripheral lymph nodes (popliteal or prefemoral), and quantitative collections of lymph were recorded for periods up to several weeks (Hall and Morris, 1965). From measurements of blood flow and lymphocyte output, it was calculated that one in every four lymphocytes entering a node in the blood migrated out of the blood vascular compartment and into the efferent lymph.

When individual lymph nodes were stimulated with antigen, the blood flow per gram increased an average of fourfold. During such immune responses, the output of lymphocytes in the efferent lymph increased by a similar order of magnitude.

When afferent lymph was collected from dermal regions, the output of lymphocytes was low (10^6 cells/h); however, when a cellular hypersensitivity lesion was produced in the skin, the output of lymphocytes increased and reached 10–20 times this value at the peak of the reaction. When the blood flow to such lesions was measured, it was found to increase by a similar order of magnitude.

We concluded that antigen, through its interaction with immunologically competent cells, causes a local increase in blood flow and in the traffic of lymphocytes through the site. The mechanism is not clear but is likely to be the same regardless of whether the site is a lymph node or any other lesion characterized by mononuclear cell infiltration.

BARRY B. HOBBS and JOHN B. HAY · Division of Experimental Pathology, Departments of Radiology and Pathology, and Institute of Immunology, Medical Sciences Building, University of Toronto, Toronto, Ontario, Canada.

ACKNOWLEDGMENTS

This work was supported by the Medical Research Council of Canada (MA-5056) and the Hellyer Foundation.

Reference

Hall, J. G., and Morris, B., 1965, The origin of the cells in the efferent lymph from a single node, *J. Exp. Med.* **121**:901.

7.4. Flow of Albumin through Renal Lymph: The Total Clearance

J. L. ATKINS, C. C. C. O'MORCHOE, and G. G. PINTER

In the dog, total renal lymph flow (TRLF) cannot be determined by a direct technique such as simple cannulation. Our technique is based on two experimentally verified premises: (1) there is no loss of albumin between renal lymphatics and thoracic duct (TD) drainage under normal conditions, and (2) the process of equilibration between plasma and renal lymph albumin-specific activities occurs at a nearly identical rate in all lymph vessels draining the kidney.

Two equivalent tracers of plasma albumin were infused, one into the left renal artery and the other into the venous outflow of the same kidney. The experimental kidney received the arterial tracer directly in a relatively high concentration, whereas all other organs were perfused equally with both tracers. This experimental arrangement set apart the lymph drainage of the left kidney by the relatively high concentration of the arterially infused tracer. The fractional contribution of the left kidney to the thoracic duct lymph albumin flow was calculated from albumin-specific activities in arterial plasma, thoracic duct, and lymph from a single cannulated renal lymphatic vessel. Since the concentrations of equilibrated albumin were similar in TD and renal lymph, the renal fraction of TD volume flow is the same as the volume flow draining from the kidney.

In hydropenic dogs, the TRLF was 0.367 ml/min per 100 g kidney weight ($\pm$0.091 SEM). In animals with ureteric occlusion, TRLF was 0.629 ($\pm$0.258 SEM). Although seemingly large, this difference was not significant, owing to the large variability of the measurements, particularly in kidneys with occluded ureters.

J. L. ATKINS, C. C. C. O'MORCHOE, and G. G. PINTER · Department of Physiology, University of Maryland, School of Medicine, Baltimore, Maryland, and Department of Anatomy, Loyola University, Stritch School of Medicine, Chicago, Illinois.

7.5. Contributions to Regional Tissue Lymph by the Local Lymph Node in Sheep

J. W. QUIN, A. D. SHANNON, and F. C. COURTICE

The simultaneous collection of afferent and efferent lymph from various regions of the body of conscious sheep has shown that the local lymph node makes significant contributions to the capillary filtrate from the regional tissues as it passes through the node. Thus protein concentrations in popliteal postnodal lymph are some 40% higher than the corresponding concentrations in prenodal lymph (Table I), in accord with previous results (Beh *et al.,* 1974). Studies with labeled proteins have demonstrated that this contribution of both albumin and immunoglobulin at the lymph node is derived from the blood plasma compartment and not by *de novo* synthesis within the node. Furthermore, the amount of protein added at the node has been shown to be positively correlated with the numbers of lymphocytes recirculating through the node, suggesting the transfer of blood plasma protein into the lymph with the passage of lymphocytes across the postcapillary endothelium (Quin and Lascelles, 1975). The differences in protein content of pre- and postnodal lymph are abolished during anesthesia in the sheep, and this finding may account for the absence of any difference reported previously for the anesthetized rabbit (Osogoe and Courtice, 1968; Roberts and Courtice, 1969).

Relatively large amounts of bilirubin are added to the capillary filtrate from regional tissues at the level of the popliteal lymph node in the conscious sheep (see Table I). In addition, the bilirubin concentrations in postnodal lymph from five other regions of the body contained 3–8 times the corresponding plasma bilrubin concentration (Quin and Shannon, 1975). In contrast, prenodal lymph from four regions always contained less bilirubin than plasma. These results, in conjunction with histological examination of regional lymph nodes, indicated that significant red cell catabolism takes place within lymph nodes in the sheep.

It is concluded that capillary filtrate from regional tissues passing through the local lymph node is altered in composition by events occurring within the resting node of the conscious sheep.

J. W. QUIN, A. D. SHANNON, F. C. COURTICE · Department of Experimental Pathology, John Curtin School of Medical Research, Australian National University, Canberra, Australia.

Table I. Lymph: Plasma Ratios for the Concentrations of Various Proteins and of Bilirubin in the Afferent and Efferent Lymph of the Popliteal Node of the Sheep

	Lymph:plasma ratio	
	Afferent popliteal[a]	Efferent popliteal[a]
Protein		
IgG_1	0.23 ± 0.05	0.45 ± 0.04
IgG_2	0.21 ± 0.03	0.41 ± 0.04
IgM	0.18 ± 0.01	0.29 ± 0.02
Albumin	0.27 ± 0.03	0.45 ± 0.03
Total protein	0.22 ± 0.04	0.37 ± 0.03
Bilirubin	0.52 ± 0.10	5.58 ± 1.15

[a] Means ± standard errors derived from six sheep in which simultaneous collections were made of afferent and efferent popliteal lymph.

References

Beh, K. J., Watson, D. L., and Lascelles, A. K., 1974, Concentrations of immunoglobulins and albumin in lymph collected from various regions of the body of the sheep, *Aust. J. Exp. Biol. Med. Sci.* **52:**81.

Osogoe, B., and Courtice, F. C., 1968, The effects of occlusion of the blood supply to the popliteal lymph node of the rabbit on the cell and protein content of the lymph and on the histology of the node, *Aust. J. Exp. Biol. Med. Sci.* **46:**515.

Quin, J. W., and Lascelles, A. K., 1975, Relationship between the recirculation of lymphocytes and protein concentration of lymph in sheep, *Aust. J. Exp. Biol. Med. Sci.* **53:**1.

Quin, J. W., and Shannon, A. D., 1975, High concentration of bilirubin in post-nodal lymph associated with red blood cell catabolism in lymph nodes of the sheep, *Lymphology* (submitted).

Roberts, J. C., and Courtice, F. C., 1969, Measurements of protein leakage in the acute and recovery stages of a thermal injury, *Aust. J. Exp. Biol. Med. Sci.* **47:**421.

7.6. Effects of Chemical and Physical Conditions on the Flow Rate of Intestinal Lymphatics

NORMAN B. ACKERMAN

Because of the importance of the lymphatic circulation as a route of cancer dissemination and of the role it plays in the inflammatory process, we have studied the dynamics of intestinal lymph flow. Using a technique described by Ackerman (1973), lymphatic vessels were cannulated in the mesentery proximal to the intestinal lymph nodes in dogs, and pooled samples were measured over 5-min collection periods.

Significant increases in lymph flow, approximately 5 times control rates, occurred during periods of elevated intraluminal pressure within the bowel and during periods of hyperperistalsis. Excessive handling and manipulation of the intestine also resulted in a significant, sevenfold rise in lymph flow. Ligation of the venous outflow of the bowel caused excessive eightfold increases in lymph flow, and even partial ligation had a marked effect. Arterial ligation or simultaneous arterial and venous ligation produced a gradual decrease in lymph flow to approximately one-third of control rates. These findings support the use of a "no touch" technique for resection of intestinal cancers, as advocated by Turnbull *et al.* (1967), but suggest the use of an early artery ligation modification. They also suggest that some routine diagnostic procedures (barium enemas, colonoscopy, sigmoidoscopy) and preoperative preparations (cleansing enemas) may be potentially harmful.

Hypothermia of the intestine to temperatures below 10°C markedly decreased lymph flow, and freezing temperatures virtually stopped all flow. Warming temperatures produced a biphasic response, initially increasing flow slightly with a later secondary fall. Increasing hydration of the animal by intravenous infusion of saline, dextrose solutions, or dextran increased lymph flow in proportion to increases in central venous pressures in preliminary experiments. Preliminary studies with diuretic agents support the thoracic duct studies of others (Szwed *et al.,* 1972) by indicating that intestinal lymph flow is affected significantly by furosemide, with a rapid, short-lived increase in flow.

NORMAN B. ACKERMAN · Department of Surgery, SUNY, Upstate Medical Center, and Veterans Hospital, Syracuse, New York.

References

Ackerman, N. B., 1973, Vascular influences on intestinal lymph flow and their relationship to operation for carcinoma of the intestine, *Surg. Gynecol. Obstet.* **137**:801.

Szwed, J. J., Kleit, S. A., and Hamburger, R. J., 1972, Effect of furosemide and chlorothiazide on the thoracic duct lymph flow in the dog, *J. Lab. Clin. Med.* **79**:693.

Turnbull, R. B., Jr., Kyle, K., Watson, F. R., and Sprath, J., 1967, Cancer of the colon, *Ann. Surg.* **166**:420.

7.7. Lymph Flow Augmentation Secondary to Rises in Serum Calcium

MAXIMO DEYSINE, MILAN MADER, ELISEO ROSARIO, and ARTHUR H. AUFSES, JR.

To investigate why increases in serum calcium produce marked thoracic duct lymph flow (TDLF) augmentations (Deysine *et al.,* 1974), this ion was injected intravenously in 0.125-mm increments in groups of five parathyroidectomized dogs. Animals were rendered apneic with intravenous pentobarbital and ventilated with a respirator.

After L-tubocurarine (0.53 mg/kg body weight) or succinylcholine chloride (0.2 mg/kg body weight), calcium produced a 100% or 333% rise in TDLF, respectively. This rules out skeletal muscle contractility as a factor in the response to calcium. Atropine (0.40 mg/kg body weight) produced a 500% increase in TDLF after calcium. Sympathetic blockage attempted by a combination of adrenalectomy, reserpinization (0.5 mg/kg body weight in three doses 24 h apart), phenoxybenzamine hydrochloride (4 mg/kg body weight infused in 45 min), and propranolol (1 mg/kg body weight infused in 30 min) significantly diminished TDLF after calcium ($P < 0.001$). An infusion of angiotensin completely abolished TDLF. While angiotensin was still being infused, calcium increased TDLF 268%. Papaverine, known to block the entrance of calcium into the cells, was able to completely block the action of calcium on TDLF (Tomiyama *et al.,* 1973). We suggest that (1) lymph propulsion changes after calcium are particularly mediated by the sympathetic system, and (2) calcium may also act by directly contracting the lymphatic channel wall.

References

Deysine, M., Mader, M., Rosario, E., and Mandell, C., 1974, Lymphatic flow alterations secondary to changes in total serum calcium levels (38303), *Proc. Soc. Exp. Biol. Med.* **147:**158.

Tomiyama, A., Takayanagi, I., and Takagi, K., 1973, Relaxation of intestinal smooth muscle and calcium movements, *J. Pharm. Pharmacol.* **25:**65.

MAXIMO DEYSINE, MILAN MADER, ELISEO ROSARIO, and ARTHUR H. AUFSES, JR. · Department of Surgery, Long Island Jewish-Hillside Medical Center, New Hyde Park, New York, and The Health Sciences Center, The State University of New York at Stony Brook, Stony Brook, New York.

7.8. Transport of Air via Lymph Vessels in Experimentally Induced Emphysema

WILLIAM P. MAHER

Emphysema other than pulmonary is defined as a swelling or inflation due to air presence in connective tissue spaces. Some considerations of the condition are as follows:

1. Air, or possibly gas elaborated by microorganisms, may forcibly penetrate eroded, torn, broken, or cut tissue margins resulting from trauma, surgery, or disease.
2. Inflation may extend from these margins to remote regions apparently unrelated to entrance portals.
3. Inflation is often extremely rapid to distant sites.

Theories proposed in an effort to explain extremely rapid-rate dispersion and remote region involvement include vascular transport, dissection through tissue spaces, and combinations of these two factors. Presently, opinion is divided regarding air distribution mechanisms.

Lymphatic patterns can be analyzed stereomicroscopically in cleared dog and human tongues previously injected with an ink–water medium (Maher and Swindle, 1966). It was considered possible that air distribution effects might be analyzed similarly. Air was injected interstitially into newborn dog tongues previously cleared by a Spalteholz method. Distribution effects were compared to ink replications of arterial, venous, and lymphatic lumina. Stereomicroscopic analysis revealed that air is transported via lymphatics in addition to connective tissue spaces. This may explain air distribution beyond boundaries provided by fascial compartments. Apparently, arteries and veins do not participate as a mechanism for the immediate transport of air or gas forcibly penetrated into connective tissues.

These pilot studies demonstrate air transport via lymphatics in a biological model (postmortem dog tongue). These observations remain to be established *in vivo;* it is hoped that this will provide an anatomicophysiological basis for clinical interpretation and subsequent treatment of emphysematous conditions.

WILLIAM P. MAHER · Department of Anatomy The Medical College of Wisconsin, and Marquette University, Milwaukee, Wisconsin.

Acknowledgment

This work was supported by the Marquette University Committee on Research.

Reference

Maher, W. P., and Swindle, P. F., 1966, Blood and lymph vessels of the tongue of dog and man, *Anat. Rec.* **154:**503.

8

Neurohumoral Control of Blood Vessels

8.1. Integrated Response of the Microvasculature to Stimulation of the CNS in the Rat

S. BAEZ, S. M. FELDMAN, and P. M. GOOTMAN

Renkin and Rosell (1962) reported specific sites for CNS control of arterioles and precapillary sphincters. Gootman *et al.* (1973) showed that all segments of precapillary microvessel and sphincter can respond to CNS stimulation. However, precapillary arterioles (metarterioles) and precapillary sphincters failed to respond to supramaximal stimulation of paravascular nerves in rat mesentery (Furness and Marshall, 1974). In the present experiment, responses of the larger consecutive segments of arterioles (Art) were measured during electrical stimulation of vasoactive CNS sites in nine rats with chronically implanted unipolar electrodes. Currents were for maximal constriction or lumen closure of precapillary sphincter (Pc sph) and/or immediately preceding metarteriole (Met): 0.08–0.15 mA (10-s trains, 100-μs pulses, 5–100 Hz). Under pentobarbital sodium (25 mg/kg, i.m.), responses of microvessels were measured by image-splitting methods in mesoappendix in six rats, cremaster in two rats, and both in one. In all experiments, stimulation resulted in blood pressure elevation (112.6 $\pm$ 17.6% to 165.2 $\pm$ 18.5% mm Hg, mean and standard deviation) and constriction of three consecutive segments of precapillary vessels and sphincter: 10.5 $\pm$ 9.3% for Art_1 (43.4 $\pm$ 8.8 μm, ID), 40.0 $\pm$ 26.6% for Art_2 (20.4 $\pm$ 3.7 μm, ID), 70.3 $\pm$ 24.6% for Met (11.4 $\pm$ 3.7 μm, ID), and 75.5 $\pm$ 20.2% for Pc sph (7.5 $\pm$ 1.3 μm, ID). Stimulation characteristically increased ($\times$3) vasomotor activity of Pc sph and Met, but infrequently increased that of larger arterioles at currents used. The data show (1) an

S. BAEZ, S. M. FELDMAN, and P. M. GOOTMAN · Albert Einstein College of Medicine, New York University, and Downstate Medical Center, Brooklyn, New York.

overall CNS influence on microcirculation; (2) a response gradient of terminal microvessels in both tissues to CNS stimulation, increasing toward the last muscular outpost of the arteriolar tree, and (3) the ability of the metarteriole and sphincter can completely close lumen to CNS stimulation and actively participate in local flow regulation, hence directly influencing exchange surface area. No evidence was found for specific CNS control of sphincters independent of arterioles.

ACKNOWLEDGMENTS

This work was supported by NIH Grants HL-06736, MH-9204, and NS-09934.

References

Furness, J. B., and Marshall, J. M., 1974, Correlation of the directly observed responses of mesenteric vessels of the rat to nerve stimulation and noradrenaline with the distribution of adrenergic nerves, *J. Physiol. (London)* **239:**75.

Gootman, P. M., Baez, S., and Feldman, S. M., 1973, Microcirculatory responses to central neural stimulation in the rat, *Am. J. Physiol.* **225:**1375.

Renkin, E., and Rosell, S., 1962, Independent sympathetic vasoconstrictor innervation of arterioles and precapillary sphincter, *Acta Physiol. Scand.* **54:**381.

8.2. Comparative Studies on Adrenergic Receptors in Different Rat Blood Vessels

BURTON M. ALTURA

During the past 5 years, we have noted that a variety of rat blood vessels, both macro- and microscopic in size, demonstrate a wide and varied sensitivity to constrictor adrenergic amines (Altura, 1971, 1972*a,b* 1975). In addition, these preliminary data indicated (1) that some of these different vessels exhibited different maximal constrictor responses to a series of α-adrenergic agonists (e.g., epinephrine, norepinephrine, phenylephrine, dopamine, α-methylnorepinephrine) and (2) that certain vessels failed to respond to tyramine, a so-called indirectly acting adrenergic amine. In view of these findings, the present studies were designed to determine whether (a) the α-adrenergic receptor may be different on different blood vessels within a mammal and (b) indirectly acting adrenergic amines (e.g., tyramine, TY; amphetamine, AMP) can contract terminal blood vessels devoid of nervous innervation, e.g., metarterioles (MT) and precapillary sphincters (PS) (Altura, 1971).

8.2.1. Methods

All of these studies were performed on either intact mesenteric microvessels from pentobarbital-anesthetized male rats or on isolated rat aortic strips. An image-splitting television microscope recording system was used for the *in vivo* observations on mesenteric arterioles (MA), MT, PS, and muscular venules (MV), similar to that described previously (Altura, 1971, 1972*a,b*, 1975). Helically cut aortic strips (AS) from male rats were set up isometrically as described previously (Altura, 1975). Complete cumulative dose–response curves (DRC) were obtained for 13 adrenergic amines on these vessels in the presence and absence of an α-adrenergic antagonist, phentolamine (PH).

8.2.2. Results

Although the relative maximal contractile responses (i.e., the intrinsic activities, IA's) for epinephrine (E) and norepinephrine (NE) are 100% on

BURTON M. ALTURA · Department of Physiology, State University of New York, Downstate Medical Center, Brooklyn, New York.

the MT, PS, and AS, the IA's for NE on the MA and MV are significantly less than E. The data indicate that not only do the relative IA's in a series of 13 adrenergic agonists significantly differ from one type of blood vessel to another but also the ED_{50}'s relative to E and NE differ. Furthermore, (1) the DRC for dopamine, octopamine, and phenylephrine do not always parallel those of E and NE on the different rat vessels, and (2) the apparent dissociation constants (i.e., apparent K_B values) of PH for the receptor–agonist complexes also differ with vessel type. In addition, (1) TY and AMP fail to contract MT and PS, and (2) the structure–activity data for catecholamines on terminal muscle are different from those on MA and AS.

8.2.3. Comments

These data support the ideas that (1) the structure–activity relationships for catecholamines and their analogues on terminal vascular muscle are probably different from that for arterial smooth muscle (Altura, 1975), (2) different types of α-adrenergic receptors may exist in different regions of the peripheral vasculature, and (3) adrenergic amines like tyramine, amphetamine, and others of this class probably contract vascular smooth muscle by a release of NE from postganglionic nerve endings in arterial walls rather than by a direct action on vascular muscle.

ACKNOWLEDGMENTS

This work was supported in part by United States Public Health Service Research Grants HL-18015 and MH-26236.

References

Altura, B. M., 1971, Chemical and humoral regulation of blood flow through the precapillary sphincter, *Microvasc. Res.* **3**:361.

Altura, B. M., 1972*a*, Can metarteriolar vessels occlude their lumens in response to vasoactive substances? *Proc. Soc. Exp. Biol. Med.* **140**:1270.

Altura, B. M., 1972*b*, Sex as a factor influencing responsiveness of arterioles to catecholamines, *Eur. J. Pharmacol.* **20**:261.

Altura, B. M., 1975, Pharmacologic effects of alpha-methyl DOPA, alpha-methylnorepinephrine and octopamine on rat arteriolar, arterial and terminal vascular smooth muscle, *Circ. Res. Suppl.* **36**: I-233.

8.3. Adrenergic Innervation of the Blood Vessels of the Spinal Cord of the Cat

E. T. ANGELAKOS, J. D. IRVIN, and J. L. OSTERHOLM

The adrenergic innervation of the extramedullary (pial) and spinal cord tissue (parenchymal) vessels was studied in cats using the formaldehyde fluorescence histochemical technique. Basically this technique involves reacting tissue monoamines with paraformaldehyde vapor for a specified time under optimal conditions of pH, relative humidity, and temperature. The specificity of this reaction is such that catecholamines can be differentiated from other monoamines including serotonin.

The extramedullary vessels were found to receive extensive adrenergic innervation in all segments, which was most abundant in the cervical region. Within the cord, autofluorescent latex injection studies and microangiography demonstrated a much greater vascularity of the gray matter compared to the white matter. A proportion of the small blood vessels within the cord was found to have adrenergic nerve terminals in close association to the vessel wall; this was more extensive in the vessels in the white than in the gray matter. The varicosities of the adrenergic fibers associated with these parenchymal vessels were smaller and less intensely fluorescent than those found in the adrenergic fibers associated with the extramedullary vessels. Pretreatment with a monoamine oxidase inhibitor (nialamide) resulted in an increase in the fluorescent intensity of the adrenergic varicosities in all vessels, while treatment with reserpine eliminated the adrenergic fluorescence. Spinal cord injury of a 500 g/cm magnitude resulted in the appearance of an increased number of catecholamine varicosities in relationship to the parenchymal microvasculature in both the white and gray matter.

As a means of delineating the origin of the catecholamine fibers supplying the spinal vessels, the effects of spinal cord transection, spinal root section, pretreatment with the peripheral ganglionic blocking agent, ecolid (chlorisondramine), and chronic bilateral adrenalectomy were studied. Seven to ten days after T_4 cord transection, there was no change in the adrenergic innervation of the extramedullary vessels above or below the cut or in the adrenergic innervation of the parenchymal vessels above the transection. However, no parenchymal fluorescence was found below the cut. Root section or ecolid pretreatment resulted in the absence of any

E. T. ANGELAKOS, J. D. IRVIN, and J. L. OSTERHOLM · Hahnemann Medical College, Philadelphia, Pennsylvania.

adrenergic fluorescence in relationship to the extramedullary vascular system, while the parenchymal vessels were normally innervated in this preparation. There was no alteration from normal in the pattern of spinal vascular fluorescence 1 wk following bilateral adrenalectomy.

It is concluded that the extramedullary blood vessels of the spinal cord of the cat receive adrenergic innervation segmentally from the peripheral adrenergic nervous system. The parenchymal vessels, on the other hand, must receive their adrenergic innervation from fibers descending within the cord, possibly as part of the bulbospinal noradrenergic system.

ACKNOWLEDGMENTS

This work was supported by NIH Grants HE-13008 and NS-10163 and by a contract from the Office of Naval Research.

8.4. Effect of CO_2 on the α-Adrenergic Receptor: A Control Mechanism for Tissue Blood Flow

FREDERICK N. MILLER, DAVID L. WIEGMAN, MICHAEL J. DEVANEY, and PATRICK D. HARRIS

The close proximity of small arteries and veins (Nicoll and Webb, 1955) and the high diffusibility of carbon dioxide (Landis and Pappenheimer, 1963) suggest to us that there is a countercurrent exchange of carbon dioxide from the small veins to the small arteries. This exchange of carbon dioxide could provide negative feedback control of the microvasculature by altering the sensitivity of the small artery to α-adrenergic stimulation. The following study was designed to determine if carbon dioxide would modify small artery response to norepinephrine.

8.4.1. Methods

In vivo concentration–response curves were obtained by closed-circuit television microscopy to quantitate the effects of norepinephrine on small arteries (70–160 μm in diameter) and small veins (130–230 μm) in the cremaster muscle of Sprague-Dawley rats.

Animals were anesthetized with urethane, 800 mg/kg, and α-chloralose, 60 mg/kg (i.p.), and the cremaster muscle, with major vessels and nerves intact, was suspended by ligatures in a bath of Krebs solution. Small artery and small vein diameters were measured every 30 s, and heart rate and blood pressure were recorded every minute. Five to seven concentrations of norepinephrine were added to the bath to obtain a complete concentration–response curve in each experiment. The ED_{50} was graphically determined for each vessel in each experiment and converted to a pD_2 value ($-\log ED_{50}$) as a measure of vessel sensitivity to norepinephrine. Three groups of animals were used with (1) a bicarbonate (B) buffered Krebs solution in the bath ($P_{CO_2} \simeq 60$), (2) a tris-bicarbonate (T-B) buffered Krebs solution ($P_{CO_2} \simeq 60$), and (3) a tris (T) buffered Krebs solution ($PCO_2 \simeq 0$).

FREDERICK N. MILLER, DAVID L. WIEGMAN, MICHAEL J. DEVANEY, and PATRICK D. HARRIS · Dalton Research Center and the Departments of Pharmacology, Physiology, and Electrical Engineering, University of Missouri, Columbia, Missouri.

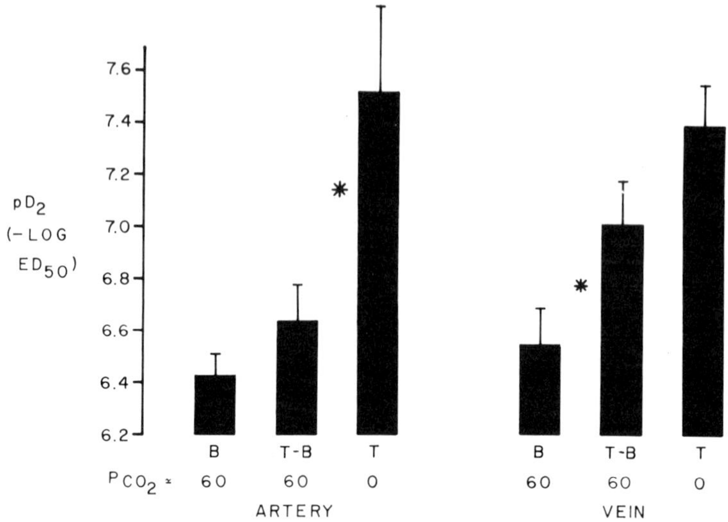

Figure 1. Small artery and vein sensitivity to norepinephrine expressed as pD_2 values ($\bar{X} \pm$ SEM). The buffer system and resulting P_{CO_2} (mm Hg) in the cremaster bath for the three groups of animals were (1) bicarbonate (B), $P_{CO_2} \simeq 60$ ($N = 10$); (2) tris-bicarbonate (T-B), $P_{CO_2} \simeq 60$ ($N = 8$); and (3) tris (T), $P_{CO_2} \simeq 0$ ($N = 8$).

8.4.2. Results

In both the artery and the vein, the greatest sensitivity occurred with $P_{CO_2} \simeq 0$ (T group in Fig. 1). The pD_2 values were 7.5 ± 0.33 in the artery and 7.4 ± 0.16 in the vein. These vessels were about 10 times less sensitive with $P_{CO_2} \simeq 60$ (B group in Fig. 1). In the vein, there was a statistically significant difference between the two $P_{CO_2} \simeq 60$ groups (B and T-B groups). In the artery, there was no statistical difference between the two high CO_2 groups (B and T-B groups).

8.4.3. Conclusion

Our data indicate that CO_2 is not the only factor involved in the decrease in norepinephrine sensitivity in the vein. However, in the artery, decreased sensitivity to norepinephrine can be attributed to the presence of CO_2. These data are consistent with our hypothesis that countercurrent exchange of CO_2 provides a signal for control of the microvasculature. As an example for the operation of this control system, increased tissue metabolism would increase venous P_{CO_2}, which would increase the countercurrent exchange of carbon dioxide from the small vein to the small artery. Increased levels of carbon dioxide in the artery would give decreased sensitivity of the α-adrenergic receptor. Thus the small artery would dilate, even though there were constant levels of circulating catecholamines and/or nerve activity. This dilation would increase blood flow and nutrient supply to the metabolizing tissue. In this manner, countercurrent exchange of carbon dioxide would provide a negative feedback mechanism for local control of tissue blood flow.

ACKNOWLEDGMENTS

This research was supported in part by United States Public Health Service Grants HL 12614, HL 53252, HL 05810, and HL 20422 from the National Heart and Lung Institute.

References

Landis, E. M., and Pappenheimer, J. R., 1963, Exchange of substances through the capillary walls, in: *Handbook of Physiology,* Section 2: Circulation, Vol. II (W. F. Hamilton and P. Dow, eds.), pp. 1018–1019, American Physiological Society, Washington, D.C.

Nicoll, P. A., and Webb, R. L., 1955, Vascular patterns and active vasomotion as determiners of flow through minute vessels, *Angiology* **6:**291.

8.5. Effects of α and β Blockade on Oxygen Supply to Rat Brain and Muscle

J. A. LIPP and HARVEY R. WEISS

A comparison of a tissue highly innervated with α and β receptors (muscle) was made to a lesser innervated tissue (brain) to determine how resting α and β tone regulates oxygen supply. The β blocking agent, propranolol, shifts the oxyhemoglobin dissociation curve, unloading oxygen at the tissue (Agostoni *et al.*, 1973). The effect of α and β blockade on blood flow, tissue oxygen tension (Po_2), and small vessel blood volume was investigated in the brain and biceps brachii muscle of 75 anesthetized rats. Tissue Po_2 and tissue perfusion were measured polarographically. Small vessel blood volume was determined with $^{59}FeCl_3$ and used to calculate open capillary density. Propranolol or phenoxybenzamine was given in a dose of 2 mg/kg.

Phenoxybenzamine caused a slight decrease in blood pressure with no change in heart rate. Tissue perfusion in the cortex did not change, while muscle blood flow increased significantly. Brain Po_2 decreased significantly, while there was no change in muscle Po_2. There was no significant change in small vessel blood volume. This is in agreement with Honig *et al.* (1970), who reported no change in open capillary density with acute denervation. With propranolol there was a significant decrease in heart rate and no effect on blood pressure. There was no change in blood flow in either tissue. The Po_2 of the brain and muscle did not change. There was no signficant change in small vessel blood volume. The data were analyzed by the Krogh model for metabolism changes.

No resting α or β tone was observed in the cortex. Propranolol did not affect blood flow, Po_2, or small vessel blood volume, but showed a calculated increase in metabolism which could be attributed to increased oxygen unloading at the tissue. Phenoxybenzamine increased muscle blood flow but not brain blood flow, indicating that brain is less innervated than muscle. As small vessel blood volume did not increase, the α tone is not on precapillary sphincters, but on arterioles. Phenoxybenzamine caused a calculated increase in metabolism of the brain. Muscle metabolism increased, showing that oxygen consumption in small animals is flow dependent (Whalen *et al.*, 1973; Honig *et al.*, 1971).

J. A. LIPP and HARVEY R. WEISS · Department of Physiology, CMDNJ-Rutgers Medical School, Piscataway, New Jersey.

ACKNOWLEDGMENTS

This study was supported in part by USPHS-16134 and by a grant-in-aid from the American Heart Association, New Jersey Affiliate.

References

Agostoni, A., Berfasconi, C., Gerli, G. C., Luzzana, M., and Rossi-Bernardi, L., 1973, Oxygen affinity and electrolyte distribution of human blood: Changes induced by propranolol, *Science* **182:**300.

Honig, C. R., Frierson, J. L., and Patterson, J. L., 1970, Comparison of neural controls of resistance and capillary density in resting muscle, *Am. J. Physiol.* **218:**937.

Honig, C. R., Frierson, J. L., and Nelson, C. N., 1971, O_2 transport and $\dot{V}O_2$ in resting muscle: Significance for tissue capillary exchange, *Am. J. Physiol.* **220:**357.

Whalen, W. J., Buerk, D., and Thuning, C. A., 1973, Blood flow limited oxygen consumption in resting skeletal muscle, *Am. J. Physiol.* **224:**763.

8.6. Evidence for Increased β-Adrenergic Receptor Function in Isolated Perfused Carotid Artery from Cold-Acclimated Rabbits

STEPHEN F. FLAIM and ARNOLD C. L. HSIEH

Honda *et al.* (1962) found that auricular blood vessels of cold-acclimated rabbits responded less to systemically infused catecholamine (CH). Owen (1972) attributed this to a reduced sensitivity to norepinephrine of the vascular smooth muscle of the rabbit central ear artery. Recent studies have shown that a similar alteration occurs in the carotid artery of cold-acclimated rabbits (Flaim and Hsieh, 1975). In this study, an attempt has been made to determine if this altered response is related to a potentiation of the activity of the β-adrenergic receptor.

Two groups of rabbits which had been temperature acclimated for a period of 13 months were used. The control group (WA) was held at 30°C and the experimental group (CA) was held at 5°C. Animals were sacrificed and segments of carotid artery were excised and mounted in a chamber by cannulation of the inflow and outflow ends. The segments were perfused with a series of solutions with known drug concentrations, and maximum values for hydraulic resistance (R) were electrically calculated.

Segments from each group were exposed to a series of CHs (epinephrine, E; norepinephrine, NE; phenylephrine, PH within a dose range of 3.2×10^{-5} mg/ml to 4.0×10^{-3} mg/ml. Regression equations for the responses of each group to each CH were calculated and compared as follows. E: $Y_c = 0.300X_c + 1.373 \pm 0.016$ ($n = 17$); $Y_w = 0.288X_w + 1.327 \pm 0.014$ ($n = 18$). NE: $Y_c = 0.299X_c + 1.297 \pm 0.009$ ($n = 15$); $Y_w = 0.289X_w + 1.309 \pm 0.011$ ($n = 15$). PH: $Y_c = 0.389X_c + 1.454 \pm 0.013$ ($n = 12$); $Y_w = 0.354X_w + 1.387 \pm 0.012$ ($n = 12$). Y is $\log R/R_0$ and X is the log dose of CH. The CA group showed a decreased sensitivity to PH ($p < 0.05$) and to NE ($p < 0.005$) with no change in response to E ($p > 0.25$). The response of a second group of arteries to stimulation with NE in the presence of the β-blocking agent, propranolol (3.6×10^{-5} mg/ml), was obtained. In the presence of β-blockade, the altered response to NE previously seen in the CA group was eliminated (Fig. 1).

STEPHEN F. FLAIM · The Division of Cardiology, Milton S. Hershey Medical Center, Pennsylvania State University, Hershey, Pennsylvania. ARNOLD C. L. HSIEH · Department of Human Physiology, School of Medicine, University of California, Davis, California.

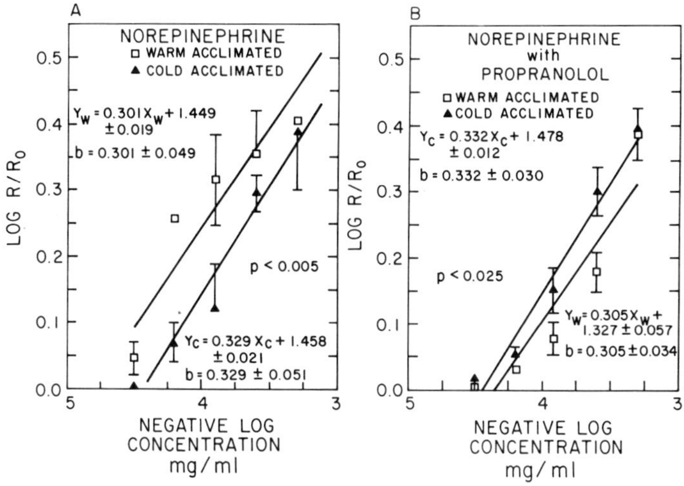

Figure 1. Regression lines showing the responses of the warm-acclimated and cold-acclimated groups to norepinephrine (panel A) and to norepinephrine in the presence of the β-adrenergic blocking agent, propranolol (panel B).

In summary, these data indicate that cold acclimation results in an increased β-adrenergic receptor function in the vascular smooth muscle of rabbit carotid artery.

ACKNOWLEDGMENT

This study was supported in part by the United States Public Health Service, National Heart and Lung Institute Grant HL-14780-02.

References

Flaim, S. F., and Hsieh, A. C. L., 1975, Reduced sensitivity to norepinephrine in isolated, perfused carotid artery from cold-acclimated rabbits, *Fed. Proc.* **34(3)**:477.

Honda, N., Judy, W. V., and Carlson, L. D., 1962, Effects of adrenaline and noradrenaline on ear vessels in cold- and warm-adapted rabbits, *J. Appl. Physiol.* **17**:754.

Owen, T. L., 1972, Norepinephrine sensitivity of ear artery strips from cold- and warm-acclimated rabbits, doctoral dissertation, Department of Human Physiology, School of Medicine, University of California at Davis.

8.7. Catecholamines in Low Flow States

E. N. TERRY, R. H. CLAUSS, L. ROUEN, and W. REDISCH

In a model developed to study relationships between catecholamines and vasomotion (Terry *et al.*, 1973), animals were bled, producing hypovolemia and a "shock syndrome." Effects of catecholamines and interference with their activity under controlled conditions in low flow states were studied.

Drugs and doses used were as follows: dibenzylene, 5 mg/kg; Kö 592, a β-blocking agent, 20 mg/kg and 0.3 mg/kg; and α-methyl-p-tyrosine (AMPT), 100 mg/kg.

Animals were bled to a mean systemic pressure of about 35 mm Hg, maintained in this hypovolemic state for about 3 h, and then reinfused over a period of 30 min. Drugs were administered either before or after reinfusion. All parameters were recorded at 15-min intervals throughout 1 h prior to and after reinfusion.

Plasma catecholamine values were very high, particularly in the dibenzylene group, where tachycardia was also pronounced. Central venous pressures were relatively low except in the group treated with β-blocking agents. Effects of drug administration before reinfusion of blood seemed to be more on perfusion, while drug administration after reinfusion seemed to affect flow to a greater extent. Other parameters were not influenced by the timing of drug administration.

The present study seems to confirm the small arteriolar level control of perfusion of microvessels (Cardon *et al.*, 1970; Algire and Merwin, 1955). Subsequent to bleeding and an increase in catecholamine levels, perfusion of exchange vessels drops to a very low level, persisting over at least 3 h. Presumed regulation through "precapillary sphincters" (Mellander, 1971; Chambers and Zweifach, 1944) would imply an initial short-lasting decrease of perfusion, followed by a sustained increase in perfusion with accumulation of local metabolites (Cobbold *et al.*, 1963; Lewis and Mellander, 1962). Interference with catecholamine activity resulted in increased perfusion, not necessarily paralleled by equal flow changes. Tachycardia, pronounced with dibenzylene (Hackel *et al.*, 1964), adversely affects the myocardium. AMPT seemed to provide the best all-round protection against adverse manifestations of hypovolemia in this model (Clauss *et al.*, 1969).

E. N. TERRY, R. H. CLAUSS, L. ROUEN, and W. REDISCH · Departments of Medicine and Surgery, New York Medical College Metropolitan Hospital Center, New York, N.Y.

References

Algire, G. H., and Merwin, R. M., 1955, Vascular patterns in tissues and grafts within transparent chambers in mice, *Angiology* **6**:311.

Cardon, S. Z., Oestermayer, S. F., and Bloch, E. H., 1970, Effect of oxygen on cyclic red blood cell flow in anaesthetized mammalian striated muscle as determined by microscopy, *Microvasc. Res.* **2**:67.

Chambers, R., and Zweifach, B. W., 1944, Topography and function of the mesenteric circulation, *Am. J. Anat.* **75**:173.

Clauss, R. H., Terry, E. N., and Redisch, W., 1969, Inhibition of vasoconstrictive responses to hypovolemic shock by alpha-methyl-tyrosine, *Circulation* **39**:58.

Cobbold, A., Folkow, B., Kjellmer, I., and Mellander, S., 1963, Nervous and local chemical control of precapillary sphincters in skeletal muscle as measured by changes in filtration coefficient, *Acta. Physiol. Scand.* **57**:180.

Hackel, D. B., Martin, A. M., Spach, M. S., and Sieker, R. O., 1964, Hemorrhagic shock in dogs, *Arch. Pathol.* **77**:575.

Lewis, D. H., and Mellander, S., 1962, Competitive effects of sympathetic control and tissue metabolites on resistance and capacitance vessels and capillary filtration in skeletal muscle, *Acta Physiol. Scand.* **56**:162.

Mellander, S., 1971, Interaction of local and nervous factors in vascular control, *Angiology* **8**:187.

Terry, E. N., Clauss, R. H., Rouen, L. R., and Redisch, W., 1973, Catecholamines and vasomotion, *VASA* **15:3**;222.

8.8. Effect of Steroids on Human Venous Smooth Muscle *in Vivo* and *in Vitro*

NORMAN BARWIN

Women, during pregnancy or oral contraceptive therapy, have increased incidence of varicose veins and thromboembolic disease (Goodrich and Wood, 1964), occurring sometimes before the uterus is large enough to mechanically obstruct venous flow. Humoral factors may be involved (Mullane, 1952).

8.8.1. Method

Human femoral and superficial epigastric vein segments were obtained postmortem. Longitudinal strips, 1.0 wide by 4.5 cm long, were mounted in a 50-ml organ bath perfused with isotonic Krebs solution (15–20 ml/min). Field stimulation (20–30 V, A.C.) was applied through stainless steel electrodes (10 s every 5 min), and the resulting isometric contractions were recorded. Perfusion with the experimental perfusate was for a period of 2 h preceded and followed by periods of perfusion with control perfusate. In some experiments, control perfusion extended over the whole period. Estradiol, 17β and progesterone were first dissolved in polyethylene glycol and diluted to 10, 1, or 0.1 μg/ml in Krebs solution. Control solutions all contained a corresponding amount of polyethylene glycol.

Increased distensibility in forearm and calf was greater during pregnancy than oral contraceptive therapy, although both were significant.

8.8.2. Discussion

Venous distensibility increased progressively during pregnancy or oral contraceptive therapy. After 30 wk of oral contraceptive therapy, the increase of venous distensibility was not as marked. In pregnant patients, the changes in venous distensibility were reversible by the 8-wk postnatal period.

Increased venous distensibility also indicated that the tone in the

NORMAN BARWIN · Department of Physiology, The Queen's University of Belfast, and Department of Obstetrics and Gynecology, Ottawa University, Ottawa General Hospital, Ottawa, Ontario, Canada.

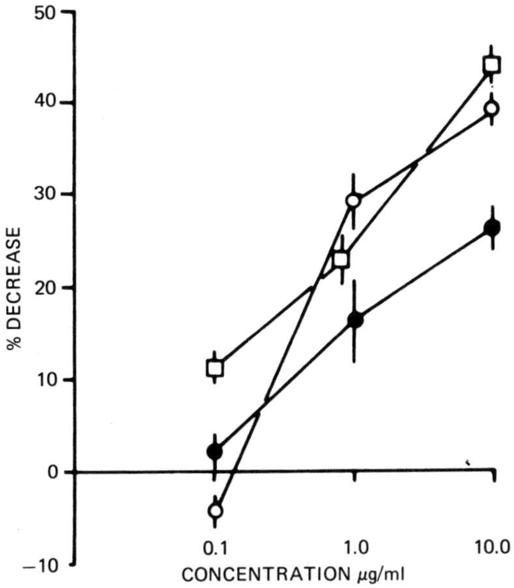

Figure 1. Percent decrease in the amplitude of contraction of human venous muscle when exposed for 2 h to estradiol-17B (●) progesterone (○) and an equal parts mixture of the steroids (□) in concentrations of 0.1, 1.0, and 10 μg/ml. Vertical lines represent ± 1 SEM.

capacity vessels fell during pregnancy and oral contraceptive therapy, possibly because of decreased venous tone resulting from the direct action of the sex steroids on the vessels. This is supported by the *in vitro* experiments where both estrogens and progesterone reduced the response of venous smooth muscle to electrical stimulus.

References

Goodrich, S. M., and Wood, J. E., 1964, Peripheral venous distensibility and velocity of venous blood flow during pregnancy or during oral contraceptive therapy, *Am. J. Obstet. Gynecol.* **90:**740.

Mullane, D. J., 1952, Varicose veins of pregnancy, *Am. J. Obstet. Gynecol.* **63:**620.

8.9. Direct Contractile and Metabolic Actions of Nitroglycerine on the Heart

R. L. COULSON and K. M. BOROW

Considerable controversy exists over the mechanism of action of nitroglycerine (Honig *et al.*, 1960; Mason and Braunwald, 1965). The usual view is that normal vessels dilate (Herman *et al.*, 1971), diseased coronaries do not (Gorlin *et al.*, 1959), and metabolic demands of the myocardium are reduced secondary to peripheral vascular actions (Williams *et al.*, 1965).

8.9.1. Methods

The method of Coulson and Rusy (1973) was used in experiments on 11 isolated rabbit hearts electrically paced and retrogradely constant flow-perfused at 25°C with modified Krebs-Henseleit solution containing 10 mM pyruvate. Left ventricles (LVs) contracted isovolumically against a volume-controlled latex balloon. Hearts were suspended in a Dewar flask calorimeter. Heat production (H, mW), oxygen consumption ($\dot{V}$, μl/s), and mechanical performance ($s^{-1} \int \text{pressure} \cdot dt$) ($P$, mm Hg) were measured at various points on the ascending limb of the Starling curve. At the apex of the Starling curve where P was optimal ($P_o t$), nitroglycerine (GTN) (0.12 mg/liter) was introduced to the perfusate and measurements were repeated at all control volumes.

8.9.2. Results

Since coronary perfusion rate was constant throughout experiments, perfusion pressure directly reflected coronary vascular tone. Comparative regression analysis determined that GTN caused a vasodilation which was independent of mechanical performance. Extravascular support, coronary resistance dependent on mechanical activity, was not altered, although mechanical activity declined (see Fig. 1) because of a fall in contractility.

Energetic parameters were altered by changing LV volume, and similar regression analysis was performed on the relationships between heat and mechanical performance (Smith, 1972) and heat and oxygen consumption.

R. L. COULSON and K. M. BOROW · Cardiology Section, Temple University Health Sciences Center, Philadelphia, Pennsylvania.

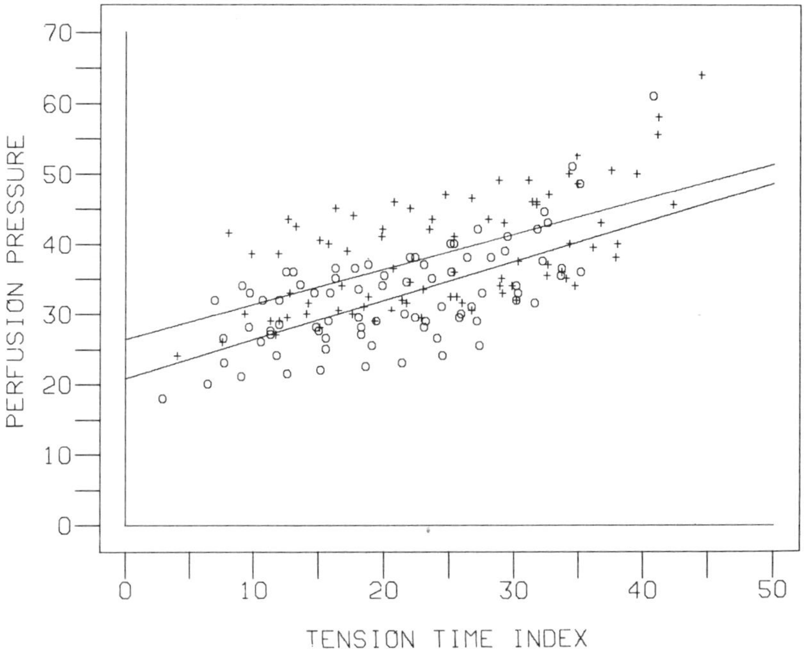

Figure 1. Comparative regression analysis of coronary perfusion pressure (mm Hg) upon tension–time index (mm Hg). Upper curve is through control data (+). Control regression $y = 26.44 \pm 1.10 + 0.50 \pm 0.08 \times X$ ($n = 81, r = 0.59, p < 0.01$). Lower curve is through GTN data (O). GTN regression $Y = 20.67 \pm 1.62 + 0.57 \pm 0.07 \times X$ ($n = 81$, r 0.62, $p < 0.01$). The intercepts (coronary vascular tone) are significantly different ($p <$ 0.01). The slopes (extravascular support) are not different ($p > 0.10$). The tension–time index was determined as the product of heart rate and the per beat time integral of left ventricular developed pressure.

8.9.3. Discussion

Nitroglycerine (0.12 mg/liter caused a fall in vascular tone. There was a fall in extravascular support secondary to the decline in P_0t, but this accounted for a reduction in coronary resistance at P_0t which was only about one-half the drop in vascular tone.

Overall mechanical force production became more efficient due to the fall in P-independent energy expenditure. The fall in contractility resulted in lower tension maintenance costs.

Control values of the calorific equivalent of oxygen (CEO) (19.71 mJ/ μl: O_2) indicated oxidation of both carbohydrates and fats (carbohydrates $\cong 20$, fatty acids $\cong 17$). The presence of a control anaerobic element (2.21 mW) suggests that glycogen from the heart's own store was utilized. Any fat metabolism must have come from internal stores since the perfusate contained only pyruvate.

After GTN, the CEO reflected carbohydrate metabolism (20.16 mJ/μl: O_2). The anaerobic component was gone (0.04 mW), suggesting that metabolism was dependent on the perfusate pyruvate.

The difference data represent metabolic activity abolished by GTN and show 2.17 mW of anaerobic activity abolished. The CEO abolished (16.59 mJ/μl: O_2) is consistent with fatty acid.

References

Coulson, R. L., and Rusy, B. F., 1973, A system for assessing mechanical performance, heat production, and oxygen utilization of isolated perfused whole hearts, *Cardiovasc. Res.* **7:**859.

Gorlin, R., Brachfeld, N., Macleod, C., and Bopp, R., 1959, Effect of nitroglycerine on the coronary circulation in patients with coronary artery disease or increased left ventricular work, *Circulation* **19:**705.

Herman, A. G., Bogaert, M. G., and Schaepdryver, A. F., 1971, Effect of Nitroglycerine at different degrees of contraction of the rabbit aortic strip. *Arch. Int. Pharmacodyn. Ther.* **190:**407.

Honig, C. R., Tenney, S. M., and Gable, P. V., 1960, The mechanism of cardiovascular action on nitroglycerine, *Am. J. Med.* **39:**910.

Mason, D. T., and Braunwald, E., 1965, The effect of nitroglycerine and amyl nitrite on arteriolar and venous tone in the human forearm, *Circulation* **32:**755.

Smith, I. C. H., 1972, Energetics of activation in frog and toad muscle, *J. Physiol. (London)* **220:**583.

Williams, J. F., Jr., Glick, G., and Braunwald, E., 1965, Studies on cardiac dimensions in intact unanesthetized man. V. Effects of nitroglycerine, *Circulation* **32:**767.

II

Blood Flow in Special Tissues

9

Pulmonary Circulation

9.1. Biomicroscopic Investigations on the Connection between the Capillary Bed and the Larger Vessels of the Lungs of Some Reptiles

I. WILLNOW and R. WILLNOW

There are fundamental differences in the topography of the pulmonary capillary bed in reptiles compared with amphibians. The microscopic differences can be related to macroscopic differences in the topography of the larger vessels. In amphibians, the large arteries remain as far as possible under the pleura, and the large veins are situated toward the interior of the lung; this is central differentiation.

In reptiles, all large vessels are under the pleura; here there is subpleural differentiation. The arteries enter the parenchyma from the pleural side, as in amphibians. Small arteries, arterioles, and precapillaries are surrounded by a space, optically vacant. This space consists of periarterial and lymph spaces which diminish and disappear as the arteries approach the capillaries. The precapillaries turn gradually into capillaries without marked distinction. The postcapillaries are short and branched. They are much more meandering and of varying caliber. But there is a fundamental difference from the amphibians, for in reptiles the postcapillaries do not tend toward the interior, but, like the precapillaries, keep to the surface of the lung.

So it is in all complicated regions of the lung with respiratory capillaries. In the terminal thin-walled sac of snakes, the capillarization is only nutritive or there are no capillaries at all. In the lungs of amphibians, there is only a respiratory capillarization.

The differences in venous topography indicate a fundamental difference in structure between amphibian and reptile lung. Further, although there is no real difference as regards small vein and precapillary topography, there are basic differences in the distribution of capillaries.

I. WILLNOW and R. WILLNOW · Vital Mikroskopische Abteilung, Institut für Anatomie, Freie Universität Berlin, Germany.

9.2. Pulmonary Capillary Filtration Coefficient and Permeability to HRP in Dogs

JAMES C. HOGG, RENE P. MICHEL, and SADAYKI INOUE

The radii of the pores in the alveolar capillary membrane were estimated by using the equation of Landis and Pappenheimer (1963):

$$\left\{\frac{(1 - a_w/r)^2[1 - 2.10(a_w/r) + 2.09(a_w/r)^3 - 0.95(a_w/r)^5]}{(1 - a_s/r)^2[1 - 2.10(a_s/r) + 2.09(a_s/r)^3 - 0.95(a_s/r)^5]}\right\} - \frac{D_s}{D_w} = \frac{D_s 8nK_F\Delta\pi}{RT\dot{m}}$$

where r is mean pore radius, a_w and a_s are radii of the water and test molecule (HRP), and D_w and D_s are free diffusion coefficients of water. The general graphic solution was obtained for the left-hand side of this equation by substituting a series of values for r. The specific solution of the right-hand side was obtained experimentally under steady-state conditions in ten dogs. In these experiments, the filtration coefficient K_F was obtained by dividing fluid movement (f_m) across the capillary by the pressure (ΔP) across its wall; f_m was obtained by assuming that right duct lymphatic (RDL) flow represents 30% of lung lymph. ΔP was determined by calculating capillary hydrostatic pressure ($\bar{\text{P}}$cap) from pulmonary artery ($\bar{\text{P}}$a) and wedge ($\bar{\text{P}}$w) pressures, estimating vascular (Πcap) and interstitial (Πis) oncotic pressures by measuring the protein concentration of plasma and lung lymph and assuming that the interstitial hydrostatic pressure $\bar{\text{P}}$is was −10 mm Hg. The pressures obtained ± SE were $\bar{\text{P}}$a 13.14 ± 0.71, $\bar{\text{P}}$w 3.91 ± 1.37, $\bar{\text{P}}$cap 7.2 ± 0.32, Πcap 16.91 ± 1.23, Πis 11.12 ± 1.52. When HRP concentrations in blood and lymph were constant, HRP flux was calculated ([HRP] $\times f_m$). The contribution of HRP to the osmotic pressure difference across the capillary membrane (Π_{HRP}) was calculated from the van't Hoff equation, and pore radius was estimated by plotting the solution obtained for the right-hand side of the equation in each experiment on the graphic solution and reading off the appropriate value for r. We estimate that K_F is 0.0071 ± 0.0021 ml/min/mm Hg/100 g of wet lung, that pore radius is 29.7 ± 1.1 Å, and that the pores occupy 10^{-6} of 1% of capillary surface area. We observed peroxidase in pinocytotic vesicles and between endothelial cells but were unable to trace it all the way through

JAMES C. HOGG, RENE P. MICHEL, and SADAYKI INOUE · Department of Pathology, McGill University, Montreal, Quebec, Canada.

pores. Visualization of HRP with the electron microscope was dose dependent and required a total dose of more than 100 mg per kilogram of body weight.

Reference

Landis, E. M., and Pappenheimer, J. R., 1963, Exchange of substances through the capillary walls, in: *Handbook of Physiology,* Section 2: Circulation, Vol. II (W. F. Hamilton and P. Dow, eds.), p. 961, American Physiological Society, Washington, D.C.

9.3. Weight vs. Electrode Detection of Outflow Response of Isolated Perfused Dog Lung to Osmotic Solutes

ARTHUR B. RITTER and WILLIAM PERL

In experiments on the weight-monitored, isolated, perfused, papaverine-vasodilated dog lung (Perl *et al.*, 1975), we have inserted a fast-responding silver–silver chloride electrode into the lung outflow on the weighing platform. The purpose was to measure time-dependent outflow concentrations of various chlorides simultaneously with the osmotically induced weight transients. When the osmotic test solute was not a chloride (urea, glucose), the sensitivity of the electrodes was sufficient to measure the baseline dilution of resident chloride (Effros, 1974).

In an edematous lung (185 g drained wet weight) at a (low) perfusate flow of 10 ml/s, the start of the weight decrease in response to a step-function increment of approximately 10 mosM NaCl preceded the start of the electrode response by about 6 s (Fig. 1). In an isogravimetric (relatively dry) lung, the start of both responses was close to synchronous. The osmotically induced fluid ΔW_{osm} entering the vascular volume should travel with the NaCl increment ΔC that induced it, if the vascular volume is very distensible (high compliance). Since ΔW_{osm} and ΔC travel together and the electrode is located at the edge of the weighing platform, both weight response and electrode response should start together. This situation is presumed to obtain in the isogravimetric lung. The edematous lung result is then presumed to arise from indistensibility (low compliance) of the vascular volume. In this case, ΔW_{osm} enters the vascular volume and "instantaneously" pushes an equal increment of vascular fluid off the weighing platform by incompressible piston action and starts the weight response. ΔW_{OSM} and ΔC, traveling together, arrive at the edge of the weighing platform later to start the electrode response. The flow × delay time indicates that the initial sites of fluid entry into the vascular volume occur at about 50 ml from the venous exit. No detectable hydrostatic pressure change (less than approximately 1 mm Hg) occurred throughout the osmotic maneuver.

ARTHUR B. RITTER · Department of Chemistry and Chemical Engineering, Stevens Institute of Technology, Hoboken, New Jersey. WILLIAM PERL · Department of Medicine, New Jersey Medical School, College of Medicine and Dentistry of New Jersey, Newark, New Jersey.

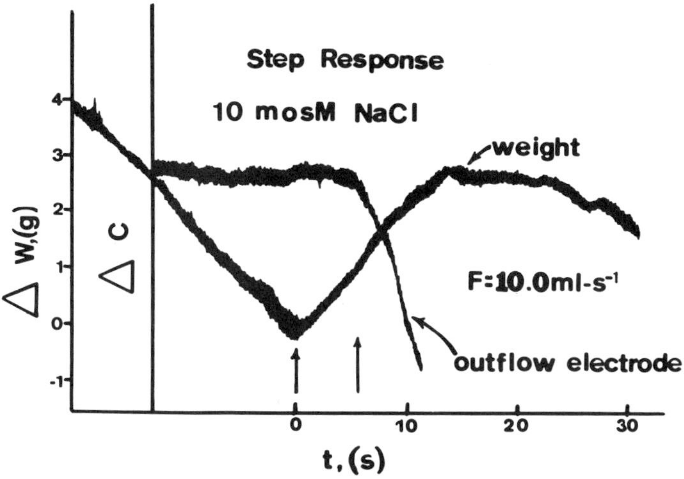

Figure 1. Response of weight increment $\Delta W(t)$ and outflow concentration increment $\Delta C(t)$ of NaCl of isolated, perfused, papaverine-vasodilated dog lung to 10 mosM step change of NaCl, showing timing delay. Weight response starts at first arrow followed approximately 6 s later by outflow electrode response (second arrow). Perfusate flow 10 ml s^{-1}, lung weight (drained, wet) 185 g. Outflow electrode response went off scale at t = 12 s.

ACKNOWLEDGMENTS

This work was supported in part by USPHS Grants HL-12879 and HL-12974, NSF Grant GK42083, and the UPTAM program at Stevens Institute of Technology.

References

Effros, R. M., 1974, Osmotic extraction of hypotonic fluid from the lungs, *J. Clin. Invest.* **54**:935.

Perl, W., Chowdhury, P., and Chinard, F. P., 1975, Reflection coefficients of dog lung endothelium to small hydrophilic solutes, *Am. J. Physiol.* **228**:797.

9.4. Pulmonary Extraction of 5-Hydroxytryptamine: Antagonism by Imipramine in the Intact Animal

MORRIS D. KERSTEIN, LESLIE H. CRONAU, C. NORMAL GILLIS, and SAMUEL MANDEL

The lungs of several species of animals including man are capable of removing 5-hydroxytryptamine (5-HT) and norepinephrine (NE) from pulmonary blood (Gillis, 1973; Heineman and Fishman, 1969). It has been shown that removal of these amines in man is quantitatively altered in the state of pulmonary hypertension and following cardiopulmonary bypass (Gillis *et al.,* 1972). In the perfused rabbit lung, it has been shown that several drugs including imipramine will inhibit the uptake of 5-HT (Gillis *et al.,* 1972; Iwasawa and Gillis, 1974). The present study was undertaken for two purposes: (1) to demonstrate that the removal of 5-HT and NE occurs in the intact dog in a similar manner as in man and (2) to demonstrate that the pulmonary removal of 5-HT can be inhibited by imipramine in the intact animal as can be demonstrated *in vitro.*

9.4.1. Materials and Methods

The extraction of 5-HT by lung vasculature in the intact animal was studied utilizing the differential uptake of [^{14}C]5-HT and [^{3}H]NE.

Imipramine, a known inhibitor of 5-HT removal by the lung *in vitro,* was studied to determine inhibition of uptake. Samples of blood were simultaneously withdrawn from the pulmonary artery (PA) and the left atrium (LA) for 30 s. Radioactivity of the supernatant was determined by liquid scintillation spectrometry after being deproteinized with perchloric acid. Extraction was taken as the difference of total isotope between the PA and LA samples.

9.4.2. Results

In 17 animals 75.3% ± 2.6 SEM of [^{14}C]5-HT was removed in a single passage through the lung; 23.8% of [^{3}H]NE was removed. In 11

MORRIS, D. KERSTEIN, LESLIE H. CRONAU, C. NORMAL GILLIS, and SAMUEL MANDEL · West Haven Veterans Administration Hospital, Department of Surgery and Anesthesia, Yale University School of Medicine, New Haven, Connecticut.

animals, imipramine (1.07–20.9 mg/kg) inhibited lung extraction of 5-HT by 3.8–99.5%. Removal was inhibited in a dose-dependent fashion.

9.4.3. Conclusion

1. Both 5-HT and NE are removed from blood during a single passage through the pulmonary vasculature of the dog. 5-HT is removed to a greater degree than is NE.
2. The degrees of extraction of 5-HT and NE are similar to those we have previously determined in man.
3. In the intact dog, imipramine inhibits the uptake of 5-HT by the lung in a dose-dependent manner.

References

Gillis, C. N., 1973, Metabolism of vasoactive hormones by lung, *Anesthesiology* **39:**626.

Gillis, C. N., Greene, N. M., Cronau, L. H., and Hammond, G. L., 1972, Pulmonary extraction of 5-hydroxytryptamine before and after cardiopulmonary bypass in man, *Circ. Res.* **30:**666.

Heinemann, H. O., and Fishman, A. P., 1969, Nonrespiratory functions of mammalian lung, *Physiol. Rev.* **49:**1.

Iwasawa, Y., and Gillis, C. N., 1974, Pharmacological analysis of norepinephrine and 5-hydroxytryptamine removal from the pulmonary circulation: Differentiation of uptake sites for each amine, *J. Pharmacol. Exp. Ther.* **188:**386.

9.5. Pulmonary Microcirculation during Lethal Hypovolemia in the Cat

MELVIN M. NEWMAN

In order to photograph the microcirculation with the least amount of physiological disturbance, the following limitations were placed on the experimental study: (1) the animals should be breathing spontaneously under light anesthesia to eliminate any artifacts from artificial respiration; (2) the animals should be breathing room air to eliminate any toxic effects from high inspired oxygen concentrations; (3) the lung should be allowed to remain as nearly as possible in its normal anatomical situation, to eliminate any changes due to stretching or torsion; and (4) the animal should be allowed to die in shock, to eliminate any effects caused by transfused blood, saline, or colloidal solutions. Cats were chosen because of convenient size and the absence of portal congestion seen in the dog shock model.

An airtight thoracic window, developed from the work of Terry (1939), Krahl (1964), and Wagner and Filley (1965), was inserted in the left chest wall of cats under sodium pentobarbital anesthesia. Spontaneous respiration of room air was resumed after negative pleural pressure was restored. Alveoli on the surface of the left lower lobe were monitored by color cinemicrography with reflected light through a Leitz Ultropak objective. Cats were bled until mean aortic pressure fell to 60–70 mm Hg (average 24.8 mm/kg blood loss). Survival time was 25–180 min. All cats showed marked tachypnea, a fall in arterial P_{CO_2} and pH, a rise in arterial P_{O_2}, and a marked increase in base deficit (Astrup) (Table I).

The chief changes in the microcirculation were a gradual decrease in the number of alveolar capillaries being perfused and aggregation (sludging) of red cells. Interstitial edema and hemorrhage occurred only in areas of local trauma.

In conclusion, observations of the capillary blood flow in the lungs of cats dying with hypovolemia contradict the original hypothesis that the lung is the primary target organ in shock. It seems more likely that the lung is the target organ of resuscitative treatment.

MELVIN M. NEWMAN · Department of Surgery, University of Colorado Medical Center, Denver, Colorado.

Table I. Pulmonary Microcirculation (17 Cats)

	Control. BP (mm Hg)		Shock BP (mm Hg)		Control Pa (mm Hg)		Shock Pa (maximum)	
	Systolic	Diastolic	Systolic	Diastolic	Systolic	Diastolic	Systolic	Diastolic
Average	149.6	99.5	88.9	46.0	28.9	15.5	31.3	16.2
Standard deviation	27.4	26.6	12.0	6.5	6.3	5.7	6.1	5.1
Standard error	6.0	5.80	2.61	1.42	1.5	1.4	1.6	1.4

	Blood removed (ml/kg)	Survival time (min)
Average	25.3	157.9
Standard deviation	5.5	95.4
Standard error	1.2	20.8

	Control Po_2	1 h shock Po_2	Control Pco_2	1 h shock Pco_2	Control pH	1 h shock pH	Control base excess (mM/liter)	Shock base excess (mM/liter)
Average	66.1	79.2	26.3	17.5	7.429	7.366	−7.175	−17.5
Standard deviation	9.9	11.1	5.1	4.95	0.05	1.177	2.297	4.8
Standard error	2.2	2.5	1.1	1.1	0.01	0.039	0.514	1.1

ACKNOWLEDGMENT

This work was carried out at the Colorado General Hospital with funds from Grant No. HL 13904 from the National Institutes of Health, U.S. Department of Health, Education, and Welfare.

References

Krahl, V. E., 1964, *In vivo* microscopy of the rabbit's lung, *Bibl. Anat.* **4**:400.

Terry, R. J., 1939, A thoracic window for observation of the lung in a living animal, *Science* **90**:43.

Wagner, W. W. Jr., and Filley, G. E., 1965, Microscopic observations of the lung *in vivo*, *Vasc. Dis.* **2**:229.

10

Myocardial Blood Flow

10.1. Microcirculation in the Ventricle of the Dog and Turtle

HARALD TILLMANNS, SHIGEAKI IKEDA, HERBERT HANSEN, JONNALAGEDDA S. M. SARMA, and RICHARD J. BING

It is generally agreed that coronary inflow is mainly diastolic and coronary sinus outflow mainly systolic (Gregg, 1962). To locate this phase shift, phasic red cell velocity and diameters of coronary arterioles, capillaries, and venules were measured in the beating turtle and dog heart using high-speed cinematography (400 frames/s) with transillumination of the left ventricle. A 20-gauge needle, containing a small quartz rod and a mirror angled at 45°, was inserted underneath the superficial layer of the myocardium to transmit heat-filtered light from a pulsating xenon arc through the ventricular muscle toward the objective of an infinity-corrected microscope. In recent experiments, a floating, counterbalanced focus keeper was used to maintain the focal distance between the moving heart and the stationary objective of the microscope. Red cell velocity was determined by frame-to-frame analysis of red cell progression using a reference scale (Tillich *et al.*, 1971; Bing *et al.*, 1972).

In the turtle and dog, peak arteriolar red cell velocity occured in unison with left coronary artery inflow, and the capillary and venule flow pattern followed that of the coronary sinus (Fig. 1). The inside diameters of arterioles, capillaries, and venules in the turtle and dog ventricle all declined about 34% during systole; capillary diameters were in the range of those observed by others (Bassingthwaighte *et al.*, 1974). Capillary arrangement appeared to be predominantly parallel and concurrent, as

HARALD TILLMANNS, SHIGEAKI IKEDA, HERBERT HANSEN, JONNALAGEDDA S. M. SARMA, and RICHARD J. BING · Lehrstuhl für Kardiologie, Medizinsche Klinik Heidelberg, Germany, Huntington Memorial Hospital and California Institute of Technology, Pasadena, California and University of Southern California, Los Angeles, Californa.

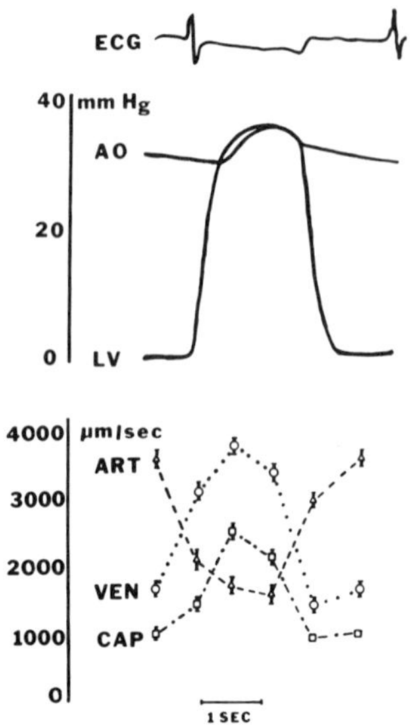

Figure 1. Red cell velocity in the turtle ventricle.

described by other investigators (Bassingthwaighte *et al.,* 1974); however, capillary loops with countercurrent flow were occasionally observed.

The data on microvascular phasic red cell velocity are consistent with the macroobservations of reduced coronary artery inflow and enhanced coronary sinus outflow during ventricular contraction. The results demonstrate that the shift in the flow pattern occurs at the transition from arterioles to capillaries.

References

Bassingthwaighte, J. B., Yipintosoi, T., and Harvey, R. B., 1974, Microvasculature of the dog left ventricular myocardium, *Microvasc. Res.* **7**:229.

Bing, R. J., Wayland, H., Rickart, A., and Hellberg, K., 1972, Studies on the coronary microcirculation by direct visualization, in: *Myocardial Blood Flow in Man* (A. Maseri, ed.), pp. 23–34, Minerva Medica, Torino, Italy.

Fox. C. C., and Hutchins, G. M., 1972, Architecture of the human ventricular myocardium, *Johns Hopkins Med. J.* **130**:289.

Gregg, D. E., 1962, Physical determinants of coronary flow, in: *Handbook of Physiology,* Section 2: Circulation, Vol. II (W. F. Hamilton and P. Dow, eds.), pp. 1533–1536, American Physiological Society, Washington, D.C.

Reynolds, S. R. M., Kirsch, M., and Bing, R. J., 1958, Functional capillary beds in the beating, KCl-arrested and KCl-arrested perfused myocardium of the dog, *Circ. Res.* **6:**600.

Sobin, S. S., and Tremer, H. M., 1972, Diameter of myocardial capillaries (abst.), *Microvasc. Res.* **4:**330.

Tillich, G., Mendoza, L., and Bing, R. J., 1971, Total and nutritional coronary flow, *Circ. Res.* **28:**148 (Suppl. 1).

10.2. Temporal Heterogeneity of Myocardial Perfusion

FRANCOIS SESTIER, RICHARD R. MILDENBERGER, and GERALD A. KLASSEN

Heterogeneity in myocardinal perfusion has been observed by several investigators (Klassen, 1971; Yipintsoi *et al.,* 1973; Utley *et al.,* 1974). This study was designed to verify if, under conditions of a steady state, with autoregulation intact, there are changes in both space and time of local coronary perfusion.

10.2.1. Methods

Four varieties of radioactive microspheres (^{125}I, ^{141}Ce, ^{85}Sr, and ^{95}Nb) were injected into the pump-perfused left coronary artery of 20-kg open-chest mongrel dogs. Two modes of injection were employed: SIM, when all four varieties of microspheres were injected simultaneously, and SEQ, when injections were made sequentially at intervals of 15–20 s. The average transit time of our system from injection to deposition of microspheres was less than 2 s. After sacrifice, the perfused myocardium was divided into 600-mg sections, each containing at least 2000 microspheres of each type. Differential counting allowed computation of flow per gram of each section for each isotope.

10.2.2. Results

The mean variance of flow/g for each section after SIM was ±0.005 $ml \cdot min^{-1} \cdot g^{-1}$ and was assumed to represent the overall experimental error. After SEQ, the section's mean variance of flow/g was ±0.029, this difference being significant ($p < 0.025$) when tested by a three-factors analysis of variance. Plotting changes in regional flow after SEQ on a time axis suggests a periodicity of flow change of from 30 to 90 s (Fig. 1): it seems that subendocardial (ENDO) and neighboring subepicardial (EPI) sections may have a different periodicity and/or be out of phase.

FRANCOIS SESTIER, RICHARD R. MILDENBERGER, and GERALD A. KLASSEN
Cardiovascular Division, Royal Victoria Hospital, and McGill University Clinic, Montreal, Quebec, Canada.

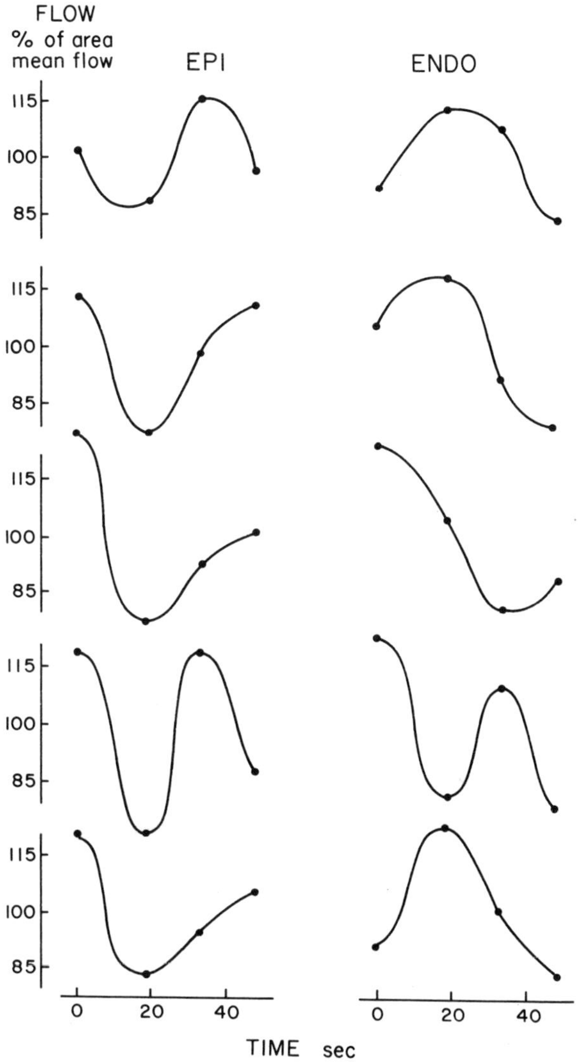

Figure 1. Sequential injection of four varieties of microspheres. Flow ($ml \cdot min^{-1} \cdot g^{-1}$) for five different subepicardial areas (left) and neighboring subendocardial areas (right), expressed as a percentage of the mean flow of the area, is plotted against time on the abscissa. A periodicity of from 30 to 90 s appears to be present.

10.2.3. Conclusion

These data suggest that cyclic changes in regional blood flow do occur and that these variations occur in both the spatial and the temporal domain.

References

Klassen, G. A., 1971/1972, Coronary artery disease, a cause of heterogenous myocardial perfusion, *Cardiology* **56:**343.

Utley, J., Carlson, E. L., Hoffman, J. I. E., Martinez, H. M., and Buckberg, G. C., 1974, Total and regional myocardial blood flow measurements with 25 μ, 15 μ, 9 μ, and filtered 1–10 μ, diameter microspheres and antipyrine in dogs and sheep, *Circ. Res.* **34:**391.

Yipintsoi, T., Dobbs, W. A., Scanlon, P. D., Knopp, T. J., and Bassingthwaighte, J. B., 1973, Regional distribution of diffusible tracers and carbonized microspheres in the left ventricle of isolated dog hearts, *Circ. Res.* **33:**573.

10.3. A New Model for Assessing Myocardial Function

COLIN E. BAYLISS, FLORA B. CRAWFORD, and BAFFOUR NSAFOAH

Research in normal and disturbed cardiac physiology has been handicapped by an inability to control and directly measure several interacting components of myocardial function. A useful model would permit direct measurements of tension, relaxation, and perfusibility free of the phasic effects of fiber shortening. Models described previously (Shelburne *et al.*, 1967; Blesa *et al.*, 1970) have not incorporated continuous parabiotic perfusion.

A new model (Fig. 1) consists of an isolated, electrically stimulated rabbit heart interventricular septum contracting isometrically against a tension transducer. It is perfused by heated, heparinized, diluted blood pumped at 1 ml/g tissue/min from the ear artery to the ear vein of an awake rabbit. A shunt can be opened to disconnect the parabiotic rabbit from the circuit if desired. A 20-ml reservoir proximal to the pump supplies blood in the presence of ear artery spasm. Carbon dioxide is added to the rabbit's inspired air as needed to maintain constant P_{CO_2} in the circuit. Each preparation acts as its own control.

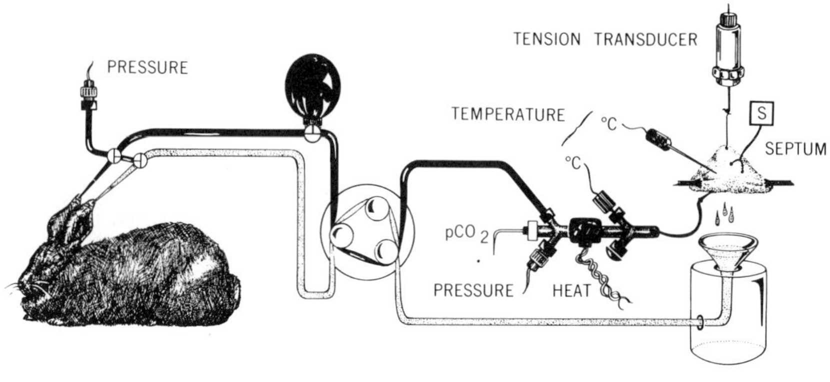

Figure 1. Diagram of model for assessing myocardial function. Arterial circuit, including reservoir and perfusion manifold, black; venous return circuit, stippled.

COLIN E. BAYLISS, FLORA B. CRAWFORD, and BAFFOUR NSAFOAH · Department of Surgery, University of Toronto, Toronto, Ontario, Canada.

Table I. Performance Characteristics of 58 Control Preparations (Mean ± SD)[a]

Contractility:	
T_{max}	13.7 ± 6.7 g
dF/dt_{max}	94 ± 63 g/s
TPT	268 ± 83 ms
Relaxation:	
T_{rest}	6.5 ± 1.6 g
$-dF/dt_{max}$	66 ± 52 g/s
RT	558 ± 172 ms
Perfusibility:	
$\bar{C}$	11.2 ± 3.4 μl/g/min/mm Hg

[a] Abbreviations: T_{max}, maximum developed tension; dF/dt_{max}, maximum rate of rise of tension; TPT, time to peak tension; T_{rest}, resting tension; $-dF/dt_{max}$, maximum rate of relaxation; RT, relaxation time; $\bar{C}$, mean conductance or flow per unit pressure.

Table II. Status of the Parabiotic Rabbit in 58 Control Preparations (Mean ± SD)[a]

ph	7.45 ± 0.05
Pco_2	37.5 ± 3.9 mm Hg
Base excess	+2.2 ± 2.8 meq/liter
Po_2	89 ± 6 mm Hg
Normal hematocrit	37.3 ± 2.9%
Diluted hematocrit	31.7 ± 2.6%
Mean arterial pressure	89 ± 9 mm Hg

[a] Values for arterial blood.

Tables I and II summarize the performance characteristics of the septa and the status of the parabiotic rabbits in 58 control preparations.

The new model is simple, clearly defined, and adaptable to a variety of investigations requiring physiologically perfused, working myocardium.

ACKNOWLEDGMENTS

This work was supported by a grant from the Ontario Heart Foundation. Colin E. Bayliss is a Scholar of the Medical Research Council of Canada.

References

Blesa, E. S., Langer, G. A., Brady, A. J., and Serena, S. D., 1970, Potassium exchange in rat ventricular myocardium: Its relation to rate of stimulation, *Am. J. Physiol.* **219:**747.

Shelburne, J. C., Serena, S. D., and Langer, G. A., 1967, The rate–tension staircase in rabbit ventricular muscle: Relation to ionic exchange, *Am. J. Physiol.* **213:**1115.

10.4. Washout and Washin Behavior of the Myocardial Extracellular Space: Significance for Evaluation of Capillary Permeability and Interstitial Space Concentrations of Metabolites

H. KAMMERMEIER and B. KAMMERMEIER

Washout or tissue clearance functions of radioactive tracers are commonly used for evaluation of capillary permeability data. However, detailed studies indicate that washout takes place not according to monoexponential functions but according to multiexponential ones, even with a substance such as inulin or sucrose which ought to be distributed in the extracellular space exclusively.

By control experiments consisting of comparative determinations of the interstitial space or residual activity of the heart, integration of the respective exponentials, and use of common methods (estimation of tissue activity), two different exponentials can be identified that are attributed to the interstitial space of the isolated perfused heart.

In further experiments, the rate of uptake of tracers was determined by integration of washout kinetics of hearts exposed to the tracers for different periods. Rate constants of uptake calculated from those data are close to those of the washout. The time constants of both are unexpectedly low (0.4–0.6 and 0.08–0.18 min^{-1}, respectively). Calculation of the permeability surface–area product from the faster component yields values (0.05–0.12 ml/min) appreciably lower than those published so far (0.1–0.4 ml/min; e.g. *cf.* Yipintsoi *et al.,* 1969.

According to calculations of myocardial capillary transfer rates from the data and experiments with labeled substrates, these findings show that in the myocardium (1) capillary transfer of substrates can be limited and determined by capillary permeability and (2) interstitial concentrations of substrates and metabolites can differ appreciably from those of plasma.

Reference

Yipintsoi, T., Tancredi, R., Richmond, D., and Bassingthwaighte, J. B., 1969, in: *Capillary Permeability* (C. Crone, ed.), p. 153, Munksgaard, Copenhagen.

H. KAMMERMEIER and B. KAMMERMEIER · Department of Physiology, Medical Faculty, Technical University of Aachen, Germany.

10.5. Changes in Coronary Vessels Induced by Repeated Hypothalamic Stimulation

B. BLUM, J. ISRAELI, and H. M. ASKENASY

Anginalike alterations in the ECG and myocardial necrotic pathology are induced in patients by cerebral irritative lesions (Cropp and Manning, 1960). These seem to be characteristic when the hypothalamus is specifically involved, as is illustrated by a number of cases including hypothalamic tumor case and by hypothalamic stimulation experiments in cats and in monkeys. We have shown that repeated hypothalamic stimulations may induce foci of myocardial necrosis in such cases (Melville *et al.,* 1963). In relatively healthy animals, the hypothalamic stimulation causes the appearance of a tall T wave; in animals with some preceding ECG abnormalities, the T wave becomes inverted. The difference between these signs is emphasized by the observation that oxytocin fully protects against the latter only. If the irritative stimulations are continued, the T wave may finally become irreversibly inverted. If such animals are left for about 24 h, minute disseminated infarcts may be found in their myocardium. On the other hand, autopsies carried out during the still reversible stage reveal typical subendocardial hemorrhages. Similar human cases also show such bleeding into the heart muscle or into the subendocardium. These can be found, in fact, even without any sign of myocardial necrosis. In some cases, however, a close association between the hemorrhages and necrosis of the myocardium is detectable. Apparently the hemorrhagic episode activates a sequence of events including hemostasis by thrombus formation, and, subsequently, myocardial ischemia and necrosis (Copley. 1974; Lehr and Chau, 1973). The role of the hemorrhages in the early reversible stage is emphasized as a possible cause for the initiation of some of the necrosis.

References

Copley, A. L., 1974, Bleeding time, other *in vivo* tests and the arrest of hemorrhage, *Thromb. Res.* **4:**1.

Cropp, G. J., and Manning, G. W., 1960, Electrocardiographic changes simulating myocardial ischemia and infarction associated with spontaneous intracranial hemorrhage, *Circulation* **22:**25.

B. BLUM, J. ISRAELI, and H. M. ASKENASY · The Sackler School of Medicine of Tel Aviv University, Tel Aviv, Israel.

Lehr, D., and Chau, R., 1973, Changes of the cardiac electrolyte content during development and healing of experimental myocardial infarction, in: *Recent Developments in the Study of Cardiac Structure and Metabolism* (N. S. Dhalla, ed.), University Park Press, Baltimore.

Melville, K. I., Blum, B., Shister, H., and Silver, D., 1963, *Am. J. Cardiol.* **12:**781.

10.6. Microangiographic Reevaluation of the Human Intramyocardial Vasculature

H. SUORANTA and M. KORMANO

The human myocardium is considered to contain two types of penetrating arteries—short vessels terminating after branching within the myocardium (class A vessels) and long vessels supplying the endocardium (class B vessels, Estes *et al.,* 1966*a,b*). Class B vessels are considered to form a subendocardial plexus of anastomosing arteries, the significance of which was advocated by the classical description of Fulton (1963*a,b*). Simple categorical division of myocardial arteries has been found inadequate in experimental work (Grayson *et al.,* 1974). Review of the literature also failed to provide convincing illustrative evidence of such clear-cut vascular categories in the human heart. Although the existence of arterial connections and their increase in ischemic heart disease are well documented (Baroldi and Scomazzoni, 1967), an extensive subendocardial network (Fulton, 1963*a,b*; Estes *et al.,* 1966*a,b*) has not been well demonstrated in the photomicrographs of the recent literature (Rissanen, 1973). We have tried to reevaluate the morphology of these vascular arrangements, which may be significant in relation to ischemic heart disease.

10.6.1. Materials and Methods

A microangiographic analysis of 12 human autopsy hearts of varying age (4–86 yr) was performed. Both coronary artery orifices were cannulated and the arteries were flushed with saline and infused with a 10% saline suspension of Micropaque (Damancy and Co.) for 1 h using 120–150 mm Hg pressure. Formalin-fixed hearts were cut transversally from apex to base into 1-cm slices which were radiographed. Pieces of posterior, anterior, and interventricular parts of these were embedded in paraffin wax. One-millimeter serial sections were cut both transversally and parallel to the endocardial surface and studied with histological and high-resolution microradiographic techniques described elsewhere in detail (Kormano and Suoranta, 1971).

H. SUORANTA and M. KORMANO · Department of Diagnostic Radiology, University of Helsinki, and Department of Diagnostic Radiology, University of Turku, Finland.

10.6.2. Results and Conclusions

Variation exists among the arteries which penetrate the myocardium, but all give branches during their course. The larger ones tend to supply the subendocardial layers. Capillary filling was most extensive near epicardial and endocardial surfaces, probably because of lack of tissue counterpressure. The course of subendocardial blood vessels was irregular because of the presence of papillary muscles and trabecular columns. Superimposition of vessels in thick slices gave an impression of a rich anastomosing subendocardial network. Careful stereoradiographic and thin-section microradiography failed to show essential difference between the subendocardial layer and the rest of the myocardium. The adult pattern of intramyocardial blood vessel architecture was already present at the age of 4 yr.

In a quantitative study, Fulton (1963*b*) was able to find only an average of six arterial anastomoses in the "subendocardial plexus" of healthy left ventricles. We also conclude that in the normal left ventricle the so-called subendocardial plexus is substantially less extensive than could be concluded from the work of Estes *et al.* (1966*b*).

ACKNOWLEDGMENT

This work was supported by the Sigrid Juselius Foundation, Helsinki, Finland.

References

Baroldi, G., and Scomazzoni, G., 1967, *Coronary Circulation in the Normal and the Pathologic Heart,* Office of the Surgeon General, Department of the Army, Washington, D.C.

Estes, E. H., Entman, M. L., Dixon, H. B., and Hackel, D. B., 1966*a*, The vascular supply of the left ventricular wall, *Am. Heart, J.* **71**:58.

Estes, E. H., Dalton, F. M., Entman, M. L., Dixon, H. B., and Hackel, D. B., 1966*b*, The anatomy and blood supply of the papillary muscles of the left ventricle, *Am. Heart J.* **71**:356.

Fulton, W. F. M., 1963*a*, Arterial anastomoses in the coronary circulation. I. Anatomical features in normal and diseased hearts demonstrated by stereoradiography, *Scot. Med. J.* **8**:420.

Fulton, W. F. M., 1963*b*, Arterial anastomoses in the coronary circulation. II. Distribution, enumeration and measurement of coronary arterial anastomoses in health and disease, *Scot. Med. J.* **8**:466.

Grayson, J., Davidson, J. W., Fitzgerald-Finch, A., and Scott, C., 1974, The functional morphology of the coronary microcirculation in the dog, *Microvasc. Res.* **8**:20.

Kormano, M., and Suoranta, H., 1971, Microvascular organization of the adult human testis, *Anat. Rec.* **170**:31.

Rissanen, V., 1973, Microvasculature in the left ventricular wall of the human heart, *Angiology* **24**:345.

10.7. Predictive Value of Myocardial Scanning for Coronary Artery Bypass Surgery

W. J. KOSTUK and M. J. CHAMBERLAIN

Coronary angiography cannot measure regional myocardial perfusion at the capillary level, and the left ventricular angiogram cannot distinguish between reversible and irreversible myocardial dysfunction. This is becoming more important because of the increasing number of patients being considered for aortocoronary bypass grafts. Delivering additional blood to heavily scarred myocardium is of no value. Regional myocardial perfusion as measured by the labeled albumin particle technique (Ashburn *et al.*, 1971) is considered capable of distinguishing scarred myocardium and ischemic but viable myocardium. Forty-three patients who underwent coronary artery bypass surgery were evaluated 2 wk postoperatively to assess the relative contribution of the bypass graft to regional myocardial perfusion. Moreover, on the basis of the postoperative study, an attempt was made at predicting the outcome of individual patients.

Following selective angiography, microspheres of human serum albumin labeled with ^{99m}Tc were injected into the grafted artery, while ^{131}I-labeled macroaggregates of human serum albumin were injected into the aortocoronary bypass graft. The myocardial distribution of these small (20–30 μm), biodegradable ($T_{1/2}$ = 3–5 h) particles was visualized with a rectilinear scanner.

Of the 18 patients who also had a normal preoperative myocardial perfusion scan, the scan remained normal in 17, while one patient, with occlusion of both his graft and the grafted artery, showed a large perfusion defect postoperatively. The grafted artery was often associated with a myocardial perfusion defect, although in 22 patients the aortocoronary bypass graft perfused the defect, resulting in an overall normal myocardial perfusion pattern. In nine patients, both the grafted vessel and the graft supplied the same region. In three patients in whom both a pre- and postoperative scan were obtained, the myocardial perfusion of the grafted vessel was improved.

Of the 43 patients, nine have had angina pectoris in the follow-up period (range 1–18 months, mean 5.5 months). Of the 34 patients who had a completely normal scan or who had improved myocardial perfusion of the grafted vessel, only four (11.7%) have had angina pectoris. One of

W. J. KOSTUK and M. J. CHAMBERLAIN, · Department of Medicine, University Hospital and University of Western Ontario, London, Ontario, Canada.

these patients had occluded his graft, and his myocardial perfusion remained normal via the native vessel. On the other hand, 55% (five of nine) of those with an abnormal scan at the 2-wk postoperative study continued to have angina pectoris. Two of the nine patients in this group had occluded their grafts, while in the others, in spite of patent bypass graft, myocardial perfusion was not altered as a result of surgery.

Labeled microspheres reflect the perfusion of myocardium beyond the major arteries and thus may be valuable in the avoidance of surgery on prospective candidates whose myocardium is beyond salvage. Moreover, if an aortocoronary bypass maintains perfusion, the patient notes symptomatic improvement.

ACKNOWLEDGMENT

This work was supported by the Ontario Heart Foundation.

Reference

Ashburn, W. L., Braunwald, E., Simon, A. L., Peterson, K. L., and Gault, J. H., 1971, Myocardial perfusion imaging with radioactive labelled particles injected directly into the coronary circulation of patients with coronary artery disease, *Circulation* **44:**851.

10.8. Myocardial Perfusion Defects in Patients with Valvular Heart Disease

W. J. KOSTUK and M. J. CHAMBERLAIN

During the course of assessing regional myocardial perfusion in patients with coronary artery disease, we have encountered patients with valvular heart disease and normal coronary arteries in whom the myocardial perfusion pattern was abnormal.

Following hemodynamic measurements and appropriate angiograms in 40 patients with valvular disease and normal coronary arteries angiographically, macroaggregates of human serum albumin labeled with ^{131}I were injected into the right coronary artery, while ^{99m}Tc microspheres of human serum albumin were injected into the left coronary artery as described by Ashburn *et al.* (1971). The myocardial distribution of the small (20–30 μm), biodegradable ($T_{1/2}$ = 3–5 h) particles was imaged and displayed simultaneously using a rectilinear scanner.

Eighteen patients had predominant mitral valve disease, 18 had predominant aortic valve disease, and four had significant involvement of both the aortic and mitral valves. The perfusion pattern in patients with mitral stenosis consisted of a normal left ventricular perfusion, with an increase in activity of the right coronary artery indicating an augmented perfusion to the right ventricular wall. Patients with mitral insufficiency in addition to an increased perfusion of the right ventricle showed an increase in their left ventricular size together with an uneven, patchy distribution of the labeled albumin particles throughout the ventricle. An abnormal myocardial perfusion scan was related to the severity of the mitral valve disease (judged hemodynamically and angiographically) in that patients with moderate and severe disease showed these changes while those with mild disease did not. In patients with aortic valve disease, the changes were limited to the left coronary artery perfusion—a decrease in the perfusion of the left ventricular myocardium. Again, as the severity of the obstruction and/or incompetence increased, the left ventricular myocardial perfusion was more likely to be abnormal.

In patients with aortic disease and/or mitral insufficiency, the electrocardiographic changes and the left ventricular myocardial perfusion were related. Only one of six patients with a normal ECG had an abnormal scan, while three of six patients with left ventricular hypertrophy alone

W. J. KOSTUK and M. J. CHAMBERLAIN · Department of Medicine, University Hospital and University of Western Ontario, London, Ontario, Canada.

had abnormal scans; nine of twelve patients with left ventricular hypertrophy and "strain" pattern exhibited abnormal left ventricular perfusion. The patchy, uneven distribution indicates that the ST segment depression may be related to inadequate left ventricular perfusion and underlying myocardial damage. Five of six patients with miscellaneous changes (left bundle branch block, ST and T wave abnormalities alone) had abnormal myocardial perfusion.

The extent of myocardial perfusion abnormalities may have some bearing on operative risk and the initial postoperative course. All six patients who had mitral valve commissurotomy had an uneventful postoperative course, while three of the four patients who had mitral valve replacement for mitral incompetence had considerable difficulty with left ventricular failure in the early postoperative course. Of the seven patients who had aortic valve replacement, three with abnormal myocardial perfusion had left ventricular failure in the early postoperative period. On the other hand, the four patients who did extremely well postoperatively had normal myocardial perfusion images preoperatively.

Myocardial perfusion abnormalities are common in patients with valvular heart disease in spite of normal coronary arteries. The degree of abnormality is related to the severity of the valvular dysfunction as well as to the electrocardiographic abnormality. The severity of the left ventricular myocardial perfusion abnormality may have some bearing on the operative risk and the initial postoperative course.

ACKNOWLEDGMENT

This work was supported by the Ontario Heart Foundation.

Reference

Ashburn, W. J., Braunwald, E., Simon, A. L., Peterson, K. L., and Gault, J. H., 1971, Myocardial perfusion imaging with radioactive labelled particles injected directly into the coronary circulation of patients with coronary artery disease, *Circulation* **44**:851.

10.9. Myocardial Perfusion Abnormalities in Patients with Cardiomyopathy

W. J. KOSTUK and M. J. CHAMBERLAIN

The diagnosis of cardiomyopathy is made only when other diagnostic considerations have been excluded. To assess myocardial perfusion in this protean disorder, labeled particles of human serum albumin were injected selectively into the coronary arteries of 17 patients with cardiomyopathy. At the time of diagnostic coronary angiography, ^{131}I-labeled macroaggregates of human serum albumin and ^{99m}Tc-labeled human serum albumin microspheres were injected into the right and left coronary arteries, respectively, similar to the procedure described by Ashburn *et al.* (1971). Following the radioactive emboli, no significant electrocardiographic or aortic pressure changes occurred. The myocardial distribution of these labeled particles was visualized with a rectilinear scanner.

All ten patients with congestive cardiomyopathy (dilated left ventricle with an elevated end-diastolic pressure and a depressed ejection fraction) exhibited abnormal myocardial perfusion scans, consisting of an increase in activity over the right atrium and ventricle, together with an enlarged left ventricular chamber which showed a diffuse, patchy distribution of radioactivity extending to the free margin of the ventricle (Fig. 1). These myocardial perfusion scans likely represent the pathology found in this idiopathic disorder, i.e., intramural fibrosis which is mainly interstitial and perivascular in location, rather than replacement fibrosis involving all the cardiac chambers (Roberts and Ferrans, 1974). Transmural myocardial scarring, on the other hand, is uncommon. One patient, however, showed perfusion deficit localized to the septum and adjacent anterior left ventricular wall. Three of six patients with hypertrophic cardiomyopathy with or without obstruction (gradient 0–100 mm Hg) had abnormal scans. The abnormality in this instance was localized to the hypertrophied interventricular septum. Of the three patients with normal scans, two had no outflow tract obstruction at rest or upon provocation with isoproterenol, while the third had a resting gradient of 30 mm Hg across the outflow tract. The single patient with restrictive cardiomyopathy showed a generalized, patchy, poor distribution of the labeled particles across the left ventricle. Previously we have shown that myocardial perfusion scans obtained following direct intracoronary artery injection of labeled particles

W. J. KOSTUK and M. J. CHAMBERLAIN · Department of Medicine, University Hospital and University of Western Ontario, London, Ontario, Canada.

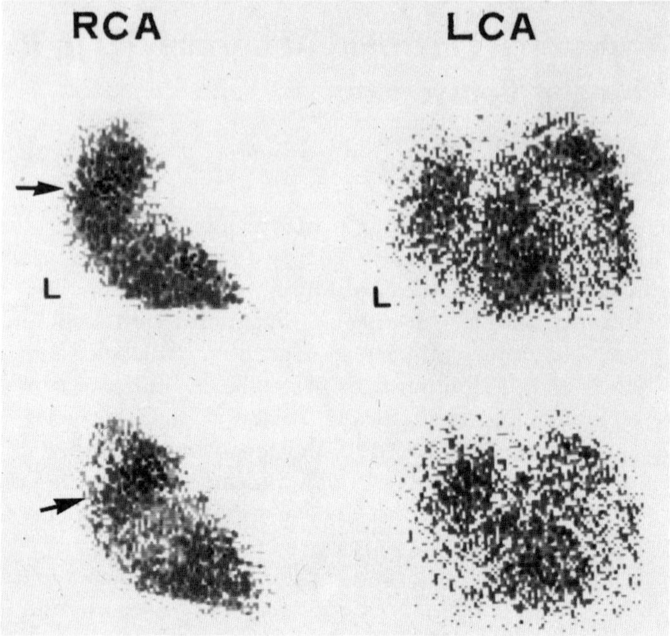

Figure 1. Myocardial perfusion scan in a patient with congestive cardiomyopathy. RCA, right coronary artery; LCA, left coronary artery. The top half (L) is the left anterior oblique view and the bottom half the anterior view. Note the increased activity (arrows) over the right heart, while the LCA shows a patchy decrease in activity which extends out to the free margin of the ventricle.

are identical to those obtained after intravenous radioactive potassium (^{43}K) at rest (Kostuk and Chamberlain, 1974). The same abnormalities in the interventricular septum in patients with hypertrohpic obstructive cardiomyopathy have been detected by both the invasive and noninvasive techniques, although the former is "cleaner," with less scatter and no background activity.

Myocardial perfusion abnormalities are quite common in patients with cardiomyopathy. The cause of the abnormalities visualized by this technique is unknown. We have not had any pathological correlations. Possibilities include fibrosis or small vessel disease. Certainly patients with congestive cardiomyopathy show scattered, patchy, interstitial fibrosis throughout their left ventricular wall. We would like to suggest that the noninvasive ^{43}K scan may be a useful screening test.

ACKNOWLEDGMENT

This work was supported by the Ontario Heart Foundation.

References

Ashburn, W. L., Braunwald, W., Simon, A. L., Peterson, K. L., and Gault, J. H., 1971, Myocardial perfusion imaging with radioactive labelled particles injected directly into the coronary circulation of patients with coronary artery disease, *Circulation* **44:**851.

Kostuk, W. J., and Chamberlain, M. J., 1974, Comparative myocardial perfusion colour scintography after intracoronary artery injection of labelled particles and peripheral injection of potassium^{43}, *Circulation* **50:**825.

Roberts, W. C., and Ferrans, V. J., 1974, Pathological aspects of certain cardiomyopathies, *Circ. Res.* **35:**828.

10.10. Fluorescence Microscopic Demonstration of Localized Myocardial Ischemia

M. KORMANO

Ischemia in the central nervous system and also in the myocardium may increase capillary permeability to trypan blue to an extent detectable to the naked eye (Meneely, 1974). Trypan blue emits red fluorescence when absorbed onto proteins used to detect extravascular distribution (Hamberger and Hamberger, 1966; Steinwall and Klatzo, 1966), which improves the sensitivity of the dye method. The fluorescence method is now widely used for the demonstration of localized ischemia and increased capillary permeability in the CNS (Olsson *et al.,* 1971) and other tissues (Kormano, 1968). In the present study, experimental myocardial ischemia was studied and comparison was made with angiographic methods.

10.10.1. Materials and Methods

The descending branch of the left coronary artery of rats was ligated, and 15 ml/kg of 1% fresh trypan blue in saline was given intravenously from 15 min to 1 month after coronary ligature. Ten minutes after injection, the animal was killed and the heart was rapidly frozen with liquid nitrogen. Fresh frozen transverse 10-μm cryostat sections were viewed with a fluorescence microscope.

In microangiographic study, the abdominal aorta is cannulated upstream, flushed with heparin–saline, and infused with 10–40% Micropaque (Damancy and Co.) suspension at a pressure of 140 mm Hg for 1 h starting either with beating heart or after cardiac standstill. Left ventricular walls were studied using microradiography and histology.

One group of experimental animals received 15 ml/kg of 25% colloidal thorium dioxide (Thorotrast, Testagar) intravenously. One minute after injection, the heart was frozen with liquid nitrogen *in situ* and 2-mm transverse sections were radiographed as described earlier in detail (Kormano, 1970).

10.10.2. Results and Conclusions

Microangiographic capillary filling within the myocardium depends on the technique used. Thus, when viscous 40% Micropaque was infused

M. KORMANO · Department of Radiology, University of Turku, Finland.

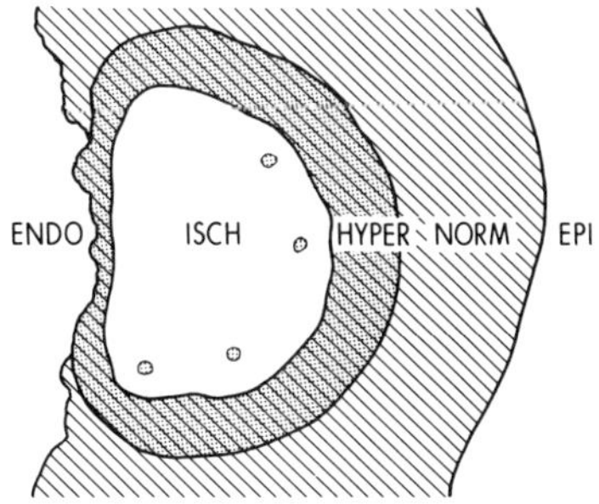

Figure 1. Schematic presentation of the intensity of trypan blue fluorescence in the experimental subendocardial myocardial infarction of the rat. ENDO, endocardial surface; ISCH, ischemic myocardium showing a few fluorescent spots (perfused vessels); HYPER, hyperemic area with extensive extravasation of dye and intense fluorescence; NORM, normal myocardium; EPI, epicardial surface.

or if infusion was started after cardiac standstill, the ischemic area was less extensively filled than normal myocardium, as reported by Grayson *et al.* (1974) with Microfil infusion. Low-viscosity (10–15%) Micropaque suspension infused with beating heart resulted in extensive retrograde capillary filling also in the ischemic area. Apparently heartbeat is necessary for maximal filling (Brown, 1965), but it also passively accumulates dye into nonperfused areas.

Distribution of Thorotrast in the myocardium represents true distribution of blood at the moment of freezing. Unfortunately, this contrast medium is no longer available and the resolution is poor.

With trypan blue fluorescence, normal myocardial capillaries show faint red fluorescence. Following recent (0–2 days) coronary ligature, an ischemic area devoid of red fluorescence was seen in 80% of animals, often only at the subendocardium (Fig. 1). Stained small arteries within the ischemic area indicated perfusion of these vessels, which, however, failed to supply blood to the surrounding capillary bed. Extensive extravasation of the dye due to hyperemia surrounded the infarct.

The red color of the trypan blue fluorescence is easily distinguished from the yellow autofluorescence. This technique is simple and gives better topographic precision than radiochemical and true physiological methods, but does not allow quantitative assessment.

Acknowledgment

This work was supported by the Sigrid Juselius Foundation, Helsinki, Finland.

References

Brown, R. E., 1965, The pattern of the microcirculatory bed in the ventricular myocardium of domestic mammals, *Am. J. Anat.* **116:**355.

Grayson, J., Davidson, J. W., Fitzgerald-Finch, A., and Scott, C., 1974, The functional morphology of the coronary microcirculation in the dog, *Microvasc. Res.* **8:**20.

Hamberger, A., and Hamberger, B., 1966, Uptake of catecholamines and penetration of trypan blue after blood–brain barrier lesions, *Z. Zellforsch.* **70:**386.

Kormano, M., 1968, Penetration of intravenous trypan blue into the rat testis and epididymis, *Acta Histochem.* **30:**133.

Kormano, M., 1970, An experimental technique of *in vivo* high resolution microangiography, *Br. J. Radiol.* **43:**180.

Meneely, G. R., 1974, The capillary factor in myocardial infarction, *Am. J. Cardiol.* **34:**581.

Olsson, Y., Crowell, R. M., and Klatzo, I., 1971, The blood–brain barrier to protein tracers in focal cerebral ischaemia and infarction caused by occlusion of the middle cerebral artery, *Acta Neuropathol.* **18:**89.

Steinwall, O., and Klatzo, J., 1966, Selective vulnerability of the blood–brain barrier in chemically induced lesions, *J. Adenopathol. Exp. Neurol.* **25:**542.

10.11. Oxygen Utilization and Coronary Vascular Reserve in the Ischemic Myocardium Following Acute Coronary Occlusion in the Dog

J. GRAYSON, C. A. SCOTT, and C. J. MORRISON

In nine dogs anesthetized with pentobarbitone sodium, the effect of acute occlusion of the anterior descending coronary artery was observed on the following: venous outflow from a cannula in the main vein draining the area; oxygen extraction ratio (OER); oxygen consumption; and conductivity increment (a measure of heat clearance) and heat production, both recorded from a heated thermocouple implanted in the ischemic area prior to occlusion.

Venous outflow and heat clearance both fell by 40%. OER rose by amounts varying between 61 and 83%. There was a consistent fall in heat production (mean 67%). However, oxygen consumption responses varied; in five experiments, there was a signficant fall (30–70%).

In three experiments, there was no significant change, and in one there was rise. Heat clearance in the infarct has been shown to be in part due to anastomotic flow from surrounding hyperemic areas through nonnutritional channels. Venous flow, which showed changes of similar magnitude to heat clearance following occlusion, might also have a component derived from surrounding hyperemic areas. Calculated oxygen consumptions, $(A_0 - V_0) \times$ flow, may therefore be overestimates of events in the infarct. Heat production always fell, and evidence suggests that heat production is closely related to oxygen consumption and to capillary flow. Falls in local capillary flow, heat production, oxygen consumption and work would seem the most likely effects in infarcting cardiac muscle. In the present investigation, perhaps the most important point is that OER was capable of relatively large changes in response to ischemic stress. In some experiments, changes from 55% to over 90% were recorded. In other experiments, the same considerations that led to overestimates of consumption, namely dilution of venous blood from the infarct by blood from surrounding hyperemic tissue, might also have led to underestimates of OER. It follows, therefore, that the ability to alter

J. GRAYSON, C. A., SCOTT, and C. J. MORRISON · Department of Physiology, University of Toronto, Toronto, Ontario, Canada.

OER might constitute an important component of coronary vascular reserve.

Reference

Grayson, J., and Lapin, B. A., 1966, Observations on the mechanisms of infarction in the dog after experimental occlusion of the coronary artery, *Lancet* **1**:1284.

10.12. Reduction of Myocardial Infarct Volume by Methylprednisolone

CLAYTON H. SHATNEY and RICHARD C. LILLEHEI

Massive doses of corticosteroids reduce the chemical indices of cardiac ischemia following acute experimental myocardial infarction (Libby *et al.*, 1973; Spath and Lefer, 1974) and thus have been assumed to decrease infarct size. This study was designed to directly measure the influence of methylprednisolone sodium succinate (MPSS) on infarct volume in experimental myocardial infarction.

Healthy, anesthetized mongrel dogs ventilated with room air underwent ligation of the distal third of the LAD coronary artery, thereby sustaining an apical infarct. Only animals with similar LAD anatomy were used. Prior to ligation, catheters were fluoroscopically inserted into the coronary sinus and aortic root, and a catheter was directly introduced into the left atrium. Dogs were then randomly placed into the control or treatment groups. One group of treated dogs received 30 mg/kg of MPSS via the left atrial catheter 15 min after infarction. Another group received

Table I. Effects of Corticosteroids in Experimental Myocardial Infarction

Group	$\overline{BP}$ (mm Hg)	CI (liters/min/m^2)	Peripheral resistance (dyn·s·cm^{-5}/m^2)	Infarct volume (%)
Control	−5	−1.65	+1746	14.5 ± 0.95 (SE)
MPSS	+8	−1.41	+1934	11.5 ± 1.52
MPSS × 2	(p = 0.06)	(p = 0.20)	(p = 0.34)	(p = 0.05)
	+6	−1.20	+1191	9.1 ± 1.48
	(p = 0.06)	(p = 0.065)	(p = 0.07)	(p < 0.0025)

30 mg/kg of MPSS 14 min after ligation and again 3 h later. Animals were monitored for 6 h and then killed, and the heart was removed. The left ventricle was dissected from the heart, weighed, sliced into 1-cm sections, and incubated in nitro blue tetrazolium solution for 15 min. Unstained tissue (no LDH) was dissected from the slices and weighed, and infarct volume was calculated. Experimental results for each group of 20 dogs are presented in Table I.

CLAYTON H. SHATNEY and RICHARD C. LILLEHEI · Department of Surgery, University of Minnesota Health Sciences Center, Minneapolis, Minnesota.

The early use of a pharmacological dose of MPSS after experimental myocardial infarction reduces the ultimate size of the infarct. The mechanism of action involves the increased perfusion pressure, the decreased afterload, and the stabilization of myocardial cellular and intracellular membranes which occur following systemic administration of MPSS (Braunwald, 1971; Chatterjee *et al.*, 1973; Spath and Lefer, 1974). These salutary effects are markedly enhanced ($p = 0.13$) by a second dose of MPSS given 3 h after the first.

References

Braunwald, E., 1971, Control of myocardial oxygen consumption: Physiologic and clinical considerations, *Am. J. Cardiol.* **27**:416.

Chatterjee, K., Parmley, W. W., Ganz, W., *et al.*, 1973, Hemodynamic and metabolic responses to vasodilator therapy in acute myocardial infarction, *Circulation* **48**:1183.

Libby, P., Maroko, P. R., *et al.*, 1973, Reduction of experimental myocardial infarction size by corticosteroid administration, *J. Clin. Invest.* **52**:599.

Spath, James A., Jr., and Lefer, A. M., 1974, Preservation of cardiac integrity by pharmacologic agents in acute myocardial ischemia, *Fed. Proc.* **33**:489.

10.13. Pathological Anatomy of the Subendocardial Vasculature after Anoxic Cardiac Arrest

S. R. K. IYENGAR

The subendocardium is the most vulnerable region to ischemic damage (Farrer-Brown, 1960; Moir and DeBra, 1967; Becker *et al.,* 1971; Estes *et al.,* 1966; Brachfeld, 1969). Subendocardial hemorrhagic necrosis has been implicated as a major factor contributing to postoperative morbidity and mortality after open heart surgery using anoxic cardiac arrest (Najafi *et al.,* 1969, 1971; Iyengar *et al.,* 1972, 1973*b*). Laboratory investigations were undertaken in our center to study the effect of anoxic cardiac arrest on the normal and hypertrophied canine left ventricle (Iyengar *et al.,* 1972, 1973*a*). Five normal dogs (group I) subjected to 60–75 min anoxic arrest developed subendocardial hemorrhage. All developed low output failure and died intraoperatively. Six dogs (group II) with left ventricular hypertrophy produced by subcoronary aortic stenosis, subjected to 50–60 min of anoxic arrest, developed extensive subendocardial hemorrhage and necrosis involving the inner third of the left ventricular wall. Four of them failed to come off bypass; two dogs developed low output failure and died within an hour after discontinuance of cardiopulmonary bypass.

Stasis in the coronary microcirculation was proposed as a major factor leading to left ventricular subendocardial hemorrhagic necrosis. When the coronary bed was flushed with a buffered Ringer solution containing glucose during anoxic arrest, the subendocardial lesion was absent or minimal (Iyengar *et al.,* 1972, 1973*a*).

Radiological examination of the coronary vessels using a gelatin–Micropaque technique similar to that described by Schlesinger (1957) and others (WHO, 1970) has proved to be a useful method of delineating the subendocardial vasculature. The normal canine myocardium shows two groups of vessels: type A, extending from epicardium to midmyocardium, and type B extending from epicardium to endocardium (Fig. 1B).

After 60 min of anoxia in dogs, type A vessels were visualized, whereas the subendocardial vasculature (type B) was conspicuously absent (Fig. 1A). Simultaneous measurement of epicardial and endocardial pH during anoxia showed a more rapid fall in the subendocardium.

When the coronary bed was flushed with a buffered Ringer solution

S. R. K. IYENGAR · Division of Thoracic and Cardiovascular Surgery, Queens University, Kingston, Ontario, Canada.

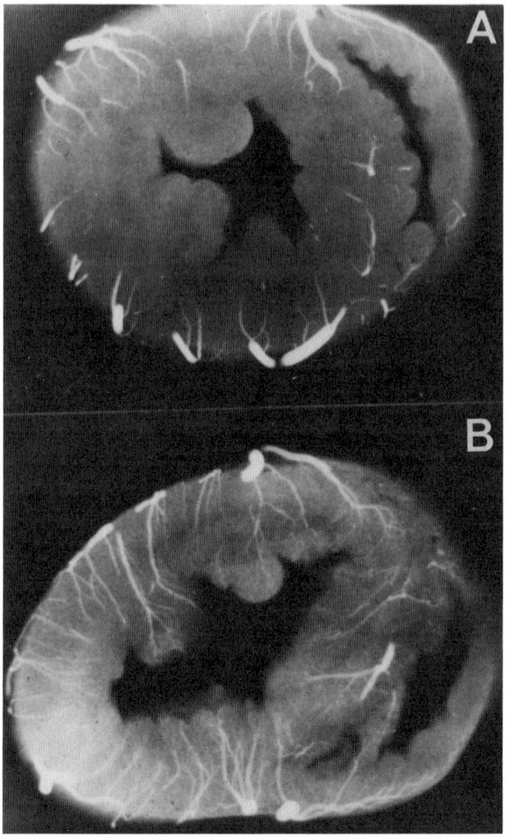

Figure 1. (A) Gelatin–Micropaque injection after 60 min of anoxic arrest. Note conspicuous absence of subendocardial vasculature (type B vessels). (B) Normal heart showing type A and type B vessels.

containing glucose during 60 min of anoxia, patency of both type A and subendocardial vasculature (type B) was well maintained.

Nonvisualization of the subendocardial vasculature (type B) correlates with the incidence of left ventricular subendocardial hemorrhagic necrosis seen in both man and dog. Whether extrinsic compression from edema or increased intramyocardial tension causes collapse of these vessels or whether there is intravascular occlusion needs to be clarified by further study.

Acknowledgment

This work was supported by the Ontario Heart Foundation, Grant No. 2-4.

References

Becker, L. C., Fortuin, N. J., and Pitt, B., 1971, Effect of ischemia and antianginal drugs on the distribution of radioactive microspheres in the canine left ventricle, *Circ. Res.* **28**:263.

Becker, R. M., Schizgal, H. M., and Dobell, A. R. C., 1973, Distribution of coronary blood flow during cardiopulmonary bypass in dogs, *Ann. Thorac. Surg.* **16**:228.

Brachfeld, N., 1969, Maintenance of cell viability, *Circulation Suppl.* **4**:202.

Estes, E. H., Entman, M. L., Dixon, H. B., and Hackel, D. B., 1966, The vascular supply of the left ventricular wall, *Am. Heart J.* **71**:58.

Farrer-Brown, G., 1960, Normal and diseased vascular pattern of myocardium of human heart, *Br. Heart J.* **30**:527.

Iyengar, S. R. K., Ramchand, S., Charrette, E. J. P., and Lynn, R. B., 1972, An experimental study of subendocardial hemorrhagic necrosis after anoxic cardiac arrest, *Ann. Thorac. Surg.* **13**:214.

Iyengar, S. R. K., Charrette, E. J. P., Iyengar, C. K. S., and Lynn, R. B., 1973*a*, An experimental model with left ventricular hypertrophy caused by subcoronary aortic stenosis in dogs, *J. Thorac. Cardiovasc. Surg.* **66**:823.

Iyengar, S. R. K., Ramchand, S., Charrette, E. J. P., Iyengar, C. K. S., and Lynn, R. B., 1973*b*, Anoxic cardiac arrest: An experimental and clinical study of its effects, *J. Thorac. Cardiovasc. Surg.* **66**:722.

Moir, T. W., and DeBra, D. W., 1967, Effect of left ventricular hypertension, ischemia and vasoactive drugs on the myocardial distribution of coronary flow, *Circ. Res.* **21**:65.

Najafi, H., Henson, D., Dye, W. S., Javid, H., Hunter, J. A., Callaghan, R., Einstein, R., and Julian, O. C., 1969, Left ventricular hemorrhagic necrosis, *Ann. Thorac. Surg.* **7**:550.

Najafi, H., Lal, R., Khahli, M., Serry, C., Rogers, A., and Haklin, M., 1971, Left ventricular hemorrhagic necrosis, *Ann. Thorac. Surg.* **12**:400.

Schlesinger, M. J., 1957, New radiographic mass for vascular injection, *Lab. Invest.* **6**:1.

World Health Organization, 1970, The Pathological Diagnosis of Acute Ischemic Heart Disease, Technical Report Series No. 441.

10.14. Metabolic Response of the Heart to Ischemic Arrest during Cardiac Surgery: Assessement by Means of Intramyocardial Carbon Dioxide Tension

GREGORY J. WILSON, WILLIAM GOLDSTEIN, and DAVID C. MacGREGOR

A continuous direct assessment of anaerobic metabolism in the myocardium has become possible by the measurement of tissue carbon dioxide tension (P_{CO_2}) using mass spectrometry. During induced ischemic arrest of the heart, intramyocardial P_{CO_2} rises in response to an accumulation of lactic acid produced by anaerobic glycolysis. Following interruption of coronary blood flow by cross-clamping of the ascending aorta, there is an early period of sustained CO_2 accumulation at a constant rate followed by a period during which the rate of rise gradually decreases to zero, creating a "plateau" in the CO_2 accumulation curve. The "transition point" (Fig. 1) between these two periods is an indicator that anaerobic metabolism is becoming inadequate to maintain cellular viability. In 24 dogs, we have examined this "transition point" as a criterion for the safe termination of ischemic arrest (MacGregor *et al.*, 1974). Total cardiopulmonary bypass with venting of the left ventricle was used, and blood temperature was controlled to keep intramyocardial temperature constant at either 38°C or 28°C. Restoration of coronary blood flow at the "transition point" of the CO_2 accumulation curve at both 38°C (range 25–35 min) and 28°C (range 44–66 min) resulted in complete functional and metabolic recovery. In contrast, reperfusion at the "plateau" at both 38°C (range 55–80 min) and 28°C (range 108–140 min) yielded only partial metabolic recovery, and at 38°C but not 28°C left ventricle ischemic rigor ("stone heart") developed (Wukasch *et al.,* 1972). These results demonstrate the usefulness of the "transition point" criterion and show the substantial metabolic variability from one heart to another. In an additional 40 dogs, the relative protection afforded by moderate hypothermia (28°C) was compared with β-adrenergic blockade (propranolol, 0.5 and 1.0 mg/kg) and both potassium and magnesium cardioplegia. Both β-blockade and chemical cardioplegia significantly delayed but did not prevent the onset of ischemic

GREGORY J. WILSON, WILLIAM GOLDSTEIN, and DAVID C. MacGREGOR Cardiovascular Laboratories, Banting Institute, University of Toronto, Toronto, Ontario, Canada.

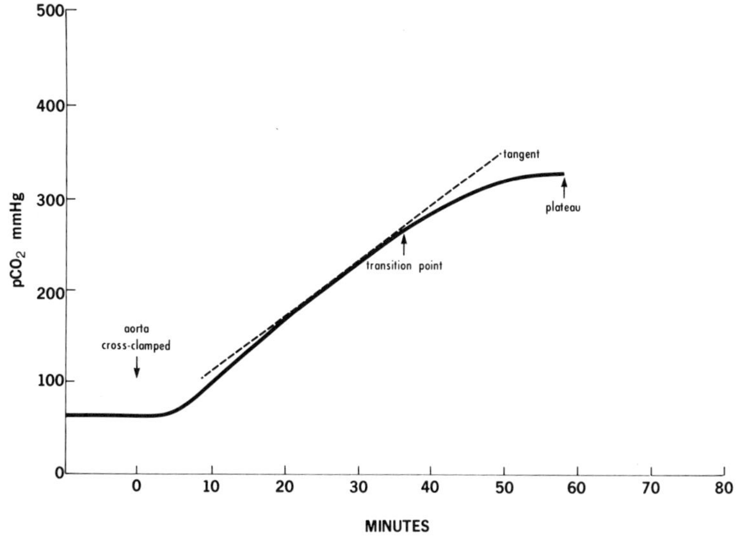

Figure 1. A typical myocardial carbon dioxide accumulation curve during induced ischemic arrest of the heart. The "transition point" is defined as the point where the curve falls below a tangent drawn through its linear portion.

rigor, whereas moderate hypothermia completely prevented this complication.

References

MacGregor, D. C., Wilson, G. J., Holness, D. E., Lixfeld, W., Yasui, H., Tanaka, S., Silver, M. D., and Gunstensen, J., 1974, Intramyocardial carbon dioxide tension: A guide to the safe period of anoxic arrest of the heart, *J. Thorac. Cardiovasc. Surg.* **68:**101.

Wukasch, D. C., Reul, G. J., Milam, J. D., Hallman, G. L., and Cooley, D. A., 1972, The "stone heart" syndrome, *Surgery* **72:**1071.

10.15. Prevention of "Stone Heart" after Anoxic Cardiac Arrest

S. R. K. IYENGAR, E. J. P. CHARRETTE, C. K. S. IYENGAR, S. WASAN, and R. B. LYNN

Ischemic contracture (stone heart) after anoxic cardiac arrest is a lethal and irreversible complication in open heart surgery (Cooley *et al.,* 1972; Katz and Tada, 1972; Wukasch *et al.,* 1972; Armstrong *et al.,* 1973; Iyengar *et al.,* 1973). Lack of energy, stasis of blood in the coronary microcirculation, metabolic acidosis secondary to anaerobic glycolysis during anoxia, and release of myocardial catecholamines appear to play the major role in the pathogenesis of ischemic myocardial injury (Iyengar *et al.,* 1972, 1973, 1975). Intermittent perfusion of the coronary bed with a buffered Ringer solution containing glucose and adrenergic blockade agents has been found to prevent the onset of stone heart in dogs subjected to 90–120 min of anoxic cardiac arrest in our laboratory (Fig. 1).

Prior to 1971, we had encountered five cases of stone heart in aortic valve replacement when anoxic arrest exceeded 50 min, in spite of moderate hypothermia (30°C) and surface cooling of the heart with ice-cold Ringer solution (Iyengar *et al.,* 1973). Based on our earlier experimental work (Iyengar *et al.,* 1972, 1973), we have been routinely using the technique of intermittent flushing of the coronary bed with a buffered Ringer solution whenever aortic cross-clamping became necessary in open heart surgery (Iyengar *et al.,* 1972, 1975). There has been no instance of stone heart, failure to come off bypass, or low output failure in 50 cases of complex valve replacements (classes III and IV) requiring 60–120 min of anoxic arrest (mean 80 min) and 35 high-risk (classes III and IV) multiple aortocoronary bypass grafts with intermittent anoxic periods totaling 50–80 min (mean 60 min). Four years of experimental and clinical experience in our center has confirmed that bloodless coronary perfusion with 800 ml Ringer solution (temperature 15–20°C) containing 200 ml low molecular weight dextran in 10% dextrose, 2 units regular insulin, 200 units heparin, 20 meq sodium bicarbonate, 8 meq KCl, and 20 mg Solucortef is a simple and effective method of myocardial protection during anoxic cardiac arrest. The perfusion is done intermittently under gravity flow in a bolus of 150–200 ml for every 10–15 min of aortic cross-clamping, into the

S. R. K. IYENGAR, E. J. P. CHARRETTE, C. K. S. IYENGAR, S. WASAN, and R. B. LYNN · Division of Thoracic and Cardiovascular Surgery and the Department of Pathology, Queen's University, Kingston, Ontario, Canada.

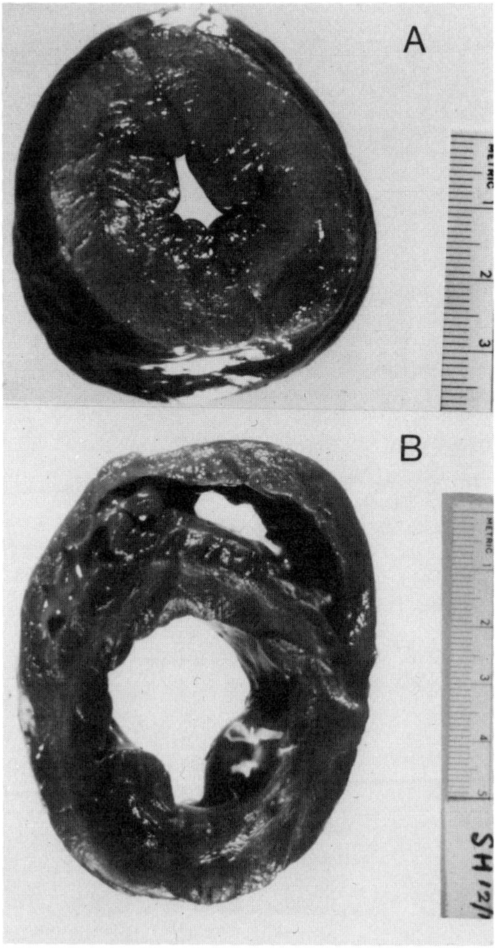

Figure 1. (A) Stone heart (control) section through middle third of the heart after 105 min of anoxic arrest showing concentric ischemic contracture of the left ventricle and marked reduction of ventricular chamber. (B) Section through middle third of the heart after 115 min of anoxic arrest and intermittent coronary flushing. Note absence of concentric contraction and normal size of ventricular chamber. The papillary muscles are well delineated.

aortic root in aortocoronary bypass or mitral valve replacement and into the coronary ostium in aortic valve replacement. The technique also permits further evaluation of metabolic and pharmacological manipulation to achieve even better protection of the myocardial cell and the coronary vasculature during anoxic cardiac arrest.

ACKNOWLEDGMENT

This work was supported by the Ontario Heart Foundation, Grant No. 2-4.

References

Armstrong, R. G., Stanford, W., Cline, R. E., and Guillebeau, J., 1973, The stone heart: Development of a canine model, with ultrastructural survey and metabolic manipulation, *Ann. Thorac. Surg.* **16:**480.

Cooley, D. A., Reid, G. J., and Wukasch, D. C., 1972, Ischemic contracture of the heart: "Stone heart," *Am. J. Cardiol.* **29:**575.

Iyengar, S. R. K., Ramchand, S., Charrette, E. J. P., and Lynn, R. B., 1972, An experimental study of subendocardial hemorrhagic necrosis after anoxic cardiac arrest, *Ann. Thorac. Surg.* **13:**214.

Iyengar, S. R. K., Ramchand, S., Charrette, E. J. P., Iyengar, C. K. S., and Lynn, R. B., 1973, Anoxic cardiac arrest: An experimental and clinical study of its effects, *J. Thorac. Cardiovasc. Surg.* **66:**722.

Iyengar, S. R. K., Charrette, E. J. P., Iyengar, C. K. S., and Lynn, R. B., 1975, Myocardial protection during anoxic cardiac arrest in aortocoronary bypass surgery, in: *Coronary Artery Medicine and Surgery,* Appleton-Century Crofts, New York.

Katz, A. M., and Tada, M., 1972, The "stone heart": A challenge to the biochemist, *Am. J. Cardiol.* **29:**578.

Wukasch, D. C., Reid, G. J., Milam, J. D., Hallman, G. L., and Cooley, D. A., 1972, The "stone heart" syndrome, *Surgery* **72:**1064.

10.16. Effect of Aprotinin on Levels of Adenine Nucleotides and Nucleosides in Postischemic Myocardium in Dogs

SYED J. MUSTAFA and THOMAS M. GLENN

Our purpose was to investigate the effectiveness of pharmacological restoration or maintenance of tissue adenine nucleotide (ANT) stores in the management of myocardial ischemia (MI). Specifically, aprotinin (APT) used to maintain the myocardial ANT pool was investigated.

10.16.1. Methods

Hemodynamic and biochemical parameters were monitored for 90 min in MI dogs with acute coronary ligation (Mustafa *et al.,* 1975).

10.16.2. Results and Discussion

Pretreatment with 10,000 kIU/kg of APT for 30 min prior to ligation resulted in significantly higher ANT than in untreated dogs, but lower than in sham animals, indicating that either the dosage of APT used was too low or the drug cannot fully maintain the total ANT pool. On the other hand, the fifteenfold increase in the sum of adenine nucleosides (ANS) was significantly lowered in APT + MI dogs, although it was still five- to sixfold higher than the control values. DeWall *et al.* (1971), using allopurinol under similar conditions, noted an improvement in contractile force and reversion of EKG changes in the ischemic myocardium. These data suggest that APT may have an influence on breakdown of ANT by affecting the purine-metabolizing enzymes or may alter the release of nucleoside(s) from the cell, which would then become available for incorporation into the nucleotide pool.

APT does not appear to have a direct effect on the levels of any of these compounds in sham animals. Further, in the present study, levels of adenosine were similar in control and APT + MI dogs. Therefore, one must assume that APT may reverse the autoregulatory ability of the heart considered to be impaired because of infarction.

Finally, the sum of ANT and ANS in control animals is higher than

SYED J. MUSTAFA and THOMAS M. GLENN · Department of Pharmacology, University of South Alabama College of Medicine Mobile, Alabama.

Table I. Effect of Aprotinin (APT) on Adenine Nucleotides and Nucleosides during Postmyocardial Infarction (MI) in Dogs[a]

	ATP	ADP	AMP	ΣATP + ADP + AMP	Hypo	Ino	Ado	ΣHypo + Ino + Ado
Sham MI + placebo	55.74[b]	16.26[b]	3.23	75.23[b]	0.64[b]	0.34[b]	0.012	0.99[c]
	±7.25	±0.56	±0.72		±0.08	±0.08	±0.005	
MI + placebo	10.49[c]	6.10[c]	4.54[c]	21.13[c]	5.57[c]	9.37[c]	0.089[c]	15.02[c]
	±1.67	±1.67	±0.28		±0.69	±1.79	±0.047	
Sham MI + APT	47.22	15.92	3.92	67.06	0.48	0.173	0.009	0.66
	±6.26	±0.85	±0.77		±0.098	±0.052	±0.002	
MI + APT	23.42[b,c]	10.24[b,c]	2.55[c]	36.21[b,c]	2.87[b,c]	3.10[b,c]	0.012[c]	5.98[b,c]
	±4.37	±0.67	±0.83		±0.37	±0.75	±0.003	

[a] Cardiac samples were analyzed for ATP by the luciferase method (Greengard, 1965*a*) and for ADP and AMP by the spectrophotometric method (Greengard, 1965*b*). Adenosine (Ado), inosine (Ino), and hypoxanthine (Hypo) were analyzed by the method of Kalckar (1947) using a Beckman model Acta III spectrophotometer. Values are expressed as nmoles/mg protein ± SE (mean of four experiments).

[b] Significant at P value of 0.05 or less between sham MI + placebo group and MI + APT group.

[c] Significant at P value of 0.05 or less between MI + placebo group and MI + APT group.

in MI and MI + APT groups. This may be explained on the basis that part of the control pool is lost into other degradative products (i.e., IMP and uric acid).

In summary, these data show that pretreatment with APT results in an improvement in the ANT pool during myocardial ischemia. These findings are supported by the hemodynamic status of the animals (Mustafa *et al.,* 1975), indicative of improved cardiac function.

ACKNOWLEDGMENT

This work was supported by Bayer AG, Pharma Forschungszentrum, West Germany.

References

DeWall, R. A., Vasko, K. A., Stanley, E. L., and Kezdi, P., 1971, Responses of ischemic myocardium to allopurinol, *Am. Heart J.* **82**:362.

Greengard, P., 1965*a*, Adenosine 5′-triphosphate: Determination by fluorometery, in: *Methods of Enzymatic Analysis* (H. V. Bergmeyer, ed.), pp. 551–555, Academic Press, New York.

Greengard, P., 1965*b*, Adenosine 5′-diphosphate and adenosine 5′-monophosphate, in: *Methods of Enzymatic Analysis* (H. V. Bergmeyer, ed.), pp. 537–577, Academic Press, New York.

Kalckar, H. M., 1947, Differential spectrophotometery of purine compounds by means of specific enzymes. I. Determination of hydroxypurine compounds. II. Determination of adenine compounds, *J. Biol. Chem.,* p. 429.

Mustafa, S. J., Miller, A. G., Tauber, P. F., Goldfarb, R. D., and Glenn, T. M., 1975, Effect of aprotinin (a protease inhibitor) on the hemodynamic and biochemical alterations associated with coronary ligation (abst.), *Fed. Proc.* **34(3)**:2848.

11

The Splanchnic Circulation

11.1. Microvascular Pressures in Innervated Rat Intestinal Muscle and Mucosa

H. GLENN BOHLEN and ROBERT W. GORE

The vasculature of the intestinal mucosa and that of muscle are in parallel. Therefore, the total pressure drop across each circuit is identical. However, structural and functional differences in the microvessels of each circuit may result in different micropressure distributions (Bohlen *et al.*, 1975; Gore and Bohlen, 1975). This possibility was tested by direct measurement of micropressures, diameters, and relative flows in the muscle and mucosal circuits of the rat's intestine. Relative pre- and postcapillary resistances within each circuit were calculated.

Micropressures and diameters were measured with a servonull transducer and TV-micrometer system, respectively. The relative flows in the muscle and mucosa were determined by intraaortic injection of microspheres (10.12 ± 0.22 μm).

The micropressure and diameter distributions measured in the muscle and mucosal circuits, when systemic arterial pressure was 100–110 mm Hg, are shown in Table I. The third-order arterioles and second-order venules are the common origin and termination of the muscle and mucosal microcirculations. Capillary pressures in the muscle were higher than in the mucosal circulation. However, $30.4 \pm 1.4\%$ of the total flow entered the muscle and $69.4 \pm 1.4\%$ entered the mucosal circuit. The relative flows were comparable to those measured in the cat intestine by Kampp and Lundgren (1967). The relative pre- and postcapillary resistances in each circuit were calculated from the pressure distributions (1A, capillary, IV) and relative blood flows. The relative precapillary resistances in the muscle and mucosa were 0.684 and 0.444, respectively. The relative postcapillary resistances were 0.448 and 0.052, respectively. Therefore, the

H. GLENN BOHLEN and ROBERT W. GORE · Department of Physiology, Arizona Medical Center, University of Arizona, Tucson, Arizona.

Table I. Micropressure and Diameter Distributions in Rat Intestinal Muscle and Mucosal Microcirculation[a]

Vessel category	Pressure (mm Hg)	Inside diameter (μm)	*N*
Muscle circuit			
First-order arteriole	44.6 ± 1.6	52.6 ± 1.8	16
Second-order arteriole	44.6 ± 2.9	29.6 ± 2.3	11
Third-order arteriole	32.4 ± 2.5	12.2 ± 0.6	14
Fifth-order arteriole	26.7 ± 2.0	8.4 ± 0.5	11
Capillary	23.8 ± 1.5	5.0 ± 0.5	8
Fourth-order venule	15.2 ± 1.2	9.9 ± 0.8	20
Second-order venule	15.7 ± 1.2	28.3 ± 5.4	10
First-order venule	10.1 ± 0.4	60.4 ± 3.6	11
Mucosal circuit			
Distributing arteriole	30.5 ± 1.7	8.3 ± 0.3	14
Capillary	13.8 ± 2.2	4.3 ± 1.1	11
Second-order mucosal venule	12.8 ± 1.5	9.3 ± 0.6	8

[a] Systemic arterial pressure was 100–110 mm Hg. Data are expressed as mean ±SE.

distribution of pre- and postcapillary resistances favored a higher capillary pressure in the muscle in the mucosal circuit, and explained the different pressure distributions in the two microvascular beds.

Acknowledgments

This work was supported by an Arizona Heart Association Fellowship and NIH Grants HL-13437, HL-05884, and HL-17421.

References

Bohlen, H. G., Hutchins, P. M., Rapela, C. E., and Green, H. D., 1975, Microvascular control in intestinal mucosa of normal and hemorrhaged rats, *Am. J. Physiol.*, **229:**1159–1164.

Gore, R. W., and Bohlen, H. G., 1975, Pressure regulation in the microcirculation, *Fed. Proc.* **34:**2031–2037.

Kampp, M., and Lundgren, O., 1967, Blood flow and flow distribution in the small intestine of the cat as analyzed by Kr^{85} wash-out technique, *Acta Physiol. Scand.* **72:**282.

11.2. Microsphere Distribution in Revascularized Intestine

CHRISTOPHER K. ZARINS and ELOF ERIKSSON

The unreliability of gross appearance in determining intestinal viability after an ischemic insult is well recognized. Radioactive microspheres have been used with a high degree of accuracy to objectively predict viability following revascularization (Zarins *et al.*, 1974; Moossa *et al.*, 1974). The behavior of microspheres in normal and revascularized rat intestine was studied by *in vivo* microscopic observation of the serosa and mesentery and compared to radioisotope activity.

Segmental intestinal ischemia of 1–6 h duration was created in ten rats. Ten minutes after revascularization, 25 ± 5 μm ^{99m}Tc-albumin microspheres were injected into the aorta and relative radioactivity was determined. Increased activity in the segment compared to normal adjacent bowel correlated with viability despite significant microcirculatory impairment on observation. Decreased activity indicated nonviability. Albumin microspheres were not visible under the microscope, and further studies were conducted with 15 ± 5 μm, 25 ± 5 μm, 35 ± 5 μm, and 50 ± 10 μm carbonized microspheres using a ^{85}Sr label. Microsphere injection caused a momentary cessation of mesenteric flow and a fall in blood pressure followed by resumption of flow and increased pressure. Microspheres lodged in arterioles according to size, with proximal arteriolar dilatation and logjamming of excess spheres (Fig. 1). Small spheres occluded distal flow, and migration of spheres continued for at least 1 h after injection. Collateral vessels restored flow to the distal bed through the arteriole or retrograde flow in the venule. Large numbers of spheres caused significant microcirculatory impairment and death.

In 15 rats, 100,000 15-μm ^{85}Sr spheres were injected after 1 h of segmental ischemia. In the noninjured intestine, microspheres were evenly distributed in 15–20 μm arterioles. In viable injured intestine, microspheres were present in increased numbers and were correlated with increased (at least twice normal) radioactivity. There was little migration and most microspheres were clumped in 30–40 μm arterioles. Significant microvascular injury was present with arteriolar and venular dilation and

CHRISTOPHER K. ZARINS · Clinical Investigation Center, Naval Regional Medical Center, San Diego, California. ELOF ERIKSSON · Department of Surgery, University of Chicago, Chicago, Illinois.

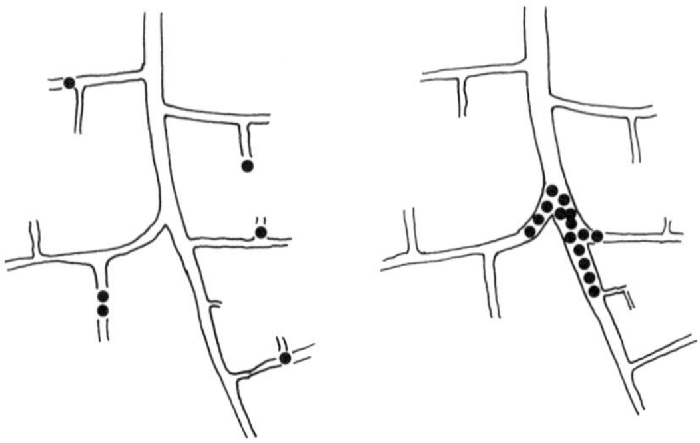

Figure 1. Microsphere distribution in normal and revascularized intestine.

venous hemorrhage. Segments with radioactivity equal to that in the normal adjacent bowel had more severe microvascular damage and clumped microspheres. Segments that were nonviable with extensive venous hemorrhage had rare microspheres and decreased radioactivity. Increased radioactivity in "hyperemic" viable segments of intestine is due to an increased number of spheres clumped in relatively large arterioles.

References

Moossa, A. R., Skinner, D. B., Zarins, C. K., and Rhodes, B. A., 1974, Preoperative evaluation of the viability of ischaemic colon in primates, *Br. J. Surg.* **61**:301.

Zarins, C. K., Skinner, D. B., Rhodes, B. A., and James, A. E., Jr., 1974, Prediction of the viability of revascularized intestine with radioactive microspheres, *Surg. Gynecol. Obstet.* **138**:576.

11.3. Microcirculation from the Villus to the Liver

HERBERT J. ROBB and CLARENCE M. JABS

In a 400-ft motion picture film, the microcirculation is detailed as it might be observed during the process of digestion.

Globules of fat are photographed as they are dispersed and broken apart by bile. The individual villus is photographed with its feeding arterioles, capillary blood flow, and central vein. Circulation is followed to the bowel wall, where one observes larger arterioles as they go to and venules as they come from the villus system. The effect of norepinephrine on the individual arteriole is noted. One can see how spasm blocks the blood flow and causes vascular stasis.

A low-magnification picture of the mesentery indicates where one can locate lymphatic vessels. High-power photographs demonstrate the lymphatic valve and individual red blood cells as they are picked up by the lymphatic system. Chylomicrons are observed in the dark-field pictures. A final scene emphasizes how lymph channels are important in removing red cells from areas of trauma.

The pancreas is photographed under progressively higher magnification using transmitted and dark-field types of illumination. Capillary blood flow is observed about the individual pancreatic acini. One can see zymogen granules at the far ends of the duct system.

The liver is photographed by transillumination. Blood flow from the hepatic artery and portal vein into the liver is observed. Blood flows about the sinussoids. This system does not narrow to a single-cell diameter as in the bowel wall. It is observed to converge again into central veins and hepatic venules.

All motion pictures are taken with the use of a horizontal camera and microscope. This technique has enabled us to hold, illuminate, and focus vessels in a more exact way for purposes of photography.

HERBERT J. ROBB · Director of Surgical Research, Wm. Beaumont Hospital, Royal Oak, Michigan; Clinical Professor of Surgery at Wayne State University, Detroit, Michigan. CLARENCE M. JABS · Research Fellow in Microcirculation, Wm. Beaumont Hospital, Royal Oak, Michigan.

11.4. Biomicroscopic Studies of Microcirculation of the Rat Intestine

R. WILLNOW and I. WILLNOW

A biomicroscopic view of the capillary bed in the intestine of the rat is presented. There are distinct relations between the microcirculation and the metabolism of the gastrointestinal tract which are significant for its functional effectiveness. The esophagus has a circulation essentially for the nutrition of the musculature, and the only important function of the organ is transporting food.

The stomach has two parts, the fundus for storage of the food and the corpus for application of gastric juice and for transportation. The corpus has a fresh red color, corresponding to a high metabolism and motor activity; the fundus is pale, corresponding to poor vascularization.

The duodenum has the highest degree of vascularization. The dense branching of all vessels shows no interrupted cylindrical patterns. No signs of resorption are to be seen, and no signs of defense, but the intense vascularization is a sign of high metabolic activity related to the supply of important volumes of digestive liquids. The color is a much more intense red than in any other part of the intestine.

Jejunum and ileum have a reduced circulation. In the aboral direction, the red color gets paler and the capillarization is not so highly developed as in the duodenum. The defensive apparatus increases according to the descent of the pH in the digestive fluid. First, lymphonodulae solitarii appear, then aggregatii. The lymph nodules have a spherical pattern of distribution of blood vessels. Therefore, the cylindrical pattern of the digestive tube is interrupted by a spherical pattern.

The cecum is comparable to the fundus of the stomach. It is an organ of storage with only the relatively small vascularization needed for the nutrition of the wall. This pattern passes over imperceptibly into the next pattern.

The colon ascendens begins with a series of several plica. The pattern of blood supply shows a distinctive character. The capillary bed originates from pairs of vessels situated subperitoneally in the bases of plica. Other parts of the colon become more and more uncharacteristic.

The testicle, epididymis, seminal vesicle, and vas deferens also have typical circulatory patterns. They are easy to investigate with incident light. Interesting too are the meandering blood vessels of the bladder, which more or less straighten depending on the filling state.

R. WILLNOW and I. WILLNOW · Vitalmikroskopische Abteilung, Institut für Anatomie, Freie Universität Berlin, Germany.

11.5. Filtration Coefficients of Single Capillaries in Rat Intestinal Muscle

ROBERT W. GORE, WILLIAM SCHOKNECHT, and H. GLENN BOHLEN

We have made direct measurements of pressures in rat intestinal muscle and mucosal capillaries (Gore and Bohlen, 1975). When arterial pressure (Pa) was 100–110 mm Hg, muscle capillary pressures averaged 23.8 ± 1.5 (SE) mm Hg, while mucosal capillary pressures averaged 13.9 ± 2 (SE) mm Hg. Mesenteric capillary pressures ranged from 30–34 mm Hg when Pa was 100–110 mm Hg (Gore, 1974; Zweifach, 1974; Landis, 1930). These data suggest that mesenteric capillaries normally filter, intestinal muscle capillaries are near fluid balance, while mucosal capillaries absorb. However, measurements of filtration coefficients and total tissue pressures ($\pi_t - P_t$), in addition to total capillary pressures ($Pc - \pi c$), are required to prove that regional differences in net fluid balance normally occur in the intestine.

Filtration coefficients (*K*) and "effective pressures" (Pe) were measured along single rat intestinal muscle capillaries. The single-occlusion method of Lee *et al.* (1971) was used. Plasma colloid osmotic pressures were measured with a membrane osmometer. Measured effective pressures (Pe) represented conditions in occluded capillaries. Therefore, previous measurements of arteriolar, capillary (Pc), and venular pressures recorded with a servonull transducer (Gore and Bohlen, 1975) were used to compute a "corrected Pe" ($P'e = Pc - P_t + \pi_t$) which reflected conditions in unoccluded capillaries. Total transmural pressures ($\Delta P = P'e - \pi c$) and fluid fluxes [$J = K(P'e - \pi c)$] were then computed as a function of capillary length. The results from 15 capillaries in five rats are shown in Table I.

A large gradient in the filtration coefficient was found between arterial capillaries [$\%(L/L_0) = 15$; $K = 0.008\ \mu m^3/\mu m^2/s/cm\ H_2O$] and venous capillaries [$\%(L/L_0) = 82$; $K = 0.115\ \mu m^3/\mu m^2/s/cm\ H_2O$]. The average *K* for all vessels was $0.05\ \mu m^3/\mu m^2/s/cm\ H_2O$. Both the gradient and the average were 2–4 times greater than previously reported for mesentery and omentum (Lee *et al.*, 1971; Zweifach and Intaglietta, 1968). The flux in arterial and venous capillaries was +0.04 and −0.81, respectively, and the average flux was $-0.23\ \mu m^3/\mu m^2/s$. In contrast to the mesentery, and contrary to our original speculation, the data imply that

ROBERT W. GORE, WILLIAM SCHOKNECHT, and H. GLENN BOHLEN · Department of Physiology, College of Medicine, University of Arizona, Tucson, Arizona.

Table I. Results of Transcapillary Fluid Exchange Studies in Single Capillaries of Rat Intestinal Muscle[a]

Percent distance along capillary measured from arteriole		15		40		64		82
[%(L/L_0)]	±	5	±	5	±	3	±	5
Total capillary length		215		270		269		234
(L_0 μm)	±	15	±	74	±	35	±	64
Measured effective pressure		20.9		21.6		20.9		19.9
(Pe = mm Hg)	±	1.0	±	1.2	±	2.1	±	1.6
Corrected Pe[a]		19.2		16.8		13.9		10.7
(P′e = mm Hg)	±	0.5	±	1.3	±	1.9	±	2.1
COP		16		16.6		15.5		16.0
(πc = mm Hg)		—	±	0.3	±	0.3	±	0.2
Total tissue pressure		−6.0		−7.0		−6.1		−7.6
($\pi_t - P_t$ = mm Hg)		—	±	1.4	±	1.8	±	2.1
Total transcapillary pressure		+3.2		+0.2		−1.6		−5.5
($\Delta P = P'e - \pi c$ = mm Hg)	±	0.5	±	1.1	±	1.8	±	2.1
Filtration coefficient		0.8		2.4		5.8		11.5
$K = 10^{-2} \mu m^3/\mu m^2/s/cm\ H_2O$	±	0.2	±	0.8	±	1.1	±	1.3
Flux		+3.7		−1.8		−16.2		−81.1
$J = 10^{-2} \mu m^3/\mu m^2/s$	±	1.5	±	1.9	±	13.1	±	31.7

[a] Data (expressed as mean ± SE) were obtained using the method of Lee *et al.* (1971). See text for explanation of Pe.

intestinal muscle capillaries are an absorptive network when systemic pressures are normal.

Acknowledgments

This work was supported by an Arizona Heart Association Fellowship and NIH Grants HL-13437, HL-17421, and HL-05884.

References

Gore, R. W., 1974, Pressures in cat mesenteric arterioles and capillaries during changes in systemic arterial blood pressure, *Circ. Res.* **34:**581.

Gore, R. W., and Bohlen, H. G., 1975, Pressure regulation in the microcirculation, *Fed. Proc.* **34:**2031–2037.

Landis, E. M., 1930, The capillary blood pressure in mammalian mesentery as determined by the micro-injection method, *Am. J. Physiol.* **93:**353.

Lee, J. S., Smaje, L. H., and Zweifach, B. W., 1971, Fluid movement in occluded single capillaries of rabbit omentum, *Circ. Res.* **28:**358.

Zweifach, B. W., 1974, Quantitative studies of microcirculatory structure and function. I. Analysis of pressure distributions in the terminal bed in cat mesentery, *Circ. Res.* **34:**843.

Zweifach, B. W., and Intaglietta, M., 1968, Mechanics of fluid movement across single capillaries in the rabbit, *Microvasc. Res.* **1:**83.

11.6. Role of Collagenase in Capillarization of Hepatic Sinusoids

KATSUYA MARUYAMA, MASAHARU TSUCHIYA, MASAYA ODA, ISAO OKAZAKI, and KAZUO FUNATSU

In a previous report, we described the process of capillarization of sinusoids (Okazaki *et al.*, 1973). In the present article, the role of collagenase in the formation process of basement membrane (BM) and the suppressive effect of glucofuranulouronic acid phenylhydrazide (GFUA) are reported.

11.6.1. Materials and Methods

Female Wistar strain rats received subcutaneous injection of 0.3 ml of 50% CCl_4 in olive oil per 100 g body weight twice a week. Rats were killed at 3, 6, and 20 wk after the initial administration of CCl_4. Light and electron microscopic observation, assay of collagenase activity (Okazaki and Maruyama, 1974), and estimation of hydroxyproline and hexosamine contents in the liver were done. Another group of rats underwent subcutaneous injection of 20 mg GFUA per 100 g body weight daily for 12 wk in addition to the administration of CCl_4. Light and electron microscopic observation and determination of hydroxyproline and hexosamine were done.

11.6.2. Results

1. In experimental hepatic fibrosis, BM formation occurs roughly parallel with the proliferation of collagen fibers.
2. Collagenase activity increases parallel with the proliferation of collagen fibers at the initial stage of hepatic fibrosis.
3. After the formation of BM, in the cirrhotic stage, collagenase activity decreases to the same level as in nontreated rat liver.

Figure 1 shows the results listed above.

4. As to the role of collagenase in the process of BM formation, two mechanisms are considered. One is that decreased collagenase

KATSUYA MARUYAMA, MASAHARU TSUCHIYA, MASAYA ODA, ISAO OKAZAKI, and KAZUO FUNATSU · Department of Internal Medicine, School of Medicine, Keio University, Tokyo, Japan.

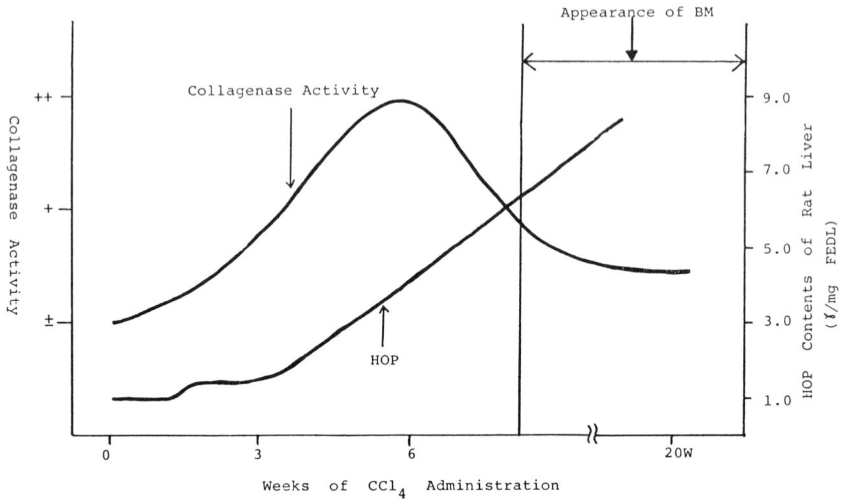

Figure 1. Changing activity of hepatic collagenase in the formation of basement membrane.

activity would result in accumulation of collagen fibers, followed by the formation of BM. Another is that decreased collagenase activity would result in decreased destruction of BM.

5. Decreased activity of collagenase as well as lysosomal enzyme is thought to have an important role in the BM formation.
6. GFUA suppresses the proliferation of collagen fibers and the formation of BM.

References

Okazaki, I., and Maruyama, K., 1974, Collagenase activity in experimental hepatic fibrosis, *Nature (London)* **252**:49.

Okazaki, I., Tsuchiya, M., Kamegaya, K., Oda, M., Maruyama, K., and Oshio, C., 1973, Capillarization of hepatic sinusoids in carbon tetrachloride-induced hepatic fibrosis, *Bibl. Anat.* **12**:476.

11.7. Effect of Diminished P_{50} on Intrahepatic Oxygen Tension as Measured in Bile

G. WATKINS and T. D. JOHNSON

A decreased P_{50} has been theorized to cause tissue hypoxia. This hypothesis has never been proven. Difficulties in part have been in the measure of tissue O_2 levels (Watkins and Thomas, 1974). A second difficulty has been in altering P_{50} without affecting other physiological moities. Acute metabolic alkalosis will lower P_{50} *in vivo* (Severinghaus, 1966). A control of isovolemic isoosmolar NaCl should mimic any changes due to the volume–ionic load itself. Oxygen tension in intrahepatic bile has been reported to rapidly and immediately reflect changes in response to alterations in oxygen delivery to the liver (Chaplin *et al.*, 1974). A study was undertaken to determine whether acute lowering of P_{50} by induced acute metabolic alkalosis diminishes biliary oxygen tension.

11.7.1. Methods

Seven mongrel dogs were anesthetized with nembutal and mechanically ventilated. Temperature and blood volumes were maintained constant. Mass spectrometer probes were used to continually and simultaneously record oxygen (Po_2) and carbon dioxide tensions in the aorta (A), portal vein (P), hepatic vein (H), and biliary radical (B). Catheters were also placed in the aorta and hepatic vein. After stabilization, 2 ml/lb of each of two solutions was infused. The isoosmolar solutions were Na_2CO_3 and NaCl. The order of infusion was random. pH, hemoglobin (Hb), and oxyhemoglobin (Sat) concentrations were measured before and 10 min after each infusion. P_{50}'s and oxygen contents (C) were calculated. Statistical analysis was performed using paired t testing.

11.7.2. Results

The results are summarized in Table I. Po_2B and Po_2H changes were immediate. Carbon dioxide was constant.

G. WATKINS and T. D. JOHNSON · University of Connecticut Health Center, Farmington, Connecticut.

Table I. Average Values of Experimental Results

	pH	Po_2A	Sat A	Hb	Sat H	Po_2H	C_A	C_H	Po_2 B	p_{50}
Steady state	7.48	88	92	19.6	63	49	25	16.9	65	26.5
Post Na_2CO_3	7.66[a]	89	95	18.0[b]	67	43	23.9	17.2	57[c]	23.0
Steady state	7.51	87	97	19.0	53	47	25.4	14.9	62	26.7
Post NaCl	7.49	91	97	16.7[a]	65[d]	50[a]	22.4	15.4	62	26.5

[a] $P < 0.01$.
[b] $P < 0.005$.
[c] $P < 0.05$.
[d] $P < 0.001$.

11.7.3. Conclusions

1. An acute decrease in P_{50} causes hepatic tissue hypoxia as measured by changes in biliary oxygen tension.
2. Acute metabolic alkalosis without organic phosphate compensation is detrimental to hepatic oxygen unloading.
3. The degree of Po_2 B change seen in this study is comparable to experimentally induced changes in oxygen delivery during moderate hypoxia, blood loss, or blood flow reduction.

References

Chaplin, H., Jr., Beutler, E., Collins, J. A., Giblett, E. R., and Polesky, H. F., 1974, Current status of red-cell preservation and availability in relation to the developing national blood policy, *N. Engl. J. Med.* **291**:68.

Severinghaus, J. W., 1966, Blood gas calculator, *J. Appl. Physiol.* **21(3)**:1108.

Watkins, G. M., and Thomas, D. D., 1974, Biliary oxygen tension: A measure of hepatic oxygen transport, *Surg. Forum* **25**:399.

11.8. Phenomenon of Intrahepatic Microcirculatory Redistribution

A. M. CHERNUKH and NATALIA Y. KOVALENKO

Using the method of contact biomicroscopy (Chernukh and Kovalenko, 1971), it was shown that after slow injection of small volumes of different substances (isotonic saline, glucose independent of its concentration, reopolyglukin, and even the blood of the same animal) into the rat portal vein, a biphasic reaction of hepatic microvessels takes place.

Three to five seconds after the injection, portal inflow was impeded in some vascular liver zones, leading to blood flow deceleration in portal venules, sinusoids, and terminal hepatic venules without corresponding hemodynamic changes in arterioles. Reduction of portal blood supply led to increased arterial hepatic flow, and the second phase of reaction began. The luminescent microvessels dilated, and the signs of blood flow deceleration in them were intensified. Zones with changed hemodynamics consisted of different numbers of simple and complex acini. They alternated with regions of parenchyma where the microcirculation remained unchanged (Fig. 1). The reaction of the hepatic microvascular bed gradually regressed, and in 30–40 min the initial microcirculatory picture was restored. Administration of the same solutions into the femoral vein or aorta caused no reaction of the liver microvessels. The occurrences described above are unique to the vessels of the portal system.

The reaction was blocked completely by pretreatment with papaverine. This may indicate that active constriction of smooth muscle cells in the system of intrahepatic portal branching initiates the phenomenon. Experiments with pharmacological blocking agents suggest that the phenomenon probably has a humoral origin. It may be connected with histophysiological peculiarities of portal smooth muscle cells which react to changes in portal blood composition and volume by increased myogenic activity (Mellander and Johansson, 1968).

A. M. CHERNUKH and NATALIA Y. KOVALENKO · Institute of General Pathology and Pathological Physiology of the USSR Academy of Medical Sciences, Moscow, USSR.

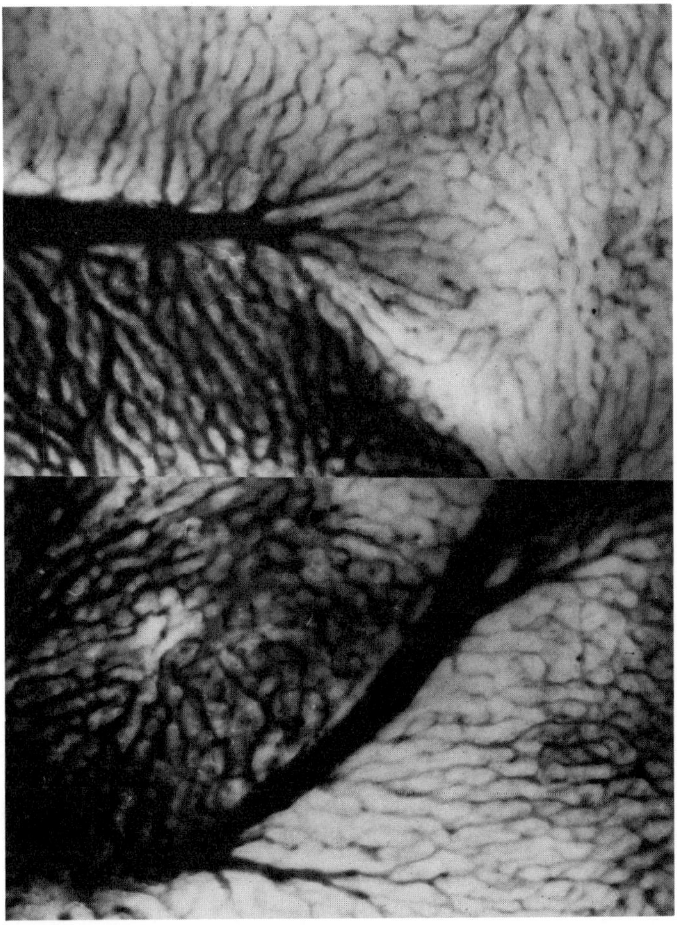

Figure 1. Intrahepatic microcirculatory redistribution in rat liver. Note the junction of zones with dilated and unchanged microvessels passing along terminal hepatic venules. Luminescent contact biomicroscopy. Microphotograph: objective ×10, ocular ×3.

References

Chernukh, A. M., and Kovalenko, N. Y., 1971, Microcirculation and permeability of the walls of microvascular bed of the rat liver in early symptoms of inflammation, in: *Proceedings of the Sixth European Conference on Microcirculation*, Aalborg, 1970, pp. 133–137, Karger, New York.

Mellander, S., and Johansson, B., 1968, Control of resistance exchange and capacitance functions in the peripheral circulation, *Pharmacol. Rev.* **20:**117.

11.9. A Flow Model of the Liver and the Microcirculatory Hepatic Unit

O. MAHRENHOLTZ and A. M. RAPPAPORT

In the liver, arterial and portal blood merge; their average pressures in a human are hepatic artery 80 torr and portal vein 12 torr. The mixed blood leaves the liver through the hepatic vein at a pressure of around 0.5 torr. A global steady-state approach, by averaging the pulsating part of the pressure in the hepatic artery, leads to

$$Q_{\mathrm{HA}}R_{\mathrm{HA}} = P_{\mathrm{HA}} - P^* \tag{1}$$
$$Q_{\mathrm{PV}}R_{\mathrm{PV}} = P_{\mathrm{PV}} - P^* \tag{2}$$
$$Q_{\mathrm{HV}}R_{\mathrm{HV}} = P^* - P_{\mathrm{HV}} \tag{3}$$

where Q, R, and P are flow rate, combined resistance, and pressure, respectively. The subscripts HA, PV, and HV stand for arterial, portal, and venous bed. Considering $Q_{\mathrm{HV}} = 1200$ ml/min, $Q_{\mathrm{HA}} = 0.3\, Q_{\mathrm{HV}}$, and $P^* = 6\, P_{\mathrm{HV}}$, one obtains the following impedances for the vascular beds: HA inflow 110, PV inflow 13, and mixed outflow 2 torr·min/liter. The arterial resistance is overestimated and a pressure reduction by intermittent flow and merging effect are found to be justified.

Rappaport (1973), through *in vivo* microscopic observations of hepatic flow, has developed a concept of microcirculatory hepatic units supplied by terminal hepatic arterioles (THA) and terminal portal venules (TPV) (Fig. 1). In the units, an intermittent flow occurs into the sinusoids controlled by sphincter activity. This activity is regulated biochemically and hormonally but appears to operate rather randomly.

Improving an engineering approach (Loch, 1969) the authors have carried out a more detailed hemodynamic study. Usually, the arteriolar flow merges into the sinusoidal and portal flow, thus partly adapting by irregular motion and jet effect the pressure differences. More important are the random opening–closing functions $\Delta(t)$ of the sphincter valves. The pressure reduction can approximately calculated as

$$\bar{P}_{\mathrm{HA}} = P_{\mathrm{HA}} \frac{1}{T} \int_0^T \Delta_{\mathrm{HA}}(t)\, dt \tag{4}$$
$$\bar{P}_{\mathrm{PV}} = P_{\mathrm{PV}} \frac{1}{T} \int_0^T \Delta_{\mathrm{PV}}(t)\, dt$$

O. MAHRENHOLTZ · Institut für Mechanik, Technische Universität Hannover, FR Germany. A. M. RAPPAPORT · Department of Physiology, University of Toronto, Toronto, Ontario, Canada.

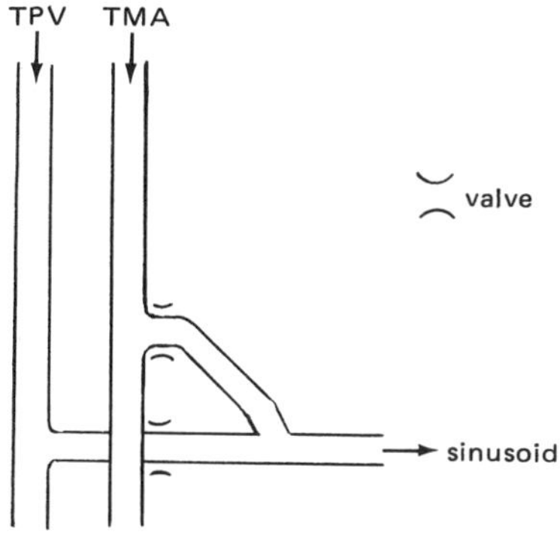

Figure 1

where $\bar{P}$ is a reduced average pressure and T is the time required for the process to become stationary. The rather complicated details show that the sinusoidal bed and its structure (ordinary capillary flow or sheet flow) are of minor importance for the hemodynamic approach but the pulsating effect due to the hepatic artery and intermittency of flow cannot be neglected.

References

Loch, L., 1969, Development of a physical model to simulate the "*in vivo*" microcirculation within the mammalian liver vascular system, B.A.Sc. thesis, University of Toronto.

Rappaport, A. M., 1973, The microcirculatory hepatic unit, *Microvasc. Res.* **6:**212.

11.10. The Isolated Perfused Liver as a Model for the Study of Disseminated Intravascular Coagulation. I. Effects of Trasylol, Heparin, and Acetylsalicylic Acid

SMILJA POPOV-CENIĆ, V. TOTOVIĆ, N. MÜLLER, and H. EGLI

Our observations on isolated perfused rat livers (Popov-Cenić *et al.,* 1973) using diluted thrombocyte-containing citrated blood as the perfusion medium have shown, as have the results of other authors (Hickman *et al.,* 1972*a,b*), that organ damage during perfusion is clearly caused mainly by an aggregation of the thrombocytes present in the perfusion medium.

In this connection, we first tested whether the changes described could be prevented by the application of a coagulation blocker such as heparin, acetylsalicylic acid (ASA), or Trasylol, and whether a normalization of organ function during perfusion could be attained by using a perfusion medium containing thrombocytes.

We were able to show using rat livers under isolated perfusion with diluted human citrated blood containing thrombocytes that thrombocyte aggregation and hypercoagulability develop in the perfusion medium. They act as a kind of "trigger mechanism" leading to an increased turnover of coagulation factors. In consequence, numerous microthromboses develop in the perfused organ, leading to blocked veins and hypoxic or ischemic organ damage. These changes can be reduced during the first hours of perfusion by addition of ASA to the medium, and reduced to some extent also by the addition of heparin. The addition of Trasylol, on the other hand, is much less effective.

References

Hickman, R., Parker, J. R., Saunders, S. J., Goodwin, N. E., and Terblanche, J., 1972*a*, Heterologous liver perfusion: A comparison of the use of livers from four different species, *Br. J. Surg.* **59**:881.

Hickman, R., Parker, J. R., Saunders, S. J., and Terblanche, J., 1972*b*, Platelet adherence in the pig liver perfused with human blood, *Transplantation* **13**:195.

Popov-Cenić, S., Totović, V., Küppers, U. and Egli, H., 1973, Liver perfusion with regard to the formation of coagulation factors and to the microcirculation disturbances, in: Seventh European Conference on Microcirculation, Aberdeen, 1972, Part II, *Bibl. Anat.* **12**:22.

SMILJA, POPOV-CENIĆ, V. TOTOVIĆ, N. MÜLLER, and H. EGLI · Institut für Experimentelle Haematologie und Bluttransfusionswesen, University of Bonn, West Germany.

11.11. Effects of Acute Hemorrhage and Carotid Artery Occlusion on Blood Flow and Its Distribution in the Wall of the Gastrointestinal Tract

C. C. CHOU, L. C. YU, and Y. M. YU

Gastric but not intestinal wall flow is redistributed away from the mucosa during norepinephrine infusion (Delaney and Grim, 1965; Ross, 1971). Regional sympathetic stimulation or hemorrhage increases or does not change intestinal villous plasma flow but decreases deep mucosal flow (Haglund and Lundgren, 1974; Svanvik, 1973). Few or no data are available on the blood flow distribution in the wall of the gastrointestinal tract in hemorrhagic hypotension and carotid artery occlusion. Therefore, we studied the flow and its distribution within the wall of the stomach, duodenum, jejunum, ileum, and colon of pentobarbital-anesthetized dogs in these two conditions. Two types of radioactive microspheres (^{141}Ce and ^{85}Sr, 15 ± 5 μm) were used; one type was injected into the left ventricle before and the other type within 10 min after rapid hemorrhage or carotid artery occlusion. The validity of the method was tested by directly measuring the venous outflow from a jejunal segment in ten experiments. Total wall flow calculated by the sphere method was significantly correlated with measured venous outflow ($p < 0.001$, $\gamma = 0.94$, $Y = 3.407 + 1.028X$, where X is venous outflow). Acute rapid hemorrhage decreased aortic pressure from 120 to 60 mm Hg, increased resistance, and decreased total wall flow in all five gastrointestinal segments, most prominently in the stomach (Table I). Only in the stomach was flow redistributed away from the mucosa. Carotid artery occlusion increased aortic pressure from 112 to 149 mm Hg, significantly increased wall flow, but did not alter resistance. In all five segments, wall flow was redistributed away from the mucosa (Table I). These studies indicate that redistribution of gut wall flow occurs only in the stomach during acute hemorrhage, but it occurs in the entire length of the gastrointestinal tract during carotid artery occlusion.

C. C. CHOU, L. C. YU, and Y. M. YU · Departments of Physiology and Medicine, Michigan State University, East Lansing, Michigan.

Table I. Effect of Acute Hemorrhage and Carotid Artery Occlusion (CAO) on Vascular Resistance, Total Wall Blood Flow ($ml \cdot min^{-1} \cdot 100\ g^{-1}$ and Its Distribution[a]

	Stomach		Duodenum		Jejunum		Ileum		Colon	
	C	E	C	E	C	E	C	E	C	E
Hemorrhage										
Resistance[b]	3.5	11.5[c]	2.3	3.1[c]	2.4	3.1[c]	2.0	3.2[c]	1.5	2.6[c]
Wall flow	48.1	8.1[c]	64.4	24.4[c]	62.6	22.8[c]	67.8	23.2[c]	89.4	27.9[c]
Mucosa (%)	81.1	71.2[c]	95.4	97.7	92.1	94.6	93.1	92.0	85.4	83.0
Submucosa (%)	12.8	15.0	2.8	1.1	5.1	3.8	2.7	2.6	6.3	7.9
Muscularis (%)	6.2	13.8[c]	1.8	1.2	2.8	1.7	4.3	5.4	8.3	9.0
CAO										
Resistance[b]	4.2	3.8	1.9	1.8	2.5	2.4	2.7	2.2	2.5	2.4
Wall flow	28.5	40.0[c]	60.8	91.8[c]	49.5	69.2[c]	52.5	80.0[c]	58.3	78.0[c]
Mucosa (%)	85.2	80.7[c]	92.7	88.0[c]	92.4	84.5[c]	88.9	81.9[c]	84.9	69.6[c]
Submucosa (%)	8.3	11.5[c]	2.5	7.0[c]	4.5	11.7[c]	2.8	8.6[c]	6.0	12.5[c]
Muscularis (%)	6.7	7.8	4.8	5.0	3.1	3.8	8.7	9.5[c]	9.1	17.9[c]

[a] Abbreviations: *C*, control; E, during acute hemorrhage ($N = 8$) or CAO ($N = 7$).
[b] Vascular resistance of the wall in mm Hg per $ml \cdot min^{-1} \cdot 100\ g^{-1}$.
[c] $P < 0.05$.

References

Delaney, J. P., and Grim, E., 1965, Experimentally induced variations in canine gastric blood flow and its distribution, *Am. J. Physiol.* **208:**353.

Haglund, U., and Lundgren, O., 1974, The small intestine in hemorrhagic shock, *Gastroenterology* **66:**625.

Ross, G., 1971, Effects of norepinephrine infusions on mesenteric arterial blood flow and its tissue distribution, *Proc. Soc. Exp. Biol. Med.* **137:**921.

Svanvik, J., 1973, Mucosal hemodynamics in the small intestine of the cat during regional sympathetic vasoconstrictor activation, *Acta Physiol. Scand.* **89:**19.

11.12. Effects of Arterial Pressure Variation on Microvascular Pressure Distribution in the Mesentery during Intravenous Infusion of Norepinephrine

DANIEL RICHARDSON and FRED COATES

The purpose of these experiments was to investigate the effects of systemic arterial pressure variations on the response of microvessels to intravenous infusion of norepinephrine (NE). Microvascular pressures (Pm) were measured by the servonull technique of Wiederhielm *et al.* (1964) in 43 rat mesenteric arterioles before and during two sequential 5–7 min infusions of 4 μg NE/kg/min. During one infusion, systemic arterial pressure (Pa) was allowed to increase in response to the NE; during the other infusion, systemic pressure was held relatively constant by use of an arterial reservoir. The infusion sequence was alternated with each succeeding vessel studied.

The constrictor effect of NE occurs to the greatest extent within the terminal arterioles of 12–15 μm inside diameter. This was evidenced by the fact that during infusion the Pm/Pa ratio decreased with vessels below this range, indicating net upstream constriction, whereas the ratio increased with larger vessels, indicating net downstream constriction.

The changes in Pm/Pa were most pronounced when systemic arterial pressure was allowed to increase during infusion. Figure 1 presents the results observed with three individual vessels that illustrate this point. Note that the increase in the Pm/Pa ratio, which indicates net downstream constriction, is much more pronounced during the infusions in which systemic pressure was allowed to increase (Pa variant). This indicates that an increase in arterial perfusion pressure has a potentiating effect on the constrictor response of NE. This notion was further evidenced by the fact that the average pressure gradient from the larger arterioles to the immediate precapillary vessels during the systemic pressure variant infusion was 1.2–1.4 times as large as the pressure gradient observed when systemic pressure remained relatively constant. Further analysis of the data showed that the degree to which the pressure gradient increased during infusion was a linear function of the change in systemic arterial

DANIEL RICHARDSON and FRED COATES · Department of Physiology and Biophysics, University of Kentucky College of Medicine, Lexington, Kentucky.

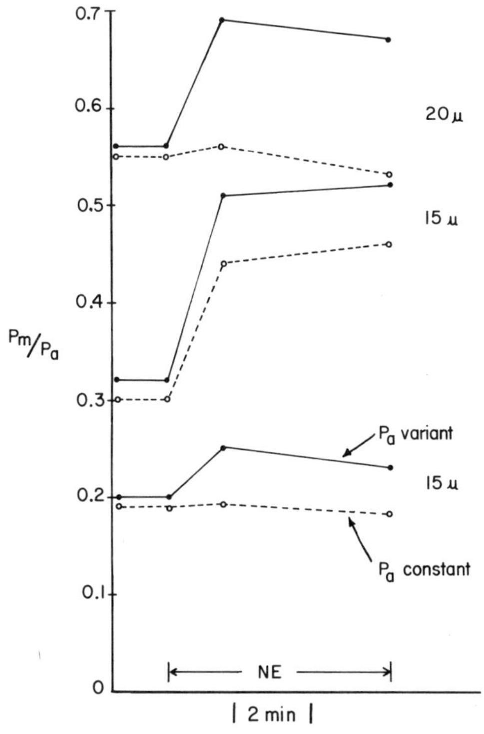

Figure 1. Effects of intravenous infusion of norepinephrine on the ratio of microvascular pressure (Pm) to systemic arterial pressure (Pa) in three different arterioles. The increase in the Pm/Pa ratio during infusion indicates net downstream constriction. Note that this is more pronounced during the Pa variant infusion, in which systemic pressure was allowed to increase.

pressure. This result is consistent with the observations of Gore (1972) which indicate that the constrictor effectiveness of NE on single microvessels is in part determined by the level of arterial perfusion pressure.

We conclude from these studies that variations in arterial pressure during intravenous infusion of norepinephrine modify the pressor effects of this catecholamine on mesenteric microvessels.

References

Gore, R. W., 1972, Wall stress: A determinant of regional differences in response of frog microvessels to norepinephrine, *Am. J. Physiol.* **222**:82.

Wiederhielm, C. A., Woodbury, J. W., Kirk, S., and Rushmer, R. F., 1964, Pulsatile pressure in the microcirculation of the frog's mesentery, *Am. J. Physiol.* **207**:173.

11.13. Mechanism of Escape from Norepinephrine Vasoconstriction in the Intestinal Circulation

P. H. GUTH, G. ROSS, and E. SMITH

The hypothesis that escape from norepinephrine-induced vasoconstriction in the intestine is due to relaxation of initially constricted vessels (Richardson and Johnson, 1969; Ross, 1971) was tested in 18 anesthetized cats. Intestinal blood flow was measured by an electromagnetic probe on the superior mesenteric artery. Intestinal submucosal and muscle arterioles and small mesenteric arteries were studied by *in vivo* microscopy (Guth and Rosenberg, 1972) using an image-splitting technique (Baez, 1966). Continuous recordings of mesenteric flow and vessel diameter were made during intramesenteric arterial infusion of NE, 1–2 μg/min for 3 min.

11.13.1. Results

Average superior mesenteric artery flow was 67.2 ± 6.6 ml/min (mean ± SE). Total mesenteric vascular resistance increased to 270 ± 56% and then escaped to 176 ± 31% of control. Microscopically, arterial constriction and escape were noted in submucosal muscle and mesenteric vessels. Results are presented in Table I.

Table I. Experimental Results (Mean ± SE)

Vessel	Number of cats	Contraction diameter (μm)	Constriction diameter (% control)	Escape diameter (% control)
Submucosal	11	41 ± 3	73 ± 5	93 ± 4
Muscle	7	35 ± 5	76 ± 5	107 ± 5
Mesenteric	7	716 ± 26	76 ± 5	95 ± 5

The constriction and escape occurred simultaneously with the mesenteric arterial flow changes in some instances, but in other instances there was a lag. Primary arteriolar dilatation was not observed during the NE infusion. Arteriovenous anastomoses were not seen.

P. H. GUTH, G. ROSS, and E. SMITH · Wadsworth VA Hospital and UCLA, Los Angeles, California.

11.13.2. Conclusion

These findings support the hypothesis that escape from NE-induced vasoconstriction is due to relaxation of initially constricted vessels.

References

Baez, S., 1966, Recording of microvascular dimensions with an image splitter television microscope, *J. Appl. Physiol.* **21:**299.

Guth, P. H., and Rosenberg, A., 1972, *In vivo* microscopy of the gastric circulation, *Am. J. Digest. Dis.* **17:**391.

Richardson, D. R., and P. C. Johnson, 1969, Comparison of autoregulatory escape and autoregulation in the intestinal vascular bed, *Am. J. Physiol.* **217:**586.

Ross, G., 1972, Escape of mesenteric vessels from adrenergic and noradrenergic vasoconstriction, *Am. J. Physiol.* **221:**1217.

11.14. *In Vivo* Study of the Effects of Acetaminophen (Paracetamol) on the Hepatic Microcirculation

A. M. RAPPAPORT and A. MacDONALD

Acetaminophen (Paracetamol), a commonly used analgesic sold over the counter, has become a frequent cause of fulminant hepatic necrosis and coma. As the necrosis always starts at the microcirculatory periphery (Fig. 1, zone 3) of the liver acini, an investigation of the microcirculatory changes was undertaken. Acetaminophen, 350 and 450 mg/kg body weight, was injected intraperitoneally into 34 and 30 mice, respectively. The microcirculation in the liver acini (Rappaport, 1973) was recorded every 6 h approximately up to 48 h, and 8 and 14 days after the injection of the drug. Already at 6 h there is sinusoidal congestion and granular flow in the terminal hepatic venules (ThV). At 12 h, flow in the terminal portal venules (TPV) and arterioles is still normal, while in zone 3 (Z_3) there is clumping of erythrocytes, edema, and congestion with hemorrhagic spots. Necrosis develops in Z_3 at 18–24 h, extends, joins the ThVs at 36 h, and surrounds the acini completely (periacinar) at 48 h. Sinusoidal flow is discontinuous and contains microthrombi. Eight to 14 days later, during repair in the perivenular area, there are still defects in the tissue and in the sinusoidal pattern. Conclusions are as follows: (1) The toxic damage to the hepatocyte caused by an arylating metabolite of acetaminophen (Mitchell *et al.*, 1973) occurs at the site of enzymatic breakdown of the drug (Z_3). (2) It disturbs the fluid exchange between the extra- and intracellular compartments and results in edema. However, the loss of plasma fluid into the tissues is not the main cause of the aggregation and clumping of erythrocytes and of microthrombi formation. (3) The resulting microcirculatory changes aggravate the damage (Clark *et al.*, 1973) and enhance the periacinar spread of hemorrhagic necrosis.

These findings are illustrated by a color movie.

A. M. RAPPAPORT and A. MacDONALD · Departments of Physiology and Pharmacology, University of Toronto, Toronto, Ontario, Canada.

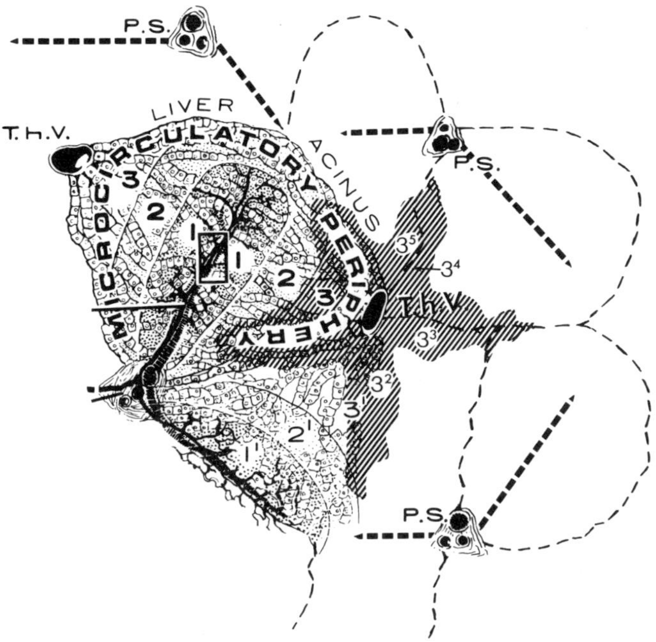

Figure 1. Blood supply of the simple liver acinus, zonal arrangements of cells, and the microcirculatory periphery. The acinus occupies adjacent sectors of neighboring hexagonal fields. Zones 1, 2, and 3 center about the terminal afferent vascular branches, bile ductules, lymph vessels, and nerves and extend into the triangular portal field, from which these branches crop out. Zones 1′, 2′, and 3′ are corresponding areas in a portion of an adjacent acinar unit. Zone 3 is the microcirculatory periphery of the acinus since its cells are as remote from their own afferent vessels as from those of the adjacent acini. The area around the terminal hepatic venule (ThV) is formed by the most peripheral portions of zone 3^{1-5} of several adjacent acini. In progressive injury to zone 3 of these acini, the damaged area assumes the shape of a starfish (heavy crosshatching around ThV). —, Boundaries of acini; **---**, afferent vessels of acini outlining the hexagons. From *Alcoholic Liver Pathology,* 1975; courtesy of the Addiction Research Foundation of Ontario.

References

Clark, R., Borirakchanyavat, V., Davidson, A. R., Thompson, R. P. H., Widdop, B., Goulding, R., and Williams, R., 1973, Hepatic damage and death from overdose of paracetamol, *Lancet* **1**:66.

Mitchell, J. R., Jollow, D. J., Potter, W. Z., Gilette, J. R., and Brodie, B. B., 1973, Acetaminophen-induced hepatic necrosis. IV. Protective role of glutathione, *J. Pharmacol. Exp. Ther.* **187**:211.

Rappaport, A. M., 1973, The microcirculatory hepatic unit, *Microvasc. Res.* **6**:212.

11.15. *In Vivo* and Electron Microscopic Study of the Splenic Microvascular System

R. S. McCUSKEY and P. A. McCUSKEY

Most *in vivo* microscopic studies of the spleen suggest that this organ has a "closed" circulation with all blood flowing within channels lined by endothelium (Knisely, 1936; Peck and Hoerr, 1951; Bloch, 1968). Electron microscopic investigations, however, suggest that the circulation within the red pulp is "open"; that is, it is not contained by endothelium but flows through a meshwork of reticular cell processes to reenter the vasculature by penetrating the endothelial wall of venous sinuses (Weiss, 1973).

In an attempt to resolve this controversy, the splenic microvasculature of the mouse and the rat was examined by *in vivo* microscopic methods (McCuskey *et al.,* 1972) and electron microscopy. The results strongly support the theory that, for the most part, the spleen has an "open" circulation. In the living spleen, blood flows from "arterial" capillaries into channels within the red pulp formed by cytoplasmic processes of reticular cells. The processes are dimensionally similar to endothelium. Where arterial capillaries empty into the red pulp, the processes of adventitial cells are in close apposition to the endothelium of the arterial capillaries. *In vivo,* this relationship frequently creates the appearance of a channel completely lined by endothelium, especially when the arterial capillary terminates in close proximity to a sinusoid or venule and the continuing channel provides a direct pathway for blood flow into the sinusoid or venule. Occasionally, arterial capillaries connect directly with sinusoids and venules. Both types of shunts are functionally significant during conditions when the red pulp is congested with mature or proliferating cells. The majority of blood leaves the red pulp by passing through apertures in the endothelium of sinusoids and venules. Many of these apertures are large enough to allow passage of erythrocytes, which are deformed in passage. Platelets transiently adhere to and plug these apertures, thereby limiting the entry of blood cells into sinusoids and venules. While the mouse spleen contains poorly developed sinusoids in comparison to the rat, the basic pattern of circulation is similar. The results were illustrated in part by a motion picture.

R. S. McCUSKEY, and P. A. McCUSKEY, · Department of Anatomy, University of Cincinnati, Cincinnati, Ohio.

ACKNOWLEDGMENTS

This work was supported by NIH Grants AM-10507 and AM-42370 and by the Southwest Ohio Heart Association.

References

Bloch, E. H., 1968, Microanatomy of living mammalian spleen *in situ*. I. Endothelium, *Anat. Rec.* **160:**520.

Knisely, M. H., 1936, Spleen studies. I. Microscopic observations of the circulatory system of living unstimulated mammalian spleens, *Anat. Rec.* **65:**23.

McCuskey, R. S., Meineke, H. A., and Townsend, S. F., 1972, Studies of the hemopoietic microenvironment. I. Changes in the microvascular system and stroma during erythropoietic regeneration and suppression in the spleens of CF_1 mice, *Blood* **39:**697.

Peck, H. M., and Hoerr, N. L., 1951, The intermediary circulation in the red pulp of the mouse spleen, *Anat. Rec.* **109:**447.

Weiss, L., 1973, The spleen, in: *Histology* (R. Greep and L. Weiss, eds.), McGraw-Hill, New York.

11.16. Experimental and Theoretical Investigations on Intrasplenic Microcirculation in Rats

P. VAUPEL, H. RUPPERT, and H. HUTTEN

The experiments were performed on 68 Sprague-Dawley rats, weight 250–350 g, anesthetized either with pentobarbitone sodium or ketamine i.p. and breathing spontaneously. Regional splenic blood flow (rSBF) was measured by means of the ^{85}Kr (β) clearance technique after an intraaortis slug injection of the dissolved indicator (0.1 ml, 1 mCi/ml). The clearance curves were evaluated utilizing a modification of the height-over-area method according to Zierler (1965), taking the deviation of the real input function from the ideal δ-function into account (Vaupel *et al.,* 1974).

In the normal and undisturbed spleen *in situ,* rSBF linearly depends on the mean arterial blood pressure (MABP) within the range of 30–140 mm Hg ($2p < 0.001$) (Fig. 1). Mean rSBF is 0.71 ml/g/min, MABP being 105 mm Hg. Considering a mean splenic weight of 0.78 g, total splenic blood flow amounts to 0.55 ml/min. In normal animals the flow was highest in the smallest ones, and it decreased steadily with body weight; this has also been proved for the guinea pig spleen (Sandberg, 1972).

After application of rigid, heat-induced spherocytes to cause total obstruction of the open circulation in the spleen due to sequestration in the perisinal meshwork of the red pulp cords, mean regional blood flow is reduced to 0.26 ml/g/min (MABP = 103 mm Hg) and is independent of MABP.

The distribution of intrasplenic blood flow between open and closed circulation depends on the size of MABP. The relative perfusion rate of the open circulation, compared with total rSBF, amounts to 72% (MABP = 80 mm Hg) and 93% (MABP = 130 mm Hg), respectively.

A progressive isovolemic hemodilution after obstruction of the perisinal meshwork results in an increase in blood flow through the closed vascular pathway, the flow being still independent of blood pressure. Hematocrit values below 27% cause blood flow dependent on pressure. This alteration of blood flow pattern may be attributed to intrasplenic hypoxia.

In tumor-bearing animals (DS carcinosarcoma in the kidney), a precipitous splenomegaly occurs (mean splenic weight being 1.4 g after 10 days) caused by a hyperplasia of the white pulp. This alteration results in

P. VAUPEL, H. RUPPERT, and H. HUTTEN · Institute of Physiology, University of Mainz, Mainz, West Germany.

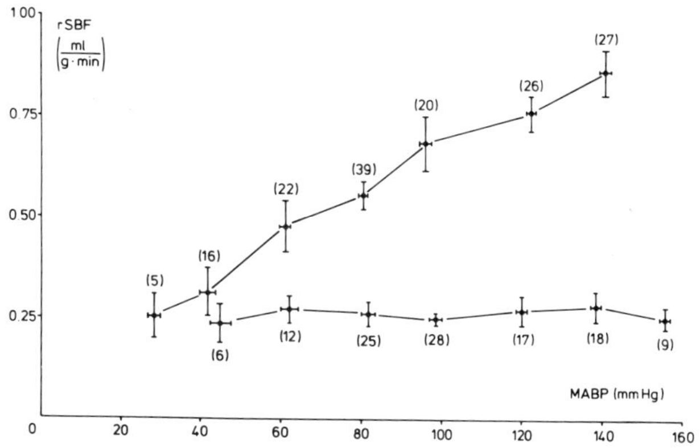

Figure 1. Regional splenic blood flow (rSBF) in the normal and undisturbed spleen *in situ* (upper curve), and after total obstruction of the open circulation by rigid spherocytes (lower curve). Values are means ± SEM.

an increase of total splenic blood flow. However, related to 1 g of splenic wet weight, rSBF has diminished.

References

Sandberg, G., 1972, Splenic blood flow in the guinea-pig measured with xenon 133, and calculation of the venous output of lymphocytes from the spleen, *Acta Physiol. Scand.* **84:**208.

Vaupel, P., Hutten, H., Wendling, P., and Braunbeck, W., 1974, Experimental and theoretical investigations on intrasplenic microcirculation in rabbits, *Res. Exp. Med.* **164:**223.

Zierler, K. L., 1965, Equations for measuring blood flow by external monitoring of radioisotopes, *Circ. Res.* **16:**309.

11.17. Neural Influences in the Humoral Regulation of the Splenic Microvasculature

F. D. REILLY and R. S. McCUSKEY

The responses of the microvasculature to many pharmacological substances may differ depending on the functional state of the nerves serving these vessels. Therefore, the influence of the nervous system on the humoral regulation of the splenic microvasculature was evaluated using *in vivo* microscopic methods (McCuskey *et al.*, 1972).

Mice were anesthetized with sodium pentobarbital (0.03 mg/g), which resulted in electrically and pharmacologically excitable sympathetic nerves. A variety of vasoactive substances were administered topically to the splenic surface of mice, some of which had been pretreated with reserpine (5 mg/kg, i.p.). These data were compared with those obtained previously in mice which had been anesthetized with urethane (2.5. mg/g) (Reilly and McCuskey, 1974). At this concentration of urethane, neural influence on the splenic microvasculature effectively was removed, thereby limiting the possibility of modification of microvascular response by direct pharmacological stimulation of the splenic nerves.

With functional sympathetic innervation, there was a significant increase in the magnitude of arteriolar constriction elicited by histamine, prostaglandins (PG) E_2 and $F_{2\alpha}$, lactic acid, and bradykinin, and of arteriolar dilatation produced by adenosine and isoproterenol. Phentolamine at high concentrations caused arteriolar vasospasms. The response elicited by isoproterenol but not adenosine was antagonized by propranolol, while the constriction produced by all substances except phentolamine and bradykinin was blocked by an α-adrenergic antagonist. Responses to several of these substances were abolished by reserpine pretreatment. The data suggested (1) that lactic acid, histamine, and PGE_2 and $PGF_{2\alpha}$ cause α-mediated arteriolar constriction by releasing stored catecholamine from sympathetic nerves; (2) that subthreshold quantities of neurotransmitter may modulate microvascular sensitivity to bradykinin, isoproterenol, adenosine, phentolamine, and PGE_2 and $PGF_{2\alpha}$ in the presence of "reactive" sympathetic nerves; (3) that the anesthetic agents used do not significantly alter the sensitivity of the contractile components of the splenic microvascular system to vasoactive substances which act directly on the vascular wall.

F. D. REILLY and R. S. McCUSKEY · Department of Anatomy, University of Cincinnati, Cincinnati, Ohio.

ACKNOWLEDGMENTS

This work was supported by NIH Grants AM-10507 and AM-42370 and by the Southwest Ohio Heart Association.

References

McCuskey, R. S., Meineke, H. A., and Townsend, S. F., 1972, Studies of the hemopoietic microenvironment. I. Changes in the microvascular system and stroma during erythropoietic regeneration and suppression in the spleens of CF mice, *Blood* **39:**697.

Reilly, F. D., and McCuskey, R. S., 1974, Regulatory mechanisms in the splenic microvascular system of mice, *Fed. Proc.* **33:**393.

11.18. The pH of Splenic Microcirculation

M. J. LEVESQUE and A. C. GROOM

The spleen is known to be responsible for the trapping and destruction of abnormal and possibly of aged red cells. Murphy stated in 1967 that the splenic pH may be as low as 6.8, a factor which according to Lacelle (1969) will enhance fragmentation and trapping of red cells.

In this investigation, the splenic pH was estimated indirectly from the washout kinetics of the spleen. This project was undertaken to provide a new technique to measure the internal pH of the spleen and to investigate the parameters responsible for the buffering capacity of the spleen.

Cat spleens *in vitro* were perfused at a constant flow rate with physiological salt solutions and buffered at pH values ranging from 6.4 to 8.1 until most of the red cells had been washed out. It was found that the fractional change in pH was exponential and parallel to the fractional change of RBC concentration in the splenic pulp. Thereafter, the pH of the outflow was constant but different and linearly related to the pH of the inflow. When the latter was less that 6.8 the pH was raised during passage through the spleen, while for an inflow pH > 6.8 the opposite effect occurred. At an inflow of 6.8 there was no change. These results suggest the following:

1. The blood of high hematocrit in the splenic pulp is bathed in fluid of pH lower than arterial blood (i.e., 6.8).
2. The spleen possesses some buffering capacity.

References

Lacelle, P. L., 1969, Alteration of deformability of the erythrocyte membrane in stored blood, *Transfusion* **9:**238.

Murphy, J. R., 1967, The influence of pH and temperature on some physical properties of normal erythrocytes and erythrocytes from patients with hereditary spherocytosis, *J. lab. Clin. Med.* **69:**758.

M. J. LEVESQUE and A. C. GROOM · Department of Biophysics, University of Western Ontario, London, Ontario, Canada.

11.19 Specific Erythropoietin-Related Changes in the Splenic Microcirculation during Hypoxic and Posthypoxic Polycythemia: Comparision with Other Organs

R. S. McCUSKEY, H. A. MEINEKE, and P. A. McCUSKY

The murine spleen is an erythropoietic organ. Significant reductions in blood flow occur in the spleens of transfused polycythemic mice (McCuskey *et al.,* 1972*a*). Restoration of an optimal microcirculation is achieved when erythropoietin (Ep) is administered (McCuskey *et al.,* 1972*b*). This response can be blocked by anti-Ep serum. Based on these data and those from experiments with genetically anemic Sl/Sl^{d} and W/W^{v} mice (McCuskey and Meineke, 1973), we have suggested that blood flow through the splenic red pulp of the mouse is regulated locally by the release of a metabolite from Ep-sensitive stem cells following stimulation by Ep. Although these data suggested that the reduction in blood flow observed during polycythemia was related to the absence of circulating Ep, it was necessary to establish firmly that these changes were not related to the transfusion of exogenous RBCs or a general microvascular response to increased circulating RBC mass, and that the restoration was not due to contaminants in the Ep preparation. As a result, the following experiments were performed.

The splenic microcirculation of polycythemic mice was examined by *in vivo* microscopy (McCuskey *et al.,* 1972*a*) after 210 h of hypoxia (erythropoietic stimulation) and also at 6 days after hypoxia (erythropoietic suppression). During the period of hypoxia, blood flow increased 30% above that of controls. Six days after hypoxia, flow was reduced to 48% of the control value. Examination of the effect of polycythemia on the microcirculation in several nonerythropoietic organs demonstrated no significant changes in blood flow in the microvasculature of pancreas, skeletal muscle, and kidney, and only slight changes in the liver. Thus these data support our hypothesis that the changes in blood flow in the murine spleen during polycythemia are specific for erythropoietic tissue; they are not the result of increased circulating RXC mass or a response to transfusion of exogenous RBCs, but are dependent on the circulating levels of Ep.

R. S. McCUSKEY, H. A. MEINEKE, and P. A. McCUSKEY · Department of Anatomy, University of Cincinnati, Cincinnati, Ohio.

ACKNOWLEDGMENTS

This work was supported by NIH Grants Am-10507 and AM-42370 and by the Southwest Ohio Heart Association.

References

McCuskey, R. S., Meineke, H. A., and Townsend, S. F., 1972*a*, Studies of the hemopoietic microenvironment. I. Changes in the microvascular system and stroma during erythropoietic regeneration and suppression in the spleens of CF_1 mice, *Blood* **39:**697.

MuCuskey, R. S., Meineke, H. A., and Kaplan, S. M., 1972*b*, Studies of the hemopoietic microenvironment. II. Effect of erythropoietin on the splenic microvasculature of polycythemic CF_1 mice, *Blood* **39:**809.

McCuskey, R. S., and Meineke, H. A., 1973, Studies of the hemopoietic microenvironment. III. Differences in the splenic microvascular system and stroma between Sl/Sl^d and W/W^v anemic mice, *Am. J. Anat.* **137:**187.

12

Blood Flow in Skeletal Muscle

12.1. Microcirculation in Skeletal Muscle: Geometry of the Capillary Vascular Network

M. J. PLYLEY and A. C. GROOM

It is well known that during their course from arteriole to venule the capillaries in skeletal muscle branch and anastomose repeatedly (Krogh, 1919; Hammersen, 1968). There appears, however, to have been little previous attempt to quantitate the extent and pattern of capillary branching, although Eriksson and Myrhage (1972) reported that the capillaries of the tenuissimus muscle of the cat were 1.015 mm long, with branches to adjacent capillaries every 0.20 mm along their length. We have studied the branching pattern of these interconnections in the sartorius muscle of the frog, vasodilated by injection of papaverine and perfused with a silicone elastomer (Microfil). Each terminal arteriole gave rise to an average of 2.71 ± 1.34 (SD) capillaries. Each capillary had a mean of 3.44 ± 1.84 (SD) interior branch points. More than 90% of capillary branchings were simple divergent or convergent bifurcations, the included angle having an approximate mean value of 60° in each case. The initial branchings were mainly divergent, but the proportion of convergences increased linearly at successive branchings along the path. Some branches anastomosed with a capillary path to which the vessel had been connected previously. The incidence of such "rejoins" rose to 35% by the third and fourth branches, maximizing interaction between adjacent capillaries and maintaining each group of vessels as a fairly distinct microvascular unit. From these numerical data, plus measurements of path and segment lengths, realistic models of the capillary network have been synthesized. The fact that the anastomoses are so extensive suggests that they may play a key role in maintaining oxygenation of muscle tissue.

M. J. PLYLEY and A. C. GROOM · Department of Biophysics, University of Western Ontario, London, Ontario, Canada.

References

Eriksson, E., and Myrhage, R., 1972, Microvascular dimensions and blood flow in skeletal muscle, *Acta Physiol. Scand.* **86:**211.

Hammersen, F., 1968, The pattern of the terminal vascular bed and the ultrastructure of capillaries in skeletal muscle, in: *Oxygen Transport in Blood and Tissue* (D. W. Lübbers, U. C. Luft, G. Thiews, and E. Witzleb, eds.), pp. 184–197, George Thieme Verlag, Stuttgart.

Krogh, A., 1919, The number and distribution of capillaries in muscles with calculations of the oxygen pressure head necessary for supplying the tissue, *J. Physiol. (London)* **52:**409.

12.2. Regions of Preferential Blood Flow in Skeletal Muscle

RONALD F. TUMA, KARL-ERIK ARFORS, and HARVEY N. MAYROVITZ

The existence of preferential areas of blood flow in skeletal muscle has been debated for many years. Zweifach and Metz (1955) described the free edge of the spinotrapezius muscle as an area of preferential blood flow. Hammersen (1970) and Eriksson and Myrhage (1972) presented evidence against the presence of these preferential areas in skeletal muscle.

In this investigation, RBC velocity in the capillaries of the tenuissimus muscle was studied during control conditions and following topical application of epinephrine. Velocity recordings were made for each visible capillary crossing a line extending from the anterior free edge of the muscle to the central artery in the midline. For analysis purposes, the muscle was divided into five segments, and the mean velocity for all capillaries in each segment was determined for five animals.

In the control state, RBC velocity in capillaries nearest the free edge of the muscle was 2.8 times faster than that in capillaries nearest the midline (see Fig. 1). Following topical application of 1×10^{-3} mg/ml epinephrine, flow was stopped in all capillaries of the muscle. Two to five minutes later, flow returned first in capillaries near the free edge, and then progressed sequentially toward the midline.

The results presented confirm the presence of a nonuniform distribution of capillary blood flow. The results of the epinephrine experiments indicate that there is also a spatial nonuniformity in the reactivity of the resistance vessels. Since metarterioles and precapillary sphincters have not been demonstrated in the tenuissimus muscle, the explanation given by Zweifach and Metz (1955) does not seem applicable in the present case. One factor which may contribute to the nonuniform distribution is the difference in the pressure to which the resistance vessels are exposed. Gore (1972) had demonstrated that reactivity of vascular smooth muscle is dependent on wall stress. Lateral branches of the transverse arteriole nearest the midline are subjected to a higher intraluminal pressure and would therefore be more reactive than similar vessels near the free edge.

RONALD F. TUMA, KARL-ERIK ARFORS, and HARVEY N. MAYROVITZ · Department of Physiology, Temple University School of Medicine, Philadelphia, Pennsylvania, and Department of Experimental Medicine, Pharmacia AB, Uppsala, Sweden.

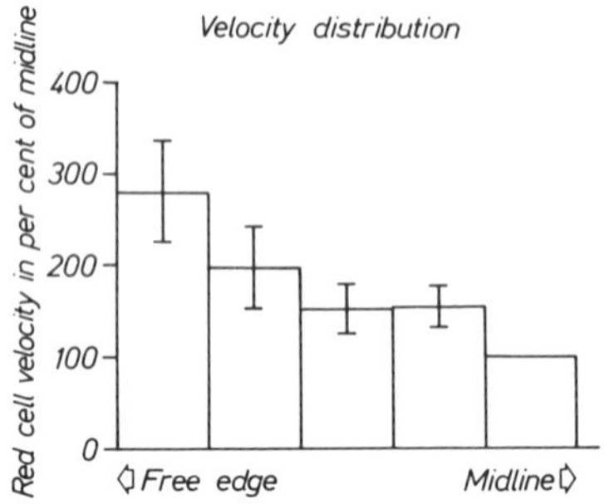

Figure 1. RBC velocity distribution. Each bar represents the mean capillary RBC velocity in one of five sections extending from the anterior free edge to the midline of the muscle.

References

Eriksson, E., and Myrhage, R., 1972, Microvascular dimensions and blood flow in skeletal muscle, *Acta Physiol. Scand.* **86:**211.

Gore, R. W., 1972, Wall stress: A determinant of regional differences in response of frog microvessels to norepinephrine, *Am. J. Physiol.* **222:**82.

Hammersen, F., 1970, The terminal vascular bed in skeletal muscle with special regard to the problem of shunts, in: *Capillary Permeability* (C. Crone and N. Lassen, eds.), pp. 351–365, Munksgaard, Copenhagen.

Zweifach, B. W., and Metz, D. B., 1955, Selective distribution of blood through the terminal vascular bed of mesenteric structure and skeletal muscle, *Angiology* **6:**282.

12.3. Distribution of Blood Flow in Microcirculation in Cat Tenuissimus Muscle

K. FRONEK and B. W. ZWEIFACH

Tenuissimus muscle has all the characteristic attributes of a skeletal muscle, and, since it consists of only several thin layers of muscle fibers, it seems to be a good object for microvascular studies. In view of the fact that muscle hemodynamics until recently were studied almost exclusively on an overall input–output relationship basis, we considered it useful to begin the microcirculatory studies by first analyzing some of the basic microcirculatory parameters and to use these to determine the viability of the tenuissimus muscle as a microvascular model.

Microspheres labeled with three different isotopes were used to study blood flow distribution. The muscle was dissected and left for 2 h under conditions simulating those during microvascular studies. Total blood flow through the dissected muscle exceeded by 25% that of the contralateral muscle (nondissected).

In the following series of experiments, the pressure, flow, velocity, and volume as a function of vessel diameter were determined by microvascular methods (Intaglietta *et al.*, 1970; Tompkins *et al.*, 1974). Arteriolar blood pressure in the tenuissimus muscle remains at a 75% level of the systemic arterial blood pressure in vessels around 50 μm, and it is about 25% of blood pressure on the arteriolar side of the capillaries. To complement these findings, we calculated the volume blood flow in arterioles by determining the flow velocity and respective diameter. Flow velocity determination in tenuissimus muscle under steady-state conditions decreases moderately with the vessel branching; as the vessel size approaches precapillaries and capillaries, there is an abrupt decrease in flow velocity (see Fig. 1). This decrease coincides with the subdivision of arterioles into several capillaries (Fronek and Zweifach, 1975).

In a subsequent series of experiments, microvascular reactivity and viability were studied by using the postocclusive reactive hyperemia test. Total inflow was measured by placing an electromagnetic flow probe around the aorta. A silastic occluder was placed distally and the arterial blood pressure was measured below the occluder by a catheter placed in the contralateral femoral artery. During the occlusion, the blood pressure

K. FRONEK and B. W. ZWEIFACH · AMES-Bioengineering, University of California, San Diego, California.

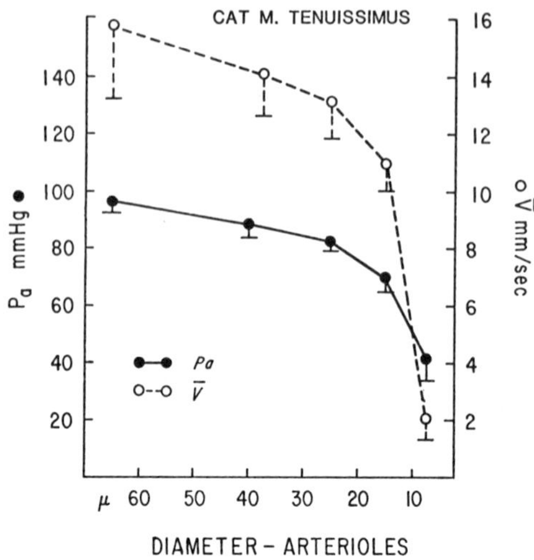

Figure 1. Pressure (Pa) and blood flow velocity ($\bar{V}$) distribution as a function of arteriolar diameter in cat tenuissimus muscle. Micropressures and blood flow velocity as a function of vessel diameter were determined simultaneously or in some instances independently. Data points represent mean values with the standard error for each set of data.

was lowered to 50 mm Hg for 1–2 min. Microvascular functions were measured simultaneously. In these experiments, the diameters of different size arterioles behave differently during the occlusion of arterial inflow. As a rule, vessels of diameters 20–30 μm, may dilate by as much as 100%, whereas larger arterioles (40–60 μm) exhibit only a moderate dimension increase by 10–25%. Summarizing the results of our experiments, we can conclude that

1. The tenuissimus muscle microvascular preparation is a viable hemodynamic model with a well-defined pressure flow and vessel diameter relationship.
2. The postocclusive reactive hyperemia response has a different response pattern in different sizes of arterioles. It seems that 20–35 μm arterioles are affected to a greater degree than are the larger feeding vessels.

Acknowledgment

This work was supported by United States Public Health Service Grant HL-10881.

References

Fronek, K., and Zweifach, B. W., 1975, Microvascular pressure distribution in skeletal muscle and the effect of vasodilation, *Am. J. Physiol.* **228**:791.

Intaglietta, M., Pawula, R. F., and Tompkins, W. R., 1970, Pressure measurement in the mammalian microvasculature, *Microvasc. Res.* **2**:212.

Tompkins, W. R., Monti, R., and Intaglietta, M., 1974, Velocity measurement by self-tracking correlator, *Rev. Sci. Instrum.* **45**:647.

12.4. Apparent Distribution of Capillary and Shunt Flow in Canine Skeletal Muscle

W. N. DURÁN and B. E. KANOY, JR.

The indicator dilution method was used to study the distribution of microvascular flow in isolated gracilis muscles perfused with blood at controlled flows. ^{125}I-iodoantipyrine (Ap), a flow-limited molecule, served as a capillary flow indicator, while ^{22}Na was used as a capillary diffusion capacity (PS) indicator, and ^{51}Cr-albumin served as an intravascular tracer. The data were analyzed according to a circulation model consisting of capillary (exchange) and shunt (nonexchange) pathways (Chien, 1971). Capillary fractional extraction (E) of Na, corrected for shunt pathways contribution, decreased as a function of plasma flow. Calculated PS-Na increased as flow was increased and tended to be independent of flow at high perfusion rates, confirming the diffusion-limited transport of Na. In a preliminary series of experiments, E-Ap varied between 0.76 and 0.85 at blood flows between 4 and 10 $ml \cdot min^{-1} \cdot 100\ g^{-1}$, the variation of E-Ap being independent of the flow rate. In subsequent experiments, E-Ap decreased from 0.95 to 0.92 as blood flow was increased from 1.6 to 21 $ml \cdot min^{-1} \cdot 100\ g^{-1}$. The difference between the two series is tentatively attributed to technical improvements in the surgical isolation of the muscles. Since E-Ap indicates the fraction of flow through the exchange network, these results show that (1) almost all of the total blood flow goes through capillaries in resting gracilis muscles; (2) if our tentative explanation is correct, subtle damage to the muscle during surgical isolation can cause a fall of E-Ap and consequently an increase in the fraction of flow through shunt and pathways; (3) variation of the number of open capillaries, rather than shift of blood from nonexchange to exchange vessels, is the main mechanism by which the microcirculation meets the metabolic needs of tissues.

ACKNOWLEDGMENTS

This work was supported by NIH Grant HL-12749 and North Carolina Heart Association Grant 1973-74-A-23.

Reference

Chien, S., 1971, A theory for the quantification of transcapillary exchange in the presence of shunt flow, *Circ. Res.* **29**:173.

W. N. DURAN and B. E. KANOY, JR. · Department of Physiology and Pharmacology, Duke University Medical Center, Durham, North Carolina.

12.5. The Microvascular Bed and Capillary Surface Area in Rat Extensor Hallucis Proprius Muscle

RHAGNAR MYRHAGE and OLGA HUDLICKÁ

The extensor hallucis proprius is a fast muscle (contraction time 20 ms) in rats, easily accessible for dissection and exposure for intravital microscopy. The muscle can be transilluminated at an adequate resolution. The population of muscle fibers is mixed—60% are white, 24% are intermediate, and 16% are red.

The vascular tree is of an irregular type; the terminal arterioles have a small number of branching straight capillaries 535 ± 25 μm (SE) long with an ID of 4.0 ± 0.08 μm at the arteriolar end and 5.5 ± 0.09 μm at the venular end. The flow is intermittent and occasionally stops for less than a minute. A small number of capillaries are significantly shorter (about 250 μm); in these, the flow is less intermittent. Intercapillary branches are rare.

The capillary/fiber ratio, as found by histochemical staining for capillary endothelium, is 1.01 ± 0.01 in the proximal part and 0.93 ± 0.02 in the distal part of the muscle.

The number of capillaries/mm^2 is 1347 ± 53 at the proximal and 1043 ± 64 at the distal end of the muscle. The corresponding cross-section area of the whole muscle is 0.51 ± 0.09 mm^2 and 0.16 ± 0.04 mm^2, respectively.

From the *in vivo* measurements, the calculated average surface area of individual capillaries was 7980 μm^2. Combining intravital microscopy with histological staining, it is possible to calculate the total capillary surface area, A, as

$$A = A_c \times \frac{L}{l_c} \times \frac{p + d}{2}$$

where A_c is the average area of individual capillaries, L is total muscle length (13.0 ± 0.5 mm), l_c is the length of the individual capillaries, and p is the number of capillaries/mm^2 at the proximal end of the muscle and d the number at the distal end.

With a muscle weight of 14.3 ± 0.52 mg, the capillary surface area is 1.6 m^2/100 g tissue—somewhat higher than the value of 0.7 m^2/100 g

RHAGNAR MYRHAGE · Laboratory of Experimental Biology, Department of Anatomy, University of Göteborg, Sweden. OLGA HUDLICKÁ · Department of Physiology, The Medical School, Birmingham, England.

tissue based on India ink perfusion of cat muscle (Pappenheimer *et al.*, 1951). The discrepancy is probably due to underestimation of the number of capillaries and to the fact that capillary length was not taken into account.

Reference

Papenheimer, J. R., Renkin, E. M., and Borrero, L. M., 1951, Filtration, diffusion and molecular sieving through peripheral capillary membranes: A contribution to the pore theory of capillary permeability, *Am. J. Physiol.* **167:**13.

12.6. Kinetics of Red Cell and Plasma Washout from the Vascular Bed of Skeletal Muscle

T. J. BOWDEN and A. C. GROOM

When skeletal muscle is perfused with a cell-free physiological salt solution, the majority of the red cells in the vascular bed are washed out extremely rapidly. However, a small fraction of the cells (approximately 1%) are washed out with a rate constant 3 orders of magnitude lower than this, as shown by Groom *et al.* (1973). These authors identified such cells as mainly reticulocytes and suggested that they adhere to the vascular walls. If this be so, the slow compartment of washout should be restricted to cells and not be present in the washout of plasma. We have therefore studied the washout of both cells and plasma in the following way. Radioactive serum albumin was injected intravenously in anesthetized cats (nembutal, 40 mg/kg) and allowed to equilibrate in the circulation for 60 min. One gastrocnemius muscle was isolated except for the artery and vein, and was perfused at 37°C with oxygenated Ringer solution containing 0.1% (w/v) sodium nitroprusside to induce maximal vasodilation. Cell and ^{125}I-albumin concentrations in serial samples of the outflow were measured and plotted semilogarithmically vs. the volume of fluid which had perfused the muscle. A slow component of plasma washout similar to that of red cells was found to be present. Such a component has been shown not to exist in the spleen (Levesque and Groom, 1975), and the difference between the two vascular beds must presumably account for the difference in plasma washout. The plasma slow compartment in skeletal muscle may be due to the trapping of plasma in the capillaries by the red cells which comprise the slow compartment.

References

Groom, A. C., Song, S. H., and Campling, B. G., 1973, Clearance of red blood cells from the vascular bed of skeletal muscle with particular reference to reticulocytes, *Microvasc. Res.* **6**:51.

Levesque, M. L., and Groom, A. C., 1975, Washout of red cells and plasma from the spleen, *Fed. Proc.* **34(3)**:385.

T. J. BOWDEN and A. C. GROOM · Department of Biophysics, University of Western Ontario, London, Ontario, Canada.

12.7. Blood Oxygen Saturation Determination in Frozen Dog Gracilis Muscle

HARVEY R. WEISS and A. K. SINHA

A new method has been developed to determine the %HbO_2 of blood in vessels as small as 12 μm in a quick-frozen tissue. A three-wavelength (560, 523, 506 nm) computational technique was developed to measure %HbO_2 independent of path length or hemoglobin concentration and to correct for light scattering. The method and its theoretical basis have been reported in detail (Sinha *et al.,* 1975). The method was tested spectroscopically and microspectroscopically in cuvettes, cut frozen blood, and blood vessels from frozen tissue against the Van Slyke technique. The three-wavelength method was also compared to a four-wavelength geometric technique (Schmidt and Niesel, 1964). The rate of freezing was shown not to influence the %HbO_2 determination. Calculations show that %HbO_2 changes due to shifts in the Hb dissociation curve resulting from freezing or variations in pH or in 2,3-DPG or Hb concentration are about 2%. A linear relation was found in all cases between our method and the Van Slyke technique in calculations of %HbO_2. The accuracy of the three-wavelength technique was 2–5% within 95% confidence limits spectroscopically and 5.6–10% microspectroscopically. The repeatability of the measurements was about 5% under all conditions. In anesthetized dogs, ten gracilis muscles were isolated. The %HbO_2 of the arteries and veins was determined by the Van Slyke technique. The muscles were then quick-frozen and a microspectroscopic analysis of vessels less than 100 μm was performed. The two methods were in excellent agreement, with a correlation coefficient of 0.987. We found similar precision and accuracy using either the three- or the four-wavelength technique. Other techniques employing more complicated measuring schemes have been developed (Gamble *et al.,* 1974; Grunewald and Lübbers, 1975). Our method is much simpler and should prove useful with any tissue where differences in venous %HbO_2 are expected.

ACKNOWLEDGMENTS

This study was supported in part by HL-16134 and a grant-in-aid of the American Heart Association, New Jersey Affiliate.

HARVEY R. WEISS and A. K. SINHA · Department of Physiology, CMDNJ-Rutgers Medical School, Piscataway, New Jersey.

References

Gamble, W. J., LaFarge, C. G., Fyler, D. C., Weisul, J., and Monroe, R. G., 1974, Regional coronary venous oxygen saturation and myocardial oxygen tension following abrupt changes in ventricular pressure in the isolated dog heart, *Circ. Res.* **34:**672.

Grunewald, W. A., and Lübbers, D. W., 1975, Die Bestimmung der intracapillären HbO_2-Sättigung mit einer Kryo-mikrofotometrischen Methode angewandt am Myokard des Kaninchens, *Pfluegers Arch.* **353:**255.

Schmidt, K., and Niesel, W., 1964. Messung der Sauerstoffsättigung des Hämaglobins an durchbluteten Geweben im reflektierten Licht mit dem Rapidspektroskop, *Pfluegers Arch.* **280:**369.

Sinha, A. K., Neubauer, J. A., Lipp, J. A., and Weiss, H. R., 1975, Oxygen saturation determination in frozen blood, *Microvasc. Res.* **10:**312.

12.8. Functional Arteriolar Vasodilatation in Striated Muscle

R. J. GORCZYNSKI and B. R. DULING

Hamster cremaster muscles were suffused with a solution equilibrated with 0% O_2 and 5% CO_2 pH 7.35 (Baez, 1973). Internal arteriolar diameter was measured during electrical stimulation of five to ten muscle fibers in order to characterize the microvascular basis of functional hyperemia. The time course of the diameter change during muscular contraction typically consisted of three phases (Fig. 1, upper trace): a latent period, an early rapid transient dilation (early peak), and a slowly developing sustained vasodilatation (late peak). The diameter change associated with the early peak ranged from 2.5 ± 0.6 to 6.7 ± 1.3 μm and that of the late peak from 3.8 ± 0.4 to 12.1 ± 1.4 μm as the contraction peak was increased from 1 to 8/s. The duration of the latent period decreased from 21.0 ± 1.3 to 6.7 ± 1.5 as contraction frequency increased from 1 to 8/s. The arteriolar responses were restricted to the immediate

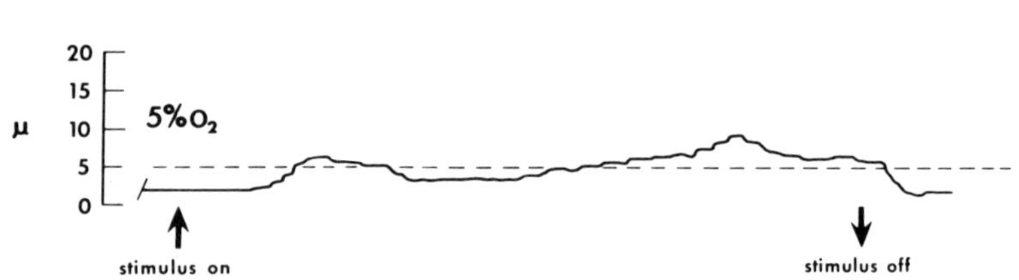

Figure 1. Typical recording of arteriolar diameter illustrating the time course of arteriolar diameter change in response to muscular contraction at a frequency of 4 contractions/s and the effect of elevated Po_2 on the response. Upper trace: Suffusion solution equilibrated with N_2 (0% O_2). Abbreviations: EP, early peak; LP, late peak. Lower trace: Suffusion solution equilibrated with 5% O_2.

R. J. GORCZYNSKI and B. R. DULING · Department of Physiology, University of Virginia School of Medicine, Charlottesville, Virginia.

vicinity of the active fibers, with no evidence of a propagated response. Elevation of suffusion solution Po_2 by equilibration with 5% O_2 (Fig. 1) caused significant increases in the latent period of 18.6 ± 3.0, 16.3 ± 3.9, and 11.0 ± 4.1 s at 2, 4, and 8 contractions/s, respectively. The magnitude of the late peak was also significantly decreased by elevated Po_2 at 2 and at 4 contractions/s, while the time required to reach the late peak was increased significantly. The phasic nature of the increase in arteriolar diameter in response to muscular contraction is consistent with the hypothesis that a corresponding two-component process links contraction to the vasodilatation observed (Mohrman *et al.,* 1973). The data suggest that changes in Po_2 play an important role in the regulation of blood flow during muscular contraction.

ACKNOWLEDGMENT

This work was supported by United States Public Health Service Research Grant HL-12792.

References

Baez, S., 1973, An open cremaster muscle preparation for the study of blood vessels by *in vivo* microscopy, *Microvasc. Res.* **5**:384.

Mohrman, D. E., Cant, J. R., and Sparks, H. V., 1973, Time course of vascular resistance and venous oxygen changes following brief tetanus of dog skeletal muscle, *Circ. Res.* **33**:323.

12.9. Blood Flow Changes Due to Compression in Contracting Muscles

SIMON RODBARD

Effects of tissue compression on blood flow have been examined in isolated hearts and limbs, and in models. Muscle compression similar to that occurring during contraction produces an initial transitory reduction in arterial inflow (hypoemia); flow then tends to return to control values (compression autoregulation). Our data indicate that muscle contraction produces the hypoemia by raising tissue pressure, thereby collapsing blood capillaries. The elevated tissue pressure pushes some tissue fluids into the capillaries; as tissue pressure falls, some of the capillaries reopen, producing the autoregulation. Removal of compression lowers tissue pressure; the capillaries open more widely and hyperemia results. Tissues then refill with ultrafiltrate, some of the capillaries tend to collapse partially, and flow returns toward initial values. The hypoemia at onset of compression and the hyperemia on removal of the compression vary with the intensity, duration, and number of compressions or contractions. Postcompression hyperemia may exceed that induced by contraction. Hyperemias (postocclusion, compression, contraction) may therefore operate through similar mechanical relationships of capillary transmural (inside minus outside) pressures.

References

Kikuchi, Y., and Rodbard, S., 1974, Autoregulatory escape and postescape hyperaemia in a capillaron model, *Cardiovasc. Res.* **8:**395.

Kira, S., and Rodbard, S., 1971, Effects of histamine and acetylcholine on the isolated perfused lung lobe, *Q. J. Exp. Physiol.* **56:**1.

Rodbard, S., and Kira, S., 1972, Lobar, airway, and pulmonary vascular effects of serotonin, *Angiology* **23:**188.

Rodbard, S., Handel, N., and Sadja, L., 1971, Flow patterns in a model of a contracting muscle, *Cardiovasc. Res.* **5:**396.

SIMON RODBARD · City of Hope Medical Center, Duarte, California.

12.10. Changes in the Capillary Density and Reactivity of the Vascular Bed in Chronically Stimulated Fast Muscles

OLGA HUDLICKÁ, MARY COTTER, and W. H. ALLUM

Chronic stimulation of fast muscles at a frequency naturally occurring in nerves to slow muscles (5–10 Hz) results in a transformation of muscles toward a slower type (Pette *et al.,* 1973), increase in the capillary density which precedes any changes in the oxidative capacity (Cotter *et al.,* 1973*a*), and growth of new capillaries (Cotter *et al.,* 1973*b*). The capillary/muscle fiber ratio after 4 wk of such stimulation approaches the high ratio in slow muscles and persists for several weeks after stimulation has been discontinued. Chronic stimulation of either fast or slow muscles at a frequency naturally occurring in nerves to fast muscles (short bursts of tetani) does not affect the capillary density.

The increase in the capillary density in muscles stimulated at "slow nerve" frequency seems to be connected with a higher demand for oxygen in the early stages of stimulation.

Resting blood flow in muscles with a higher density of capillaries resembles that of control muscles; however, the increase in blood flow in response to vasodilator stimuli (acetylcholine, isoprenaline, functional or reactive hyperemia) is considerably greater. The vessels are less responsive to vasoconstrictor stimuli such as infusion of norepinephrine or stimulation of the sympathetic nerves even if the density of adrenergic nerve fibers does not appear to be changed.

References

Cotter, M. Hudlická, O., Pette, D., Staudte, H., and Vrbova, G., 1973*a*, Changes of capillary density and enzyme pattern in fast rabbit muscles during long-term stimulation, *J. Physiol. (London)* **230**:34.

Cotter, M., Hudlická, O., and Vrbova, G., 1973*b*, Growth of capillaries during long-term activity in skeletal muscle, *Bibl. Anat.* **11**:395.

Pette, D., Smith, M. E., Staudte, H. W., and Vrbova, G., 1973, Effects of long-term electrical stimulation on some contractile and metabolic characteristics of fast rabbit muscles, *Pfluegers Arch.* **338**:257

OLGA HUDLICKÁ, MARY COTTER, and W. H. ALLUM · Department of Physiology, University of Birmingham, Birmingham, England.

12.11. Skeletal Muscle Vascular Volume Changes with Increased Venous Pressure

C. H. BAKER, R. P. MENNINGER, R. E. SCHOEN, and E. T. SUTTON

It is well known that total tissue volume increases with elevations of venous pressure (Baker, 1970; Diana and Shadur, 1973). However, the relative changes in circulating and total vascular volume in skeletal muscle and the volume of vascular area that may be mobilized have not been reported.

12.11.1. Methods

Dog gracilis muscles were removed, enclosed in a plethysmograph, and perfused at either constant inflow pressure or constant inflow. Circulating blood volumes were measured by the constant infusion technique using RBC-^{51}Cr or albumin-^{131}I (Zierler, 1962). Control venous pressure averaged 3 mm Hg and elevations (ΔPv) over the range of 5–40 mm Hg were produced. Volume changes were determined during the following ΔPv by plethysmography and by changes in total muscle radioactivity. Changes in total, active, and mobilized vascular volume were calculated. The mobilized active vascular volume (active volume change vs. total volume change) consists of vessels filled with blood which were closed off and unattainable by the indicators during the control period but which were opened by the ΔPv.

12.11.2. Results

Active vascular volumes and total vascular volumes increased with venous pressure to about 25 mm Hg, then plateaued (Fig. 1). Active vascular volumes (indicators) increased by significantly greater amounts than total vascular volumes (plethysmography). Volume changes in the constant inflow groups were doubled those in the constant pressure groups. Mobilized active volume averaged 45% of the active vascular volume change. With venous pressure elevation, there was an increase in the RBC-^{51}Cr volume to albumin-^{131}I volume ratio.

C. H. BAKER, R. P. MENNINGER, R. E. SCHOEN, and E. T. SUTTON · Department of Physiology, University of South Florida College of Medicine, Tampa, Florida.

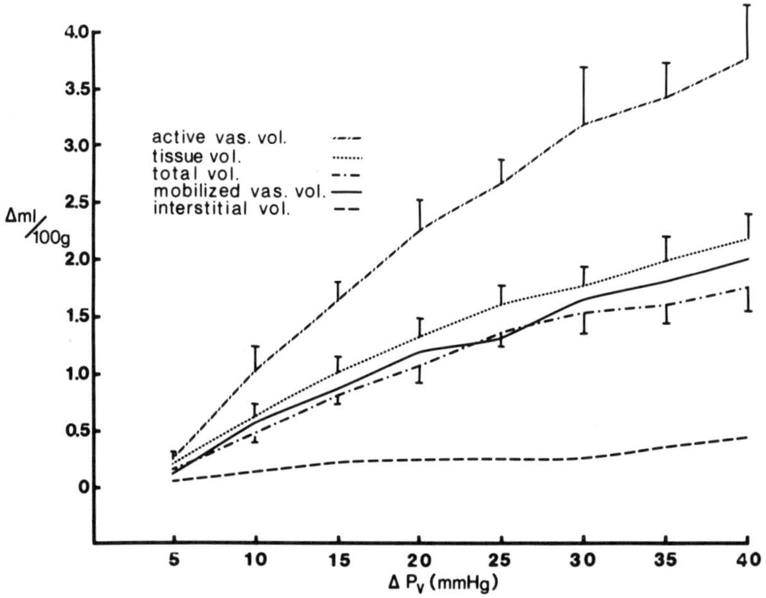

Figure 1. Mean changes in active vascular volume (RBC-^{51}Cr), total tissue volume, total vascular volume, mobilized blood volume, and extravascular volume in muscles infused at constant inflow. Brackets indicate ± 1 SEM.

12.11.3. Conclusions

The data indicate that there is a marked redistribution of blood flow in the skeletal muscle microcirculation as a result of elevated venous pressure. There is also a redistribution of red cells with respect to plasma, possibly due to a decrease in plasma skimming with red cells gaining access to vessels that previously were unattainable by them. Blood flow resistance decreased slightly with elevation of venous pressures.

ACKNOWLEDGMENTS

This work was supported by NIH Grant HL-14541 and the Suncoast Heart Association.

References

Baker, C. H., 1970, Blood flow and volume distribution with elevated venous pressure, *Am. J. Physiol.* **281**:674.

Diana, J. N., and Shadur, C. A., 1973, Effect of arterial and venous pressure on capillary pressure and vascular volume, *Am. J. Physiol.* **225**:637.

Zierler, K. L., 1962, Circulation times and the theory of indicator-dilution methods for determining blood flow and volume, in: *Handbook of Physiology* Section 2: Circulation, Vol. 1, pp. 585–615, American Physiological Society, Washington, D.C.

12.12. Flow Improvement in the Vasodilated Skeletal Muscle of the Dog by Slow Defibrinogenation with Arvin

K. LENNART APPELGREN, LENNART GUSTAVSSON, and HELGE MYRVOLD

Blood with low fibrinogen levels has a decreased *in vitro* viscosity, more so at low shear rates (Chien, 1967). A purified fraction from the venom of the Malayan pit viper, *Agkistrodon rhodostoma,* called Abott 38414 or Ancrod (Abott Laboratories, United States) or Arvin (Knoll Pharmaceutical Ltd., West Germany), given subcutaneously at 0.1 unit/kg body weight at daily intervals will cause a slow defibrinogenation in man and dog with virtually no bleeding problems (Knoll AG, 1974). The promising clinical results reported from West Germany in patients with severe arterioocclusive disease, not available to surgical treatment (e.g., see Ehrly 1975), prompted us to study the *in vivo* flow-improving effect of defibrinogenation (DF) experimentally using a well-defined vascular bed, the fully vasodilated calf muscle of the dog. Vasodilation was produced by inducing muscular work in the muscle preparation by electrical stimulation of the sciatic nerve. The muscle preparation was as described by Kjellmer (1964) and Djojosugito *et al.* (1970). Flow was measured by electromagnetic flowmeter, and flow was compared in control and DF dogs at different perfusion pressures. *In vitro* viscosities were measured by a Wells-Brookfield model LVT cone-plate viscosimeter at different shear rates.

The maximal flows in control dogs were in agreement with known values in skeletal muscle at different perfusion pressures (Djojosugito *et al.,* 1970), while flows in DF dogs were well above these values at all perfusion pressures. The assumption of an identical vascular bed in control and DF dogs is probably better at high perfusion pressures and flow rates. The relative flow increase was 100–150% at high flows–perfusion pressures in the DF dogs compared to the control dogs, while the *in vitro* viscosity was 100% above that of DF dogs in blood from the control dogs at a shear rate of 230 s^{-1}. The effect of DF was even more pronounced in the low flow rate–low perfusion pressure range, in accordance with a larger decrease seen in *in vitro* viscosity at low shear

K. LENNART APPELGREN, LENNART GUSTAVSSON, and HELGE MYRVOLD · Rheology Laboratory and Department of Surgery I, Sahlgrenska University Hospital, and University of Gøteborg Faculty of Medicine, Gøteborg, Sweden.

rates. However, the assumption of the same geometrical conditions in the vascular bed in control and DF dogs is uncertain in this flow–perfusion pressure range.

In summary, a considerable increase of flow was found in a well-defined vascular bed after slow defibrinogenation with Arvin. The relative changes in flow and viscosity were especially pronounced in the low flow rate–low perfusion rate–low shear rate range. The changes seen in this low range promise to be of special value in patients with severe arterioocclusive disease.

ACKNOWLEDGMENTS

The research grant for this investigation was kindly supplied by MEDA Pharmaceuticals Ltd., Sweden, which also provided the Arvin used in this investigation. A traveling grant for one of us (K. L. A.) is also gratefully acknowledged.

References

Chien, S., 1967, Blood viscosity: Influence of erythrocyte aggregation, *Science* **157**:829.

Djojosugito, A. M., Folkow, B., Øberg, B., and White, S., 1970, A comparison of blood viscosity measured *in vitro* and in a vascular bed, *Acta Physiol. Scand.* **78**:70.

Ehrly, A. M., 1975, Improvement of the microcirculatory properties of blood in patients with vascular diseases treated with Ancrod, in: *First World Congress for Microcirculation,* Toronto, June 15–20, 1975, Abst. 278.

Kjellmer, I., 1964, The effect of exercise on the vascular bed of skeletal muscle, *Acta Physiol. Scand.* **62**:18.

Knoll AG, 1974, Pharmacological and clinical test of the registered drug Arwin(R), Suppl. 2 to request for registration of Arwin(R) in West Germany, Knoll Pharmaceutical Ltd., March 20, 1974 (in German).

13

Microcirculation in Other Tissues

13.1. Quantitative Studies of Brain Microcirculation Using Quasilinearization Techniques

CHEN LIN CHANG, DUANE F. BRULEY, and MELVIN H. KNISELY

The dynamics of brain tissue oxygen supply have been simulated. In accordance with the long-range goal of a real time simulation of the Krogh capillary–tissue cylinder system of nonlinear, coupled, partial differential equations, the alternating-direction–implicit method combined with the quasilinearization technique was applied. The nonlinear equation resulting from the nonlinear oxygen dissociation curve for human blood is represented by a sequence of linear equations which converge quadratically to the solution of the nonlinear equation. The error of any iteration is approximately the square of the error of the preceding iteration. With inaccurate initial guesses, the transient oxygen tension profiles in the capillary–tissue system have been obtained in two or three iterations with four-digit accuracy.

Comparison of the results obtained by this technique and the digital integration explicit method (McCracken *et al.*, 1972) has been made. From this comparison, a much shorter computation time and a more stable solution are realized using quasilinearization.

Autoregulation (Bruley *et al.*, 1973) for the prevention of tissue anoxia and therefore nerve cell damage in the cerebral cortex has been studied. Distributed-parameter mathematical models were developed to simulate the Krogh capillary–tissue anatomical unit, and closed loop control schemes representing blood flow regulation and oxygen consump-

CHEN LIN CHANG · Chemical Engineering Department, Clemson University, Clemson, South Carolina. DUANE F. BRULEY · Chemical Engineering Department, Tulane University, New Orleans, Louisiana. MELVIN H. KNISELY · Anatomy Department, Medical University of South Carolina, Charleston, South Carolina.

tion rate were superimposed. The proposed control mechanisms help explain the plateaus and overshoot characteristics in the experimental curves (Bicher *et al.,* 1973) and provide insight into differences in experimental tissue response times compared with those predicted by conventional convection–diffusion mathematical models, with constant flow and oxygen consumption rates.

References

Bicher, H. I., Reneau, D. D., Bruley, D. F., and Knisely, M. H., 1973, Brain oxygen supply and neuronal activity under normal and hypoglycemia conditions, *Am. J. Physiol.* **224(2)**:275.

Bruley, D. F., Reneau, D. D., Bicher, H. I., and Knisely, M. H., 1973, Studies of cerebral tissue oxygenation and related autoregulation, *Adv. Chem. Ser.* **118**:290.

McCracken, T. A., Bruley, D. F., Reneau, D. D., Bicher, H. I., and Knisely, M. H., 1972, Systems analysis of transport processes in human brain. II. Systems studies of the simultaneous transport of oxygen, glucose and carbon dioxide in human brain, in: *Proceedings of the First Pacific Chemical Engineering Congress,* Kyoto, Japan, October 1972, p. 137.

13.2. Microangiography and Trypan Blue Fluorescence Study of Cardiac-Arrested Dog Brain

SHU-REN LIN and MARTTI KORMANO

Cardiac arrest longer than 5 min results in abnormal cerebral flow at 3–4 h after restoration of normal blood circulation as shown by prolonged arterial phase and faint venous visualization in cerebral angiography and by uneven distribution of carbon black in the microvasculature. The pathogenesis of the late deterioration of the blood flow was studied with microangiographic visualization of the brain microvascular structures and trypan blue fluorescence experiments to reveal eventual blood–brain barrier damage or local ischemic areas. Open-chest cardiac arrest of 5–10 min was produced by fibrillation of the heart, followed by defibrillation and 2–6 h resuscitation. Trypan blue (1%, 15 ml/kg in saline) was given intravenously 10 min before the circulation was stopped. Fresh frozen cryostat sections studied with fluorescence microscopy showed an increased tendency to cortical dye extravasation in cardiac-arrested dogs. No areas totally devoid of capillary fluorescence were seen, an observation supported by the microangiographic appearance of the brain capillaries. It is concluded that prolonged cardiac arrest and long-term resuscitation will cause slight blood–brain barrier damage and moderate cerebral edema but not enough to cause total ischemia. Experimentation also suggests increased vulnerability of the cortical capillaries in long-term resuscitated animals.

SHU-REN LIN and MARTTI KORMANO · University of Rochester Medical Center, Rochester, New York.

13.3. Pharmacological Control of O_2 Autoregulation in Brain Tissue

H. I. BICHER and D. F. BRULEY

The availability of oxygen throughout parenchymatous organs is far from homogeneous, oxygen tensions varying 30 or 40 mm Hg within a few micrometers. However, the Po_2 at a given microarea of cerebral tissue is remarkably constant, and can be changed only through major alterations in blood supply or the composition of respiratory gases.

By measuring physiological parameters (tissue Po_2 and neuronal firing in the same microarea of tissue, as determined using ultramicro oxygen electrodes, arterial Po_2, blood flow, and blood pressure), we have described a precisely controlled autoregulatory mechanism to maintain constant brain tissue Po_2 (Bicher *et al.,* 1973). This includes a theoretical regulating "tissue oxygen sensor," and is defined by four criteria in the physiological compensatory response elicited by a short period of anoxia:

1. Short "reoxygenation time" (time required for tissue Po_2 to return to preanoxic level).
2. Increase in cerebral blood flow.
3. Presence of an "overshoot" (peroid after reoxygenation during which tissue Po_2 is higher than baseline).
4. A period of "anoxic silence" in neuronal activity (Bicher, 1974).

All four responses can be suppressed by the α-adrenergic blocking agent phenoxybenzamine. In the present experiments, other autonomically active agents were tested. Atropine, hexamethonium, propranolol, and isoproterenol had no influence on these parameters. Phenoxybenzamine, tolazoline, and dibenamine all suppressed autoregulation. Also, a fifth autoregulation criterion, the small or nonexistent rise in brain tissue Po_2 during normoatmospheric O_2 breathing, was added as an additional test.

In another experimental series, phenoxybenzamine was infused during O_2 or 95% O_2–5% CO_2 breathing (Fig. 1). The infusion always induced a rise in tissue Po_2. It is concluded that an α-adrenergic mechanism is part of the autoregulation process, and its pharmacological

H. I. BICHER · Department of Pharmacology, University of Arkansas Medical Center, Little Rock, Arkansas. D. F. BRULEY · Department of Chemical Engineering, Tulane University, New Orleans, Louisiana.

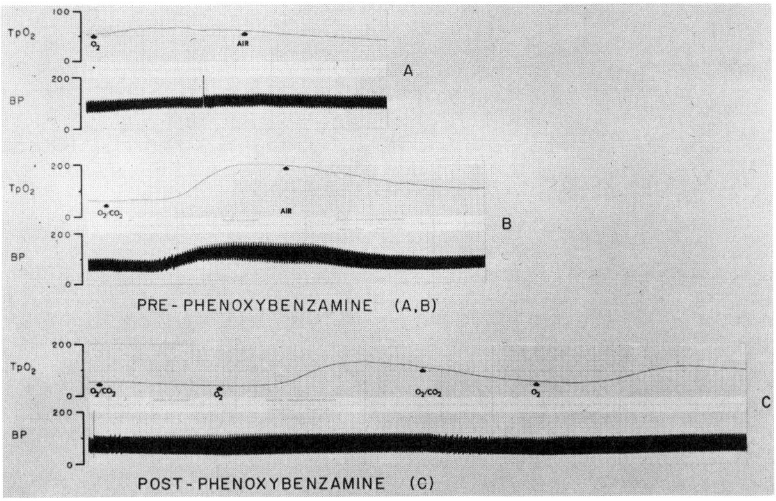

Figure 1. Effect of phenoxybenzamine on cerebral tissue Po_2. Trace A: Small tissue Po_2 rise during O_2 breathing. Trace B: Large increase in tissue Po_2 caused by 95% O_2–5% CO_2 breathing. Trace C: After phenoxybenzamine infusion, O_2 breathing rise in tissue Po_2 is larger than the preinfusion effect. Contrariwise, 95% O_2–5% CO_2 causes a fall in tissue Po_2. Time scale: 10 s between time marks (chart center).

blockade could be used to raise tissue Po_2 levels in brain with O_2 breathing at normal atmospheric pressure.

References

Bicher, H. I., 1974, Brain oxygen autoregulation: A protective reflex to hypoxia? *Microvasc. Res.* **8:**291.

Bicher, H. I., Reneau, D. D., Bruley, D. F., and Knisely, M. H., 1973, Brain oxygen supply and neuronal activity under normal and hypoglycemic conditions, *Am. J. Physiol.* **224:**275.

13.4. "Migraine"—Studies on Intravital Microcirculation: Synergism of the Action between Serotonin and Bradykinin on the Encephalic Circulation System

P. BONACCORSI

Serotonin and bradykinin are active pathogenetic elements in vascular cephalgia and in many other vascular complaints. This research aimed to investigate the possibility of vasoactive synergism between the two substances.

Guinea pigs were anesthetized with pentobarbitone sodium (15 mg/kg, i.p.); tracheostomy and intubation followed. The animals were curarized. Observations, photos, and films were made on the cortical–pial microcirculation. Sodium fluorescein (100 mg/kg) was used to check capillary permeability.

Serotonin was injected in single doses of 20, 40, and 60 mg; bradykinin was injected in doses of 4, 8, and 12 mg (into the common carotid artery). The same doses were used when the two substances were administered consecutively.

The experiments showed that apart from algogenous synergism between the two substances there is also a reinforcement of the vasoactive and hemokinetic effect.

The initial effect was mainly due to serotonin (increased viscosity, intravascular sludging, arteriolar spasms, and slowing, inversion, or mingling of arteriolar and venous blood). Then, through prolonged contact of bradykinin with the vascular endothelia, further sludging, marked vasodilatator effects (Fig. 1), and increased capillary permeability occurred, which were greater than the results obtained after administration of identical doses of the two substances separately.

It is suggested that similar phenomena may occur in serotonin discharge during a migraine headache. Pain receptors would be sensitized, even with infinitesimal doses on the order of 1 ng of bradykinin. The bradykinin is produced *in situ* because of tissue acidosis due to stagnation or to zonal ischemia or is carried from exocranial or, more frequently, immediate paracranial accumulation centers connected by vessels to the

P. BONACCORSI · Department of Otorhinolaryngology, University of Pavia, Pavia, Italy.

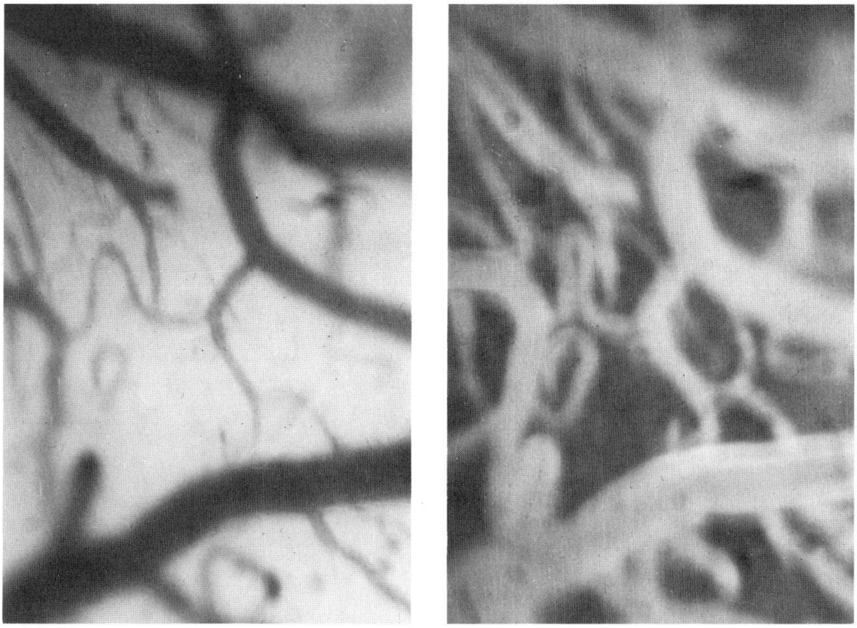

Figure 1. Left: Cortical–pial circulation system in basic conditions. Right: Maximum dilatation phase, well brought out by the intravascular fluorescence.

encephalic circulation system; because of the lower dilution involved, minimal doses are active.

These deductions relate to the success of the operation called "exocranial endonasal neurovascular decompressive ethmoidosphenectomy," described by the author. This operation aims to correct archistructural bone malformation and to restore normal hemodynamic equilibrium between the internal carotid and external carotid arteries. This occurs at the level of the circulation in the ethmoids and sphenopalatines, inosculated in the terminal branches. The operation has been performed in over 800 cases of serious vasomotor cephalgia not responding to drug therapy; there was a very high proportion of long-term recovery or definite improvement. The operation is thought to prevent the accumulation of vasoactive substances in this part of the circulation, and the "exocranial reserves" of serotonin, bradykinin, and histamine are thus eliminated.

References

Bonaccorsi, P., 1971, Ipotesi interpretative sulle modificazioni emodinamiche distrettuali del circolo della fossa cranica anteriore nella chirurgia correttiva etmoido-sfeno-settale delle cefalee vasomotorie, *Boll. Mal. Orecch. Gola Naso* **89:**43.

Bonaccorsi, P., 1972*a*, L' "Etmoidosfenectomia decompressiva neurovascolare" come trattamento chirurgico nella terapia delle cefalee a patogenesi vascolare nasale, in: *Cefalee ed Algie Cranio-facciali di Interesse Otorinolaringologico,* pp. 413–494, Arti Grafiche Pacini-Mariotti, Pisa.

Bonaccorsi, P., 1972*b*, L'etmoïdosfénectomie décompressive neurovasculaire endonasale exocranique comme thérapie chirurgique radicale de la migraine et des céphalées vaso-motrices, *Boll. Mal. Orecch. Gola Naso* **90:**169.

Bonaccorsi, P., and Dragoni, G., 1971, Radiological investigation on the ethmoidal-sphenoidal architructural alterations and the problem of the histodisreactivity of the neurovascular headaches, in: *Proceedings of the International Headache Symposium,* Sandoz, Basel.

Bonaccorsi, P., and Periti, G., 1974, L'etmoidosfenectomia decompressiva neurovascolare nelle emicranie paretiche e comiziali, *Boll. Mal. Orecch. Gola Naso* **92:**120.

13.5. Oxygen Supply to the Spinal Cord and Its Autoregulation

W. ERDMANN, W. NIX, C. HOLCOMB, G. CORSSEN, and J. H. HALSEY

Biochemical and physiological experiments in the brain cortex have demonstrated that tissue Po_2 values of 1–2 mm Hg or lower are sufficient to maintain adequate function of neuronal tissue (Erdmann *et al.,* 1973). The oxygen supply conditions of the spinal cord have so far received little attention. In this study, the tissue Po_2 of the spinal crod (TH_{10-12}) was investigated by means of microelectrodes simultaneously measuring tissue Po_2, action potential, and capillary perfusion. For this study, albino rats were anesthetized with a 79% N_2O–21% O_2 mixture, relaxed with pancuronium bromide, and artificially ventilated.

The insertion of the microelectrode into the spinal cord 0.7 mm lateral to the dorsal spinal artery involves penetration through tissue areas showing histologically different characteristics and physiological functions. Although the capillary density in the white matter is only one-fifth of that of the gray matter, mean tissue Po_2 values in the white matter are relatively high (Fig. 1). This might be due to the much lower oxygen consumption rate of the white matter. In the dorsal horn, the tissue Po_2 values range between 10 and 20 mm Hg, and marked tissue Po_2 changes in relatively short distances are perceived depending on the density of the capillary meshwork. The tissue Po_2 values in the ventral horn are even lower, ranging down to 3 mm Hg, which can be explained by the capillary density of the ventral horn being only one-tenth that of the dorsal horn (Craigie, 1920).

The autoregulatory response of the oxygen supply to the spinal cord during changes of arterial blood pressure, arterial Pco_2, and Po_2 is similar to that of the brain (Erdmann and Metzger, 1971). The autoregulation of capillary perfusion in the spinal cord to systemic blood pressure changes seems to be slower and the range smaller than in the brain. However, the gray matter is highly reactive to Pco_2. The time constant of regulation is much shorter and more accurate than that stated for the brain cortex. Unlike in the brain, there is no posthypercapnic regulative undershoot/overshoot reaction. The lack of undershoot/overshoot reaction cannot so far be explained, since this phenomenon has generally been encountered in any highly sensitive regulation circuit.

W. ERDMANN, W. NIX, C. HOLCOMB, G. CORSSEN, and J. H. HALSEY · Department of Anesthesiology, University of Alabama, Birmingham, Alabama.

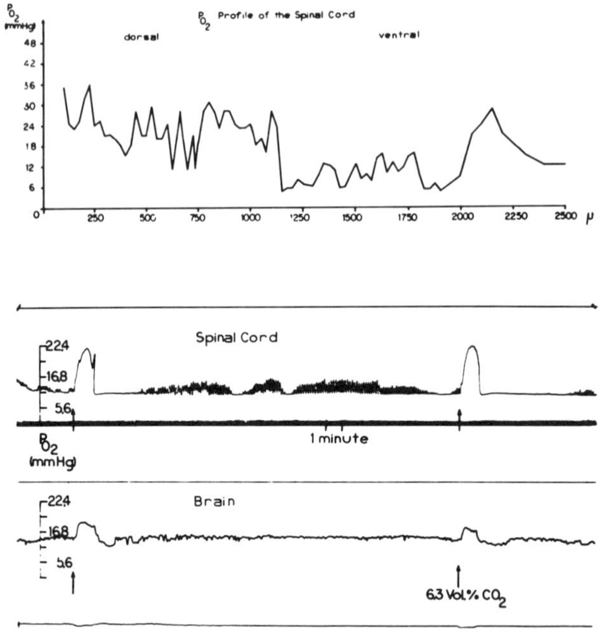

Figure 1. Upper trace: Po_2-profile of the spinal cord of the rat. Middle trace: Autoregulation (CO_2-response) of tissue-Po_2 in the spinal cora and Po_2-rhythms. Lower trace: Autoregulation (CO_2-response) of tissue-Po_2 in the brain cortex and Po_2-rhythms.

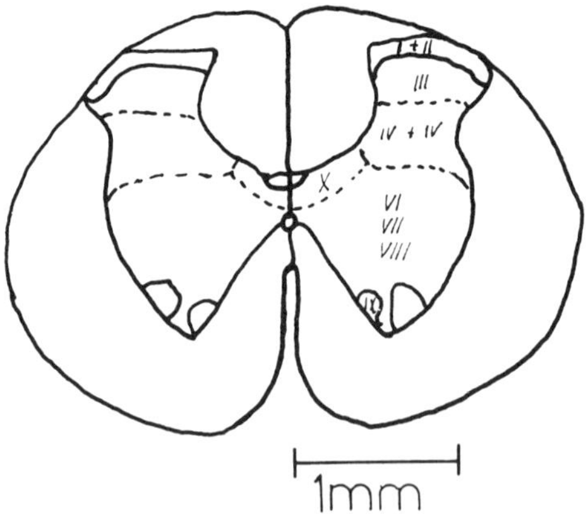

Figure 2. The structure of the spinal cord at the level of vertebra B: The electrode is inverted 0.5 cm lateral of middle line and thus measures the profile in the dorsal white matter, lamina I–VIII and then in the ventral white matter.

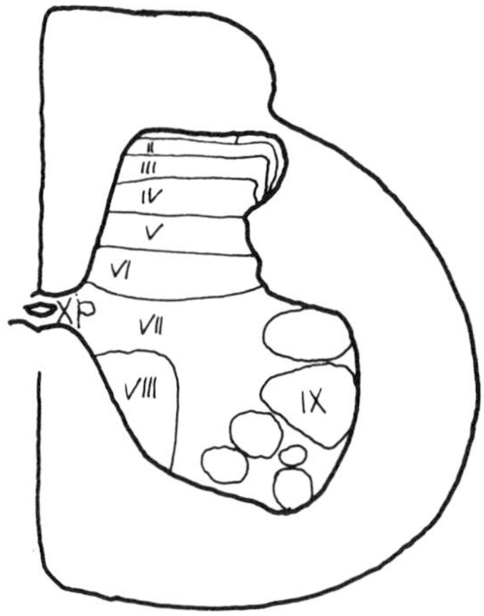

Figure 3. The structure of the spinal cord at the level of lumbar segment VII.

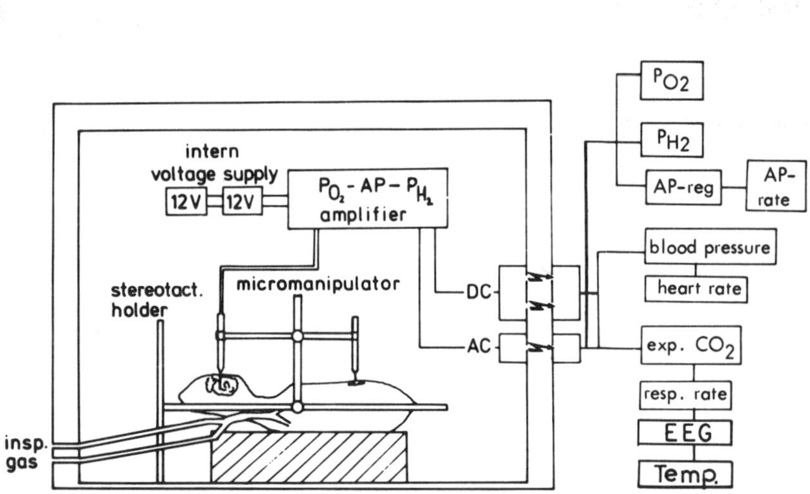

Figure 4. Experimental procedure: The experiments are performed in a shielded cage with optotelemetric transmission of the registered signals to avoid feedback noise. Besides Po_2, action potential and H_2-clearance measurement in the brain and spinal cord, the various control parameters are registered as needed.

References

Craigie, E. H., 1920, On the relative vascularity of various parts of the central nervous system of the albino rat, *J. Comp. Neurol.* **31**:429.

Erdmann, W., 1971, A quickly produced ultra-microelectrode for oxygen, H_2 clearance and action potential measurement, Mount Sinai Prize of Anesthesiology, Mount Sinai School of Medicine, New York.

Erdmann, W., and Metzger, H., 1971, Oxygen tension in microareas of the brain: Steady states of oxygen tension at arterial hyperoxia and with hypercapnia increased CBF, in: *European Conference on Microcirculation,* Aalborg, 1971 (J. Ditzel and D. H. Lewis, eds.), Karger, New York.

Erdmann, W., and Kunke, S., 1973, Changes of oxygen supply to the tissue following intravenous application of anesthetic drugs, in: *Oxygen Transport to Tissue* (H. I. Bicher and D. F. Bruley, eds.), Plenum, New York.

Erdmann, W., Kunke, S., and Krell, W., 1973, Tissue-Po_2 and cell function—An experimental study with multimicroelectrodes in the rat brain, in: *Oxygen Supply* (M. Kessler *et al.,* eds.), Urban and Schwarzenberg, Munich.

13.6. Regional Changes in Pial Blood Supply Induced by Hypothalamic Stimulation

B. BLUM, W. BEN-ARI, TAMAR YASHIN, J. ISRAELI, and H. M. ASKENASY

Blood supply to specific brain regions is controlled by autoregulatory (metabolic and pressure) and also by neuronogenic mechanisms (Ingvar and Schwartz, 1974; Langfitt and Kassel, 1968). It is still unknown what mechanisms harmonize between these two modes of regulation. However, the rich and highly sophisticated innervation revealed in this system hints at antagonistic nerve mechanisms which apparently exert close control over the regional blood supply (Edvinsson *et al.*, 1973; Hagen and Wittkowski, 1969; Iwayama *et al.*, 1972) and are possibly responsible for stability of appropriate supply under changing demands (Perl, 1962), with changes at one locus not jeopardizing supply to another locality. Our studies were designed to observe such dynamic processes in order to elucidate the brain regions involved in such a differential control of the microcirculation.

Observations on the circulation of the cat suprasylvian gyrus were made under chloralose anesthesia by means of fluorescein magnification angiography and radioactive krypton clearance and the modifications caused in it by electrical stimulation of specific sites in the lateral hypothalamus. Stimulation consisted of 12-s trains of electrical pulses 0.5 ms in duration and at a rate of 100/s. It was observed by the fluorescence technique that 1–2 s after initiation of the stimuli a capillary bed of a few square centimeters in area opened up, often with no apparent change in the diameter of the arteries or the arterioles. Sometimes the change involved just one or a few microcirculatory units. These changes lasted a few seconds. Then there occurred a rapid adaptation to the prestimulus state, sometimes even while the stimulus continued. These observations were confirmed by radioactive krypton clearances, which indicated a large increase of blood volume shunted regionally by stimulation of specific sites in the lateral hypothalamus. Our findings were in general agreement with the concept of the microcirculatory unit as an organ for the regulation of local metabolic demands (Zweifach, 1961).

B. BLUM, W. BEN-ARI, TAMAR YASHIN, J. ISRAELI, and H. M. ASKENASY · The Sackler School of Medicine, Tel Aviv University, Tel Aviv, Israel.

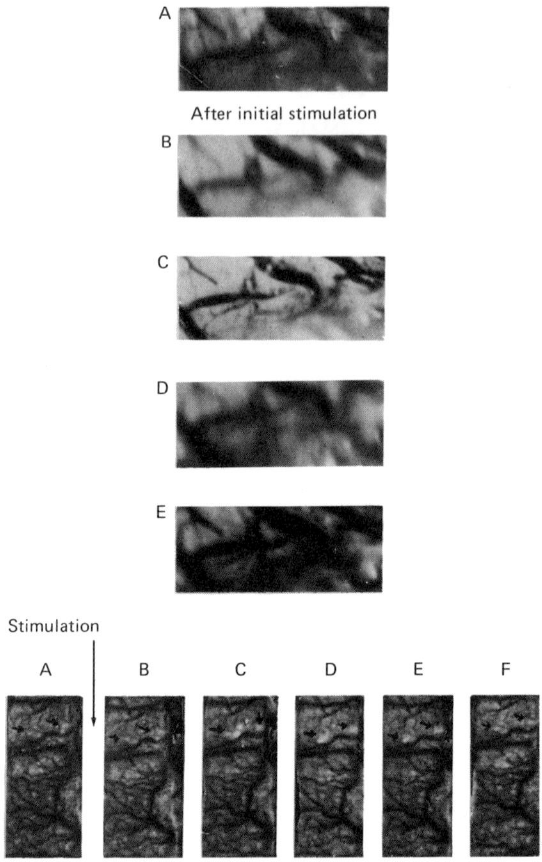

Figure 1. Fluorescence angiography photographs of the exposed brains of two cats (upper and lower) taken about 1 s apart before and after the initiation of the train stimulus. Stimulation was bihemispheric, bipolar at hypothalamic targets frontal 9.5, lateral 3, and depth 3. About $1\frac{1}{2}$ s prior to stimulation, 0.6 ml of fluorescein was injected into the lingual artery through tubing reaching from the external carotid.

Acknowledgments

Initial observations on the phenomena were made by one of the authors (B. B.) at the National Institute of Neurological Disease and Stroke, National Institute of Health, Bethesda, Maryland, in 1962.

References

Edvinsson, L., Lindvall, M., Nielsen, K. C., and Owman, C., 1973, Are brain vessels innervated also by central (non-sympathetic) adrenergic neurones? *Brain Res.* **63**:496.

Hagen, E., and Wittkowski, W., 1969, Licht und electronmikroskopische Untersuchungen zur Innervation der Piagefasse, *A. Zellforsch.* **95**:429.

Ingvar, D. H., and Schwartz, M. S., 1974, Blood flow patterns induced by speech and reading, *Brain* **97**:273.

Iwayama, T., Furness, J. B., and Burnstock, G., 1972, Dual adrenergic and cholinergic innervation of the cerebral arteries of the rat: An ultrastructure study, *Circ. Res.* **26**:635.

Langfitt, T. W., and Kassel, N. P., 1968, Cerebral vasodilation produced by brainstem stimulation: Neurovegetative control vs. autoregulation, *Am. J. Physiol.* **215**:90.

Perl, W., 1962, Heat and water distribution in body tissues and the determination of tissue blood flow by local clearance methods, *J. Theor. Biol.* **2**:201.

Zweifach, B. W., 1961, *Functional Behavior of the Microcirculation,* Thomas, Springfield, Ill.

13.7. Influence of Aminophylline on the Cerebral Blood Circulation and CSF Pressure

V. M. BERGINER

Blood vessels of the pia mater of 12 normal rabbits and of nine rabbits with dietetically induced atherosclerosis were microphotographed through a hermetic "window" in the skull. Intravenous injection of aminophylline elicited a biphasic response of the cerebral vessels: initial vasodilatation which lasted minutes followed by prolonged vasoconstriction which lasted several hours. The constriction of veins was comparably less than the constriction of arteries. Both phases depended on the dose and were less marked in the atherosclerotic rabbits than in the normal rabbits. Aminophylline decreased stasis in the cerebral vessels.

In clinical-physiological studies in 100 patients with mild acute brain concussion without local symptoms, bilateral rheoencephalography, brachial oscillography, and finger plethysmography were carried out simultaneously. These tests showed that 250 mg aminophylline i.v. removes the initial asymmetry and restores the normal tone of cerebral and peripheral vessels.

Aminophylline decreased the venous pressure (average 35.7%, $p < 0.001$), reduced CSF pressure (average 33.7%, $p < 0.001$), and decreased brain edema. The higher the initial pressure, the greater was the hypotensive effect of aminophylline.

A clinical-therapeutic double-blind trial was carried out on 220 patients: 120 patients with acute cerebrovascular accident and 100 patients with acute slight brain concussion. These were all treated with 250 mg aminophylline i.v. one or two times daily. Two-hundred patients served as nontreated controls. Aminophylline has a significantly favorable effect in the treatment of cerebral diseases in whose pathogenesis cerebral diseases dyscirculation and changes of CSF play an important role. In intracerebral hemorrhage aminophylline did not have a beneficial action.

V. M. BERGINER · Neurology Unit, Soroka Medical Center, and Ben Gurion University Hospital, Beersheva, Israel.

13.8. Electrocorticographic and Pial Microvascular Hemodynamic Correlations during Pentylenetetrazol- and Enflurane-Induced Seizures in the Cat

ROBERT R. MYERS and MARCOS INTAGLIETTA

Arteriolar diameters and venular erythrocyte velocities in the surface (pial) vessels of the cat brain were measured by television methods and correlated with changes in cerebrospinal fluid pH during pharmacologically induced electrographic grand mal seizures in the cat. Skull screws were implanted for recording the electrocorticogram, a 1-cm^2 plexiglas window was substituted for the calvarium over the left frontocentral cortex for observation of the pial microcirculation under 400 × magnification, and micro-pH probes were inserted in the surface CSF for determination of CSF pH. Arteriolar diameters were measured from the video image, and venular erythrocyte velocities were determined by cross-correlating up- and downstream erythrocyte photometric signatures.

Pentylenetetrazol-induced seizures increased arteriolar diameters up to 400% or until maximally dilated, and increased erythrocyte velocity by a factor of up to 4. These effects began during the early tonic phase of the seizure, were maximal during the early postictal period, and returned to preseizure values within 2 min after spontaneous cerebral electrical activity reappeared. The vascular effects of enflurane-induced seizures were similar but of lower magnitude since autoregulation had increased preseizure arteriolar diameters in response to enflurane-induced hypotension. Data were collected from experiments in which the mean arterial blood pressure remained constant, thereby eliminating changes in cerebral blood flow caused by variations in perfusion pressure.

High positive correlations existed between changes in CSF hydrogen ion concentration and pial hemodynamics. Increases in hydrogen ion concentration secondary to increased brain metabolism were accompanied by pial arteriolar dilatation and increased venular erythrocyte velocity.

It is concluded that the local metabolic environment of the arteriole, as reflected in CSF pH, is directly responsible for control of cerebral arteriolar diameter and hence cerebral blood flow during the seizure. Increases in systemic blood pressure secondarily increase cerebral blood flow in metabolically dilated arteries.

ROBERT R. MYERS and MARCOS INTAGLIETTA · AMES-Bioengineering, School of Medicine, University of California, San Diego, La Jolla, California.

13.9. Regional Blood Flow in Normal Skin and the Pedicle Skin Flap

CAROLINE M. YOUNG

Blood flow in the dermis of normal skin and pedicle skin flaps was estimated using an isotope clearance technique. Experiments were performed on the flank skin of the large white pig. A small volume (0.03 ml) of ^{99m}Tc was injected intradermally, and its clearance rate from the injection site was monitored by external scintillation detectors. The clearance rate of the isotope gave an indication of blood flow.

The clearance curves obtained were biexponential, with a fast and a slow component. In normal skin, the mean half clearance times (the time taken to remove 50% of the isotope) were 4 min and 20 min for the fast and slow components, respectively. Preliminary experiments on normal skin indicated that there was no variation in half clearance times across the flank.

Three pedicle skin flaps were raised on one side of the pig. The surviving length of each was divided into a distal, middle, and proximal third. Blood flow measurements were made in these three areas and equivalent areas of normal skin. For the first 10 days after a flap had been raised, there were marked changes in the half clearance times of the isotope. The greatest changes were found in the distal third of the viable flap, although similar but less marked changes were found in the middle and proximal thirds. For the first 3 days, the clearance times became longer as compared with normal skin. At later times, 3–10 days, the clearance times in the flaps were decreased.

This can be interpreted as increased blood flow, and coincided with the appearance of inflammation and edema. After 10 days, and for periods up to 1 yr, the clearance times in the flaps were again longer than in normal skin.

References

Moustafa, H. F., and Hopewell, J. H., 1974, The evaluation of an isotopic clearance technique for the measurement of skin blood flow in the pig (abst.), *Biorheology* **11**:208.

Patterson, T. J. S., 1968, The survival of skin flaps in the pig, *Br. J. Plast. Surg.* **21**:113.

CAROLINE M. YOUNG · Research Institute, Churchill Hospital, Headington, Oxford, England.

Patterson, T. J. S., and Milton, S. H., 1967, Study of the circulation in experimental skin flaps using an intra-vital dye, *Bibl. Anat.* **9**:501.

Patterson, T. J. S., Berry, R. J., Hopewell, J. W., and Wiernik, G., 1975. The effect of X-radiation on the survival of experimental skin flaps, in: *Skin Flaps* (Grabb, W. C., and Myers, M. B., eds.), Little, Brown, Boston.

13.10. Microvasculature in Open Cremaster Muscle of Mouse

T. YAMAKI, S. BAEZ, and L. R. ORKIN

Morphological and morphometric studies were carried out in the microvasculature of mouse cremaster muscle by biomicroscopy. Open cremaster muscle of male Swiss strain mice ($N = 99$) weighing 35–40 g was prepared under pentobarbital anesthesia (30 mg/kg) for microscopic observation and measurements. The femoral artery (ipsilateral) was cannulated for carbon injection in selected preparations. The vascular diameter was measured by the image-splitting method previously described (Baez, 1966).

The dimensions of the open cremaster were 14.8 ± 2.4 μm in diameter, and 110.2 ± 19.8 and 142.6 ± 37.7 μm in thickness, respectively, at the peripheral and central zone of tissue. The striated muscle fiber diameter was 54.3 ± 11.1 μm. The calculated total capillary number was 9.2×10^3, and the capillary surface area was 8.6 m^2/kg of muscle, based on analysis of 30 samples in eight mice. The measured capillary length was 580 ± 317 μm in 119 capillaries. The capillary diameters measured at the begining, middle, and end were, respectively, 5.0 ± 1.0, 5.2 ± 1.0, and 6.1 ± 1.3 μm.

Length and diameter measurements were also made on the consecutive segments of pre- and postcapillary microvessels, from arterioles of 50 μm diameter to the true capillary and from the venular end of capillaries to the collecting venules of about 70 μm. The calculated vascular volume in percent of tissue volume was $3.44 \pm 0.61\%$, of which 23.8% corresponded to precapillary and 59.7% to postcapillary microvessels. Capillary volume was 16.5% of total microvascular volume.

Previously, quantitative information concerning the vascular volume in precapillary, capillary, and postcapillary segments of the microvasculatures *in vivo* was restricted to the bat wing (Wiedeman, 1963). This study of the thin striated muscle of mouse permits, for the first time, the morphological and morphometric study of striated muscle microvasculature *in vivo*.

T. YAMAKI, S. BAEZ, and L. R. ORKIN · Albert Einstein College of Medicine, New York, N.Y.

ACKNOWLEDGMENT

This work was supported by NIH Grant HL-06736.

References

Baez, S., 1966, Recording of microvascular dimensions with an imagesplitter television microscope, *J. Appl. Physiol.* **22**:299.
Wiedeman, M. P., 1963, Dimensions of blood vessels from distributing artery to collecting vein, *Circ. Res.* **12**:366.

13.11. Childhood Asthma and Peptic Ulcer: Studies of the Lip Capillaries

JOHN A. GIUS and JOSEPH REBHUN

In previous studies, we have described changes in the lip capillaries associated with clinical conditions such as pulmonary emphysema, cancer of the lung, chronic peptic ulcer, and cigarette smoking (Gius, 1971, 1973). Peptic ulcer is reported to be 3–4 times more common in subjects with chronic obstructive lung disease than it is in normal individuals (Silen *et al.,* 1959). A relatively high incidence of duodenal ulcer disease in allergic children with bronchial asthma and hay fever has been reported (Rebhun, 1975). This study was undertaken to determine if the lip capillaries in young asthmatics with ulcer was different from those of normals.

The methods of study were similar to those described in earlier reports. The lip vessels were observed directly and photographed by means of the Leitz "Ultropak" incident light microscope. The degree of capillary deformity was graded on the scale of 1+ to 4+ and the scores were averaged. The important capillary deviations were changes in "pattern," enlargement of the venous limb, and "angiomatoid" configuration. The capillary deformity index (CD) was determined from these data.

There were 43 subjects; 28 were males and 15 were females. Their ages ranged from 8 to 18 yr. Twenty-nine had asthma. Some children with acute asthma or complications were examined in the hospital, while others were examined during a quiescent period. Treatment included ephedrine and xanthine preparations and prednisolone in three patients. Fifteen of 29 asthmatic children had abdominal pain and nine were found to have a duodenal ulcer crater on X-ray; six had prodromal X-ray signs such as duodenitis, pylorospasm, deformed bulb, and irritable cap.

18.12.1. Discussion

Allergic children often suffer from recurrent abdominal pain, which has generally been considered "functional." Gastrointestinal X-rays in a

JOHN A. GIUS and JOSEPH REBHUN · Pomona Valley Community Hospital, Pomona, California.

Table I. Severity of Asthma and Capillary Deformity

Grade of severity		CD
1+	(10)	2.1
2+	(4)	2.2
3+	(6)	2.3
4+	(9)	2.4

Table II. Asthma Patients According to Clinical Severity

Grade of clinical severity		Ulcer crater	Ulcer prodrome	No ulcer signs
1+	(10)	3	1	6
2+	(4)	2	2	—
3+	(6)	1	—	5
4+	(9)	3	3	3
29 total				

Table III. Capillary Deformity (CD) in Groups According to Diagnosis

Diagnosis	CD
No asthma, no ulcer (9)	1.8
Acute bronchitis or pneumonitis (5)	2.2
Hayfever and vasomotor rhinitis (5)	2.4
Asthma without ulcer (14)	2.1
Asthma with ulcer prodrome (6)	2.2
Asthma with ulcer crater (9)	3.0
Asthma and hay fever with ulcer crater (10)	3.1

series of private patients revealed frequent changes in the duodenum including ulcer crater as well as the prodromal signs mentioned above.

Bronchial asthma physiologically represents an obstructive type of lung disease due to allergy. In allergic diseases, the release of vasoactive substances is known to affect the small blood vessels.

Our findings suggest that patients with severe grades of bronchial asthma are likely to exhibit capillary deformity (Table I). There is no correlation between the severity of the asthma and the development of duodenal ulcer or the prodrôme signs of ulcer (Table II). However, there may be an association between the degree of capillary deformity and the appearance of the ulcer syndrome (Table III). Further studies will be required to clarify this point.

13.12.2. Conclusions

1. Children with bronchial asthma have more capillary deformity of the lip vessels than normal children.
2. The clinical severity of bronchial asthma does not appear to be related to the frequency of the peptic ulcer syndrome.
3. Children with asthma and the ulcer syndrome exhibit more capillary deformity than asthmatic children without ulcer.
4. The findings support the theory that peptic ulcer is related to changes in the microcirculation.

References

Gius, J. A., 1971, Lip capillaries in cigarette smokers with lung disease and peptic ulcer, in: *Proceedings of the Sixth European Conference on Microcirculation,* Aalborg, 1970, pp. 123–128, Karger, New York.

Gius, J. A., 1973, Chronic lung disease and peptic ulcer: Observations on the lip capillaries, in: Proceedings of the Seventh European Conference on Microcirculation, Aberdeen, 1971, Part I, *Bibl. Anat.* **11**:340.

Rebhun, J., 1975, Duodenal ulceration in allergic children, *Ann. Allergy* **34**:145.

Silen, W., Brown, W. H., and Eiseman, B., 1959, Peptic ulcer and chronic pulmonary emphysema, *Arch. Surg.* **78**:897.

13.12. Effects of Perfusion Pressure on Focal Ischemia in the Retina: Experimental and Clinical Studies

PAULO E. M. DE SOUSA RAMALHO

Vascular occlusions are common pathological findings in many diseases. Although the circulatory, hemodynamic, and clinical changes that follow vascular occlusions are known and also some of the factors involved in the recovery of the process in the retina have been reported (Dollery *et al.*, 1965; Ashton *et al.*, 1966), it is not yet possible to improve the circulation in ischemic areas rapidly and efficiently to prevent structural damage, especially in the terminal type of circulation.

Using the retina as an experimental model because of its special features, we have studied the effects of perfusion pressure (systemic blood pressure) on experimental arteriolar occlusions produced by glass microspheres (Ashton and Henkind, 1965) and fluorescein angiography (Dollery *et al.*, 1962).

The efficiency of circulation is studied by the rapidity of maximum capillary filling seen in ischemic areas after dye injection and compared to different levels of systemic blood pressure obtained by bleeding, transfusion, and administration of norepinephrine (Ramalho, 1967; Dollery *et al.*, 1968).

Over 20 small (1–3 mm) acute occlusions were studied in the pig retina. The nonperfused areas could be increased three- to fivefold by reducing the blood pressure from 100 to 40 mm Hg (mean. By increasing systemic blood pressure, these areas could be reduced considerably. It is known that acute ischemic areas are perfused retrogradely from the surrounding normally perfused capillaries.

Vasodilators have been used to improve the circulation in focal ischemias. In human branch arteriolar occlusions in the retina, it is usually difficult to recover the circulation rapidly. In our studies, we found the occluded retinal arterioles of the ischemic areas often very much dilated, reversing the A/V ratio (Fig. 1). If vasodilators are to influence, they could not possibly interfere with these maximal dilated arterioles but would dilate the normal surrounding arterioles, thus reducing the intravascular driving force to the ischemic territory.

PAULO E. M. DE SOUSA RAMALHO · Serviço de Oftalmologia, Faculdade de Medicina, Hospital de Santa Maria, University of de Lisbon, Lisbon, Portugal.

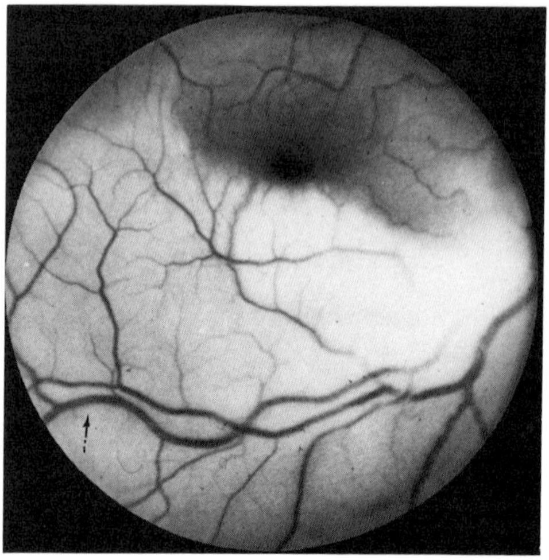

Figure 1. Right fundus photograph of a young female patient taken soon after inferior temporal arteriolar occlusion showing the ischemic area with a very much dilated (inferior temporal) arteriole which is nearly 3 times the caliber of accompanying venule (lower left).

As the increase of the systemic pressure has definite beneficial effects on focal ischemia, it would be worth trying to increase the systemic blood pressure or local intravascular pressure in order to improve the perfusion of ischemic areas.

References

Ashton, N., and Henkind, P., 1965, Experimental occlusion of retinal arterioles using graded ballotini, *Br. J. Ophthalmol.* **49:**225.

Ashton, N., Dollery, C. T., Henkind, P., Hill, D. W., Paterson, J. W., Ramalho, P. S., and Shakib, M., 1966, Focal retinal ischaemia, *Br. J. Ophthalmol.* **50:**281.

Dollery, C. T., Hodge, J. V., and Engel, M., 1962, Studies of the retinal circulation with fluorescein, *Br. J. Med.* **2:**1210.

Dollery, C. T., Ramalho, P. S., Paterson, J. W., Hill, D. W., Henkind, P., Shakib, N., and Ashton, N., 1965, Retinal microemboli, *Lancet* **1:**1303.

Dollery, C. T., Kohner, E. M., Paterson, J. W., and Ramalho, P. S., 1968, Retinal microcirculation in shock, in: *Microcirculation as Related to Shock* (D. Shepro and G. Fulton, eds.), pp. 79–91, Academic Press, New York.

Ramalho, P. S., 1967, Some aspects of acute arteriolar occlusion in the retina, Ph.D. thesis, London, University, p. 130.

Index